Endoscopic, Laparoscopic and Robotic Techniques for Foregut Disorders

Francisco Schlottmann • Mario A. Masrur
Editors

Endoscopic, Laparoscopic and Robotic Techniques for Foregut Disorders

Springer

Editors
Francisco Schlottmann
University of Buenos Aires
Ciudad Autónoma Buenos Aires
Buenos Aires, Argentina

Mario A. Masrur
Department of Surgery
University of Illinois at Chicago
Chicago, IL, USA

ISBN 978-3-032-00810-7 ISBN 978-3-032-00811-4 (eBook)
https://doi.org/10.1007/978-3-032-00811-4

This Springer imprint is published by the registered company Springer Nature Switzerland AG
The registered company address is: Gewerbestrasse 11, 6330 Cham, Switzerland

Acknowledgments

To all my family for their unconditional support, especially my mother, María Cristina, who always worked hard to give me the best possible education and remains my top admirer.

To all my co-workers at the Hospital Alemán of Buenos Aires, who make the hospital my second home.

To my lifelong surgical mentors Marco G. Patti and Daniela Molena.

To my colleague, friend, and guide Mario A. Masrur, who gave me the opportunity to learn from him at the University of Illinois at Chicago. Since then, we have been working together achieving tremendous success and joy.

To my wife Manu, who inspires and supports me every day. You are my rock, and nothing would be possible without you.

Francisco Schlottmann

To my parents, Elba and Rulo, who instilled in me the values of hard work and the importance of pursuing my dreams. Despite their limited resources, they have always supported me unconditionally and served as my first role models in life. I greatly admire their resilience and the way they overcame challenges, which continues to inspire me every day.

To my brothers, Pablo, Alejandro, Diego, and José, each of you has played a significant role in shaping the person I am today. Through your unique perspectives and examples, you have taught me invaluable lessons that I hold close to my heart.

I would also like to thank my wife, Silvana, and my son, Noah—the loves of my life. They are the reason behind everything I do. Their unwavering love and support have been my strength during the most challenging times.

I am deeply grateful to my mentors during my residency in Mendoza, particularly Dr. Sergio Bustos, who has been like a father to me. His guidance and care have been foundational in my career. I also wish to thank Dr. Pablo Omelanczuk, Dr. Jorge Nefa, and Dr. Ernesto Valerio, who taught me the fundamentals of surgery and served as exceptional role models during the early stages of my journey.

To my mentors in Chicago: Dr. Fernando Elli and Dr. Pier Giulianotti, thank you for opening the doors at UIC and providing me the opportunity to elevate my career. Your mentorship in bariatric, foregut, and robotic surgery has been instrumental in my growth.

A special acknowledgment goes to Dr. Enrico Benedetti, who has been my mentor over the past four years. His support and advice have been pivotal in advancing my academic career and achieving the successes I am fortunate to celebrate today.

To my residents and fellows: you inspire me daily to improve my teaching, refine my skills, and become a better surgeon. I learn from you every day, and for that, I am profoundly grateful.

Finally, I extend my heartfelt thanks to my dear colleague and friend, Dr. Francisco Schlottmann. Over the past few years, we have achieved remarkable progress together, including the development of this book. Despite the distance, we have built an incredible partnership, always striving for excellence and achieving great success. Here's to many more accomplishments together!

Mario A. Masrur

Contents

The original version of the book has been revised. The correction to this book can be found at https://doi.org/10.1007/978-3-032-00811-4_39

About the Editors

Francisco Schlottmann received his medical degree with honors from the University of Buenos Aires in Argentina. He then completed his general surgery residency at the Hospital Alemán of Buenos Aires. After his surgical training, he completed the Soudavar fellowship at Memorial Sloan Kettering Cancer Center, focusing his research on esophageal cancer. He then did a 2-year gastrointestinal surgery fellowship at the University of North Carolina, focusing his clinical and research activities on foregut disorders. He obtained his Master of Public Health at the University of North Carolina Gillings School of Global Public Health. He also completed a 1-year Minimally Invasive and Robotic Surgery Clinical Fellowship at the University of Illinois at Chicago. He currently serves as Clinical Instructor at the University of Illinois at Chicago and as Affiliate Professor of Surgery at the Hospital Alemán of Buenos Aires, where he also serves as the Surgical Residency Program Director. He has an active clinical and research interest in diagnostic and therapeutic endoscopic procedures as well as the surgical treatment of esophageal disorders, gastroesophageal reflux disease, obesity, esophageal cancer, and gastric cancer. He is editor of 9 books, has published over 300 journal articles, and has written more than 80 book chapters.

Mario A. Masrur is a distinguished surgeon from Mendoza, Argentina. He earned his medical degree from the College of Medicine at Universidad Nacional de Cuyo and completed his general surgery residency at Hospital Italiano de Mendoza. In 2012, he relocated to Chicago to pursue advanced training in minimally invasive and robotic surgery. He completed a fellowship in Minimally Invasive and Robotic Surgery at the University of Illinois at Chicago (UIC) from 2012 to 2014. Following his fellowship, he joined the Division of Minimally Invasive and Robotic Surgery at UI Health as faculty in 2015. He has authored over 100 peer-reviewed publications and 10 book chapters focused on minimally invasive and robotic-assisted surgery. He specializes in foregut and bariatric surgery and serves as the Director of the Bariatric Program and the Fellowship Training Program at UI Health.

Obesity

Laparoscopic Sleeve Gastrectomy

Rami Lutfi

Abstract Sleeve gastrectomy (SG) is a surgical procedure that involves a significant reduction in stomach volume, resulting in a tubular-shaped conformation of the stomach. Despite its relative simplicity, it is not easy to construct a "perfect" sleeve. Adherence to a routine and proper technique, as the surgical steps outlined in this chapter, is essential for a low incidence of complications, proper durable weight loss, and avoiding high incidence of postoperative GERD.

Keywords Obesity · Bariatric surgery · Sleeve gastrectomy · Endoscopy

Introduction

Obesity has become a worldwide epidemic, affecting around 40% of adults in the United States. There is a significant gap in the availability of weight-loss interventions, as only 1.1% of eligible obese patients undergo primary bariatric surgery. Sleeve gastrectomy (SG) is a surgical procedure that involves a significant reduction in stomach volume, resulting in a tubular-shaped conformation of the stomach. This procedure has demonstrated substantial efficacy in weight loss and the management of obesity-related comorbidities. Being capable of producing up to 60% of total weight loss (TWL) within the first postoperative year, it is the most performed bariatric procedure up to date in the US [1, 2].

The underlying mechanism of weight reduction is multifaceted, incorporating both mechanical and neurohumoral factors. Physically, the reduced capacity of stomach lumen limits food intake, thereby curbing caloric consumption.

R. Lutfi (✉)
Chicago Institute of Advanced Surgery, Chicago, IL, USA

F. Schlottmann, M. A. Masrur (eds.), *Endoscopic, Laparoscopic and Robotic Techniques for Foregut Disorders*, https://doi.org/10.1007/978-3-032-00811-4_1

Physiologically, the neurohumoral component entails the reduction of ghrelin-producing cells, leading to a disruption of the hunger signaling pathway in the central nervous system. SG can be performed as a primary procedure, as well as revisional, most commonly after gastric band removal.

In this chapter, the technical aspects of the laparoscopic approach for SG will be detailed.

Procedure Description

Patient Preparation

The patient is placed in supine position on the operative table, with arms resting on padded boards at 90 degrees abduction. 2–3 g of intravenous Cefazolin (weight adjusted) and 40 mg of Low Molecular Weight Heparin are administered for infection and thrombosis prophylaxis, respectively. Pneumatic compression devices are placed on both lower limbs prior to general anesthesia.

Communication with the anesthesia team is critical as the drapes are placed covering the patient's face. Surgeons should be made aware of any tubes inserted in the patient's nose or mouth such nasogastric tubes or temperature probes in order to prevent inadvertent stapling of such tubes.

Pneumoperitoneum and Port Placement

After aseptic and antiseptic draping and preparation of the abdomen, the peritoneal cavity is accessed carefully, preferably through the left upper quadrant, as the umbilical location is not reliable in patients with large pannus. There is a general move away from using Veress needle, especially in patients with severe obesity. One of the safest way to access the abdomen is under direct vision using a transparent tip trocar under the vision of 0-degree laparoscope at the highest point of the left mid-clavicular line.

After insufflation to 15 mmHg and switching to a 30-degree angled laparoscope, the remaining trocars are placed under direct vision, which includes a 5 and 15 mm on the patient's right side for the surgeon. A 5 mm trocar about 18 mm from the xhyphoid and to the patient left side. The liver is always retracted, using Nathanson liver retractor.

It is important to have the laparoscopy placed off the midline (3–4 cm to the patient left) in order to have an optimal angle of view of the hiatus, especially with enlarged fatty liver.

Operative Technique

Anatomy and Landmark Identification

The procedure starts with the identification of the stomach. The surgeon retracts the anterior side of the stomach with laparoscopic graspers while the assistant provides contra-traction from the omentum to allow visualization of the greater curvature and mobilization of the greater omentum. (Fig. 1).

Dissection of the Greater Curvature

Using ultrasonic or bipolar energy device, dissection begins at the junction between the antrum and the body of the stomach while keeping lateral retraction of the omentum, facilitating a more effective entry into the lesser sac. Dissection is continued superiorly until complete mobilization of the stomach fundus and visualization of the left crus is achieved. (Fig. 2).

The location of the entry point, where the first stapler will be fired, used to be a point of controversy in the first few years of the world experience with sleeve gastrectomy. It was believed that a more radical transection of the antrum would decrease the acid production of the stomach and hence the incidence of GERD. But a more radical transection complicated the ergonomics of stapling and increased the incidence of strictures at the level of incisura. It is now generally accepted that stapling should be started between 2 and 5 cm from the pylorus.

Fig. 1 Stomach retraction and mobilization of the greater omentum

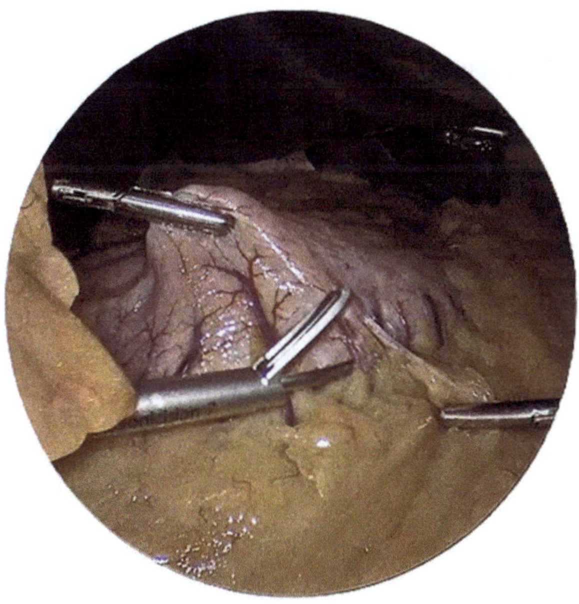

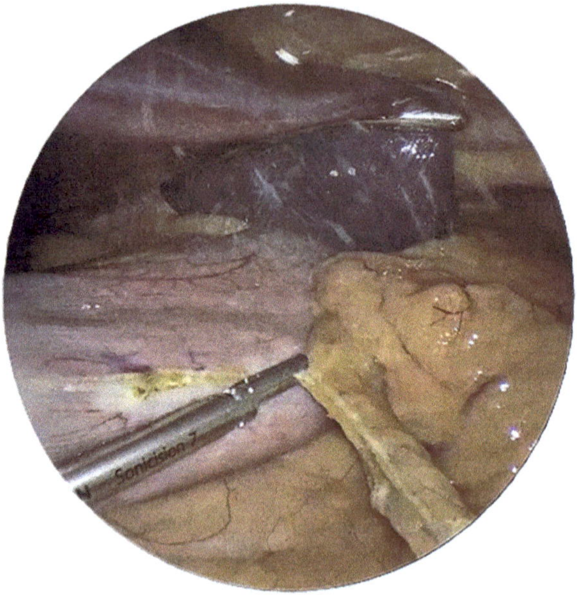

Fig. 2 Dissection of the greater omentum

It is critical to reach, expose and view the entire left crus. In this way, a complete fundectomy is ensured and avoid suboptimal weight loss or early postoperative regurgitation and/or GERD symptoms. Furthermore, this is critical for optimal posterior exposure of the hiatus and reliably rule out presence of a hiatal hernia.

Dissection of the Diaphragmatic Hiatus

The hiatus is dissected selectively when hiatal hernia present, or suspected based on preoperative symptoms, endoscopy, or visualizing a patulous hiatus anteriorly. It is important to identify any hiatal hernia in this operation due to the GERD inducing nature of the gastric sleeve. When a decision is made to dissect the hiatus, the surgeon should commit to formal repair of the crura posteriorly. Hiatal hernias can only be confidently ruled out upon posterior visualization of the crus. Having a "normal" hiatus anteriorly cannot rule out a posterior herniation.

Beginning in the left crus, using a combination of blunt and energy maneuvers, the perigastric fat tissue is excised until complete exposure of the gastroesophageal junction (GEJ) is achieved (Fig. 3). The same procedure is performed in the right crus until creation of a window posterior to the esophagus is complete (Fig. 4). Both vagus nerves need to be identified and preserved during this dissection.

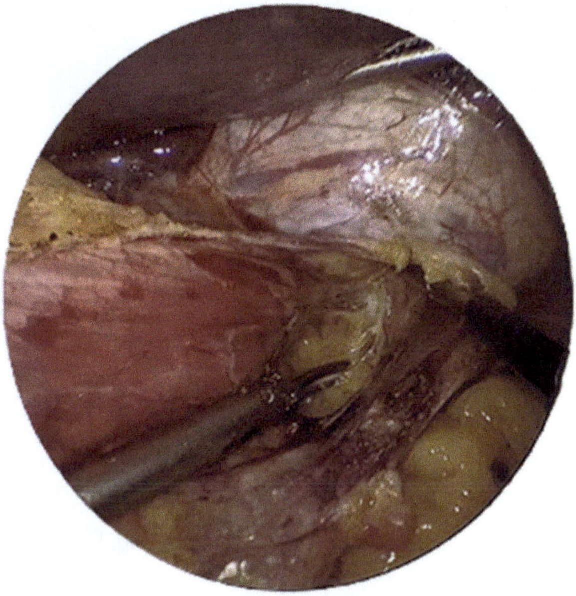

Fig. 3 Dissection of the left crus of the hiatus

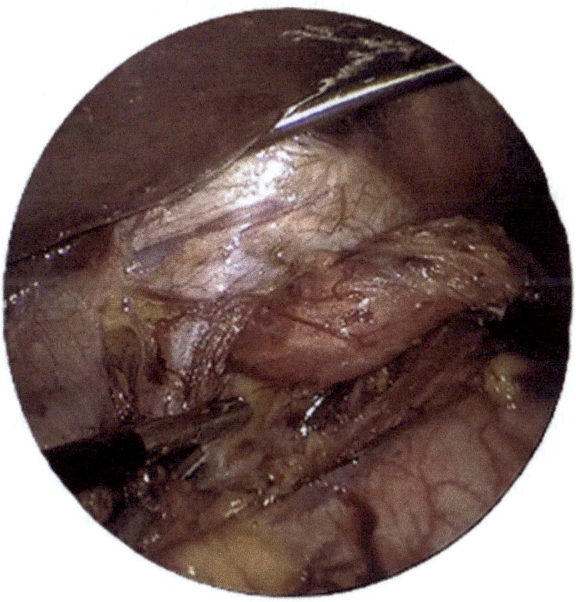

Fig. 4 Creation of the window posterior to the esophagus

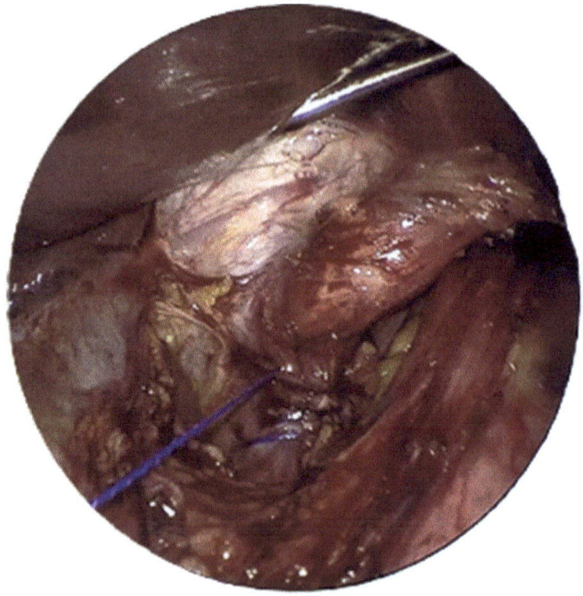

Fig. 5 Cruroplasty

A cruroplasty is performed after circumferentially clearing the esophagus and ensuring having 2–3 of the lower esophagus intraabdominally in a tension free manner This can be done using either interrupted or running non-absorbable suture in the posterior aspect of the hiatus. A non-absorbable barbed suture is preferable using a 2 layers horizontal mattress repair followed by running stitch. (Fig. 5).

Stomach Transection

A bougie is introduced orally until it reaches the distal stomach. A laparoscopic stapler is then used to transect the stomach. The use of absorbable re-inforced staplers is preferred routinely in this operation due to the unique dynamics of the gastric sleeve staple line being one of the longest staple lines we construct in GI surgery, in addition to the high-pressure nature of the resulting lumen. It is within the standard of care to reinforce with oversewing of the staple line, or to choose not to reinforce and use only buttresses material.

The first staple divides the antrum, approximately 2–5 cm proximal to the pylorus. Subsequent staples are fired sequentially, following the bougie as a guide. (Fig. 6).

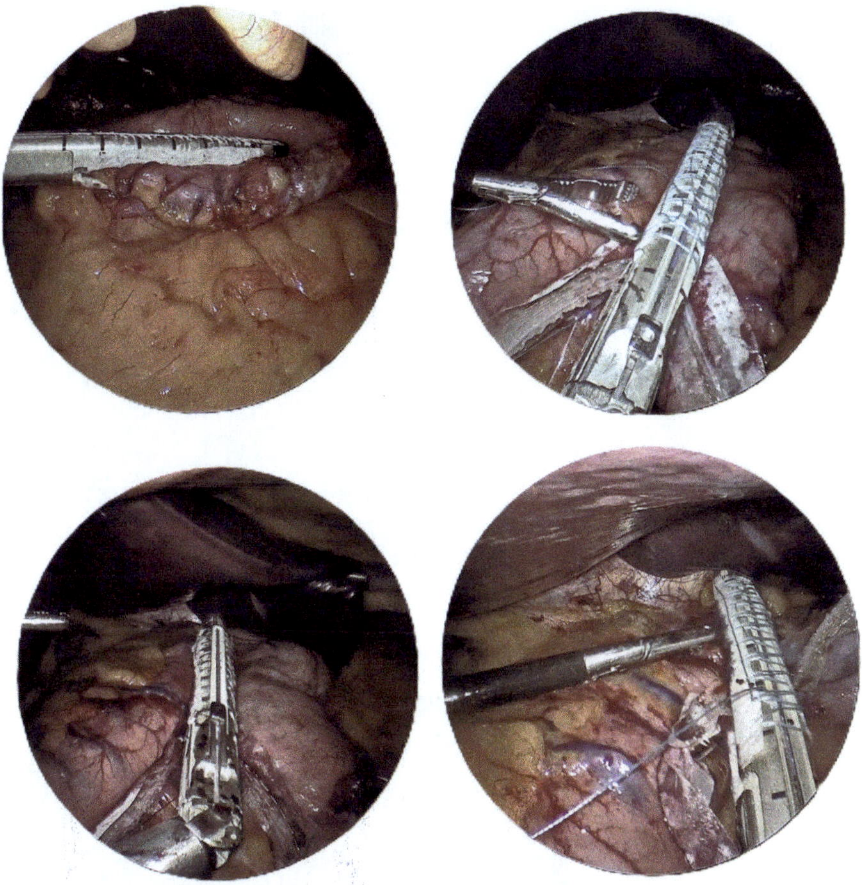

Fig. 6 Creation of sleeve gastrectomy with linear staplers

The bougie size is still not agreed upon in the surgical community. It is more important to maintain a good the distance between the bougie and the actual staplers. It is generally accepted that the bougie should be at least 40fr if the surgeon plans to stay close to it.

The final staple firing is placed approximately 1 cm lateral to the GEJ, taking care to avoid leaving a posterior pouch (Figs. 7 and 8).

While firing the staplers, it is critical to have equal retraction of the anterior and posterior gastric wall in order to prevent twisting of the staple line.

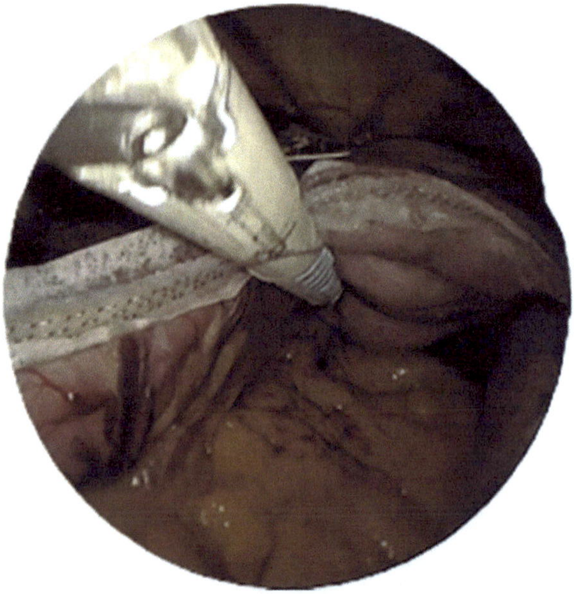

Fig. 7 Final stapler placement

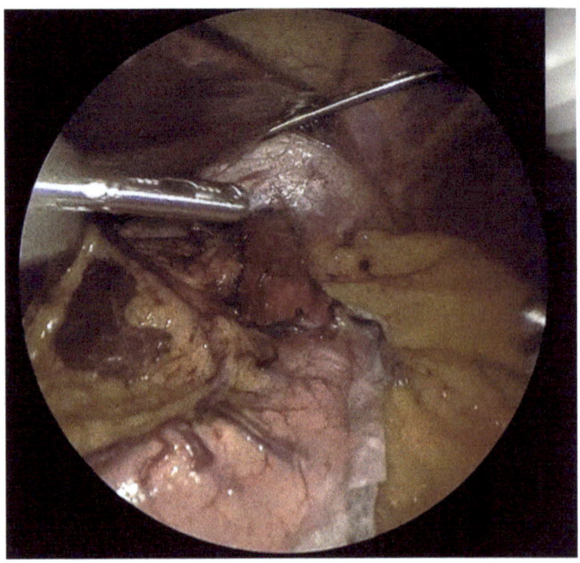

Fig. 8 Sleeve stapler line inspection

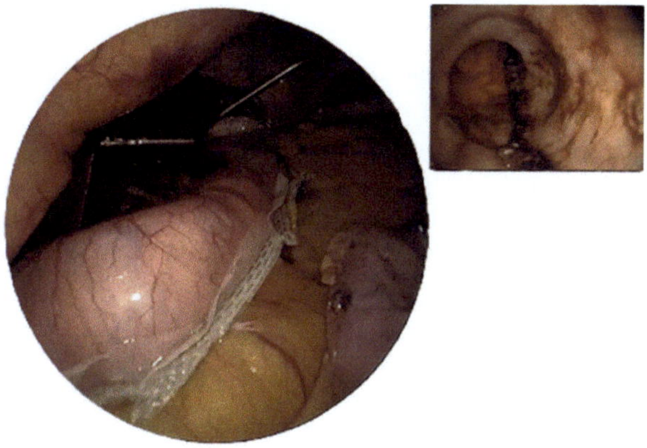

Fig. 9 Endoscopy and air leak test

EGD and Removal of the Specimen

Intraoperative endoscopy is routinely used to ensure optimal anatomy and to rule out bleeding or leak (Fig. 9).

It is also acceptable to use the bougie, to perform an air-leak test or methylene blue test.

The resected specimen is retrieved through one of the 12-millimeter port without the use of retrieval bag. Trocars are then removed, followed by closure of the remaining incisions. We recommend closing all trocar site 10 mm and above.

Conclusions

Sleeve gastrectomy is a widely performed bariatric surgical procedure globally. Despite its relative simplicity, it is not easy to construct a "perfect" sleeve. Adherence to a routine and proper technique, as the surgical steps outlined in this chapter, is essential for a low incidence of complications, proper durable weight loss, and avoiding high incidence of postoperative GERD.

References

1. Boustani P, Sheidaei A, Mokhber S, Pazouki A. Assessment of weight change patterns following roux en Y gastric bypass, one anastomosis gastric bypass and sleeve gastrectomy using change-point analysis. Sci Rep. 2024;14(1):17416. https://doi.org/10.1038/s41598-024-68480-x.
2. Estimate of Bariatric Surgery Numbers, 2011–2022. American Society for Metabolic and Bariatric Surgery. June 27, 2022. https://asmbs.org/resources/estimate-of-bariatric-surgery-numbers/. Accessed 24 Sept 2024.

Robotic Sleeve Gastrectomy

Federico Serrot and Emiliano G. Manuelli Laos

Abstract Sleeve gastrectomy (SG) is a minimally invasive bariatric procedure that has gained popularity due to its effectiveness in weight loss and improvement of obesity-related comorbidities. This technique involves the surgical removal of a significant portion of the stomach, resulting in a smaller, tubular-shaped stomach. The application of robotic surgery to this procedure offers several advantages, including enhanced precision, improved visualization, and reduced surgical trauma. By providing a comprehensive overview of the technical nuances of robotic SG, this chapter aims to contribute to the understanding and successful implementation of this procedure.

Keywords Obesity · Bariatric surgery · Sleeve gastrectomy · Robotic surgery

Introduction

Sleeve gastrectomy (SG) is a surgical procedure in which the stomach size gets significantly reduced, transforming it into a tubular shape. This procedure is highly effective for weight loss and managing obesity-related health conditions, leading to up to 25–35% total weight loss and 50–70% of the excess of weight loss within the first year after surgery and making it the most common bariatric procedure in the US [1, 2]. Weight loss after SG occurs through a combination of mechanical and hormonal factors. The reduced stomach size limits food intake, reducing calorie consumption. Additionally, the removal of ghrelin-producing cells disrupts hunger signals to the brain. SG can be performed as an initial procedure or as revision

F. Serrot (✉)
Bariatric & Metabolic Surgery, Cleveland Clinic Martin Health, Stuart, FL, USA

E. G. Manuelli Laos
Minimally Invasive & Bariatric Surgery, University of Illinois at Chicago, Chicago, IL, USA

F. Schlottmann, M. A. Masrur (eds.), *Endoscopic, Laparoscopic and Robotic Techniques for Foregut Disorders*, https://doi.org/10.1007/978-3-032-00811-4_2

surgery, often after gastric band removal or endoscopic sleeve gastroplasty. Robotic surgery has become increasingly prominent in bariatrics, with robotic sleeve gastrectomy serving as an excellent training model for its application in this field.

In this chapter, the technical aspects of the robotic approach for SG are described.

Procedure Description

Patient Preparation

The patient is positioned supine on the operating table with both arms abducted 90° and secured on padded arm boards. Prophylactic intravenous Cefazolin (2–3 g, weight-adjusted) and 5000 Units of Unfractionated Heparin are administered to mitigate the risks of postoperative infection and venous thromboembolism, respectively. Bilateral pneumatic compression devices are applied to the lower extremities prior to induction of general anesthesia. Finally, the abdomen is aseptically and antiseptically prepped and draped.

Pneumoperitoneum and Port Placement

Accessing the intraabdominal cavity and obtaining pneumoperitoneum can be accomplished in different ways. Among bariatric patients, the two most common ones are:

1. *Veress needle:* Establishing pneumoperitoneum first using a Veress needle inserted at Palmer's point, targeting an intra-abdominal pressure of 15 mmHg, followed by port placement.
2. *Optical Access Trocar:* Approximately 18–23 cm from the Xiphoid process and slightly left to the midline, an 8 m incision is performed and the individual tissue layers are divided and traversed utilizing an 8 mm Optical Access robotic trocar, with a 5 mm scope for direct visualization. The design of the coned obturator tip gives the surgeon a clear view while piercing the abdominal layers. Once intraabdominally, pneumoperitoneum is established targeting an intra-abdominal pressure of 15 mmHg. This is the technique preferred by the author of this chapter.

Once pneumoperitoneum has been established, a total of 4 trocars are placed on a straight line 18–23 cm from the Xiphoid process, commonly corresponding to the level of the umbilicus, depending on the patient's body habitus. First one is an 8 mm trocar placed slightly left to the midline (arm 2) that will be used for a 30-degree robotic camera throughout the entire case. Two extra 8 mm trocars are placed in the left side of the abdomen (arm 3 and 4), separated from each other by approximately 8 cm distance. The last trocar is 12 mm in diameter and is placed in the right upper

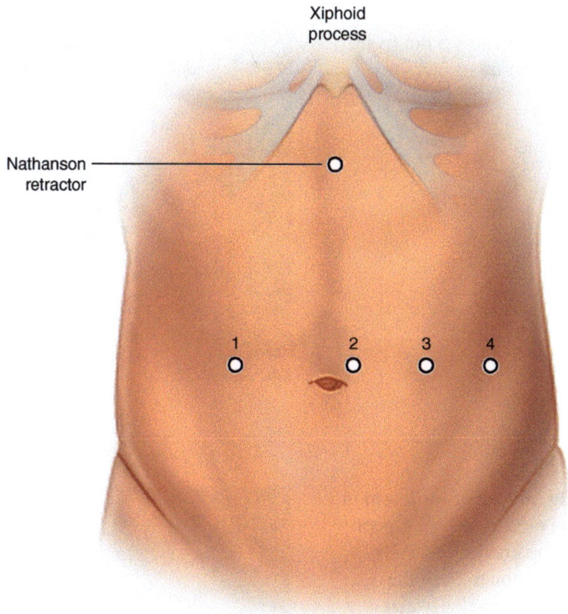

Fig. 1 Placement of trocars for robotic sleeve gastrectomy, named 1–4 for each robotic arm

quadrant (arm 1). This will be used for the stapler. Lastly, a Nathanson liver retractor is placed subxiphoid area and secured in place (Fig. 1).

Stomach Mobilization

The initial step of the procedure involves the identification and mobilization of the stomach. The anterior gastric wall is retracted using a robotic atraumatic grasper inserted in arm 1, a second robotic grasper, usually atraumatic as well, placed through arm 4 is used to retract the omentum containing the short gastric vessels, providing unobstructed access to the greater curvature. Using the Vessels sealer device through arm 3, the lesser sac is entered at the junction between Body and Antrum of the stomach where the lesser sac can be easily accessed, approximately 5 cm from the pylorus. This facilitates the mobilization of the greater omentum. (Fig. 2).

Lateral retraction of the greater omentum is maintained with the robotic grasper to optimize the exposure. The dissection is then carried superiorly until complete mobilization of the stomach fundus and visualization of the left crus are achieved. During this last step of the mobilization, arm 4 grasper usually changes from

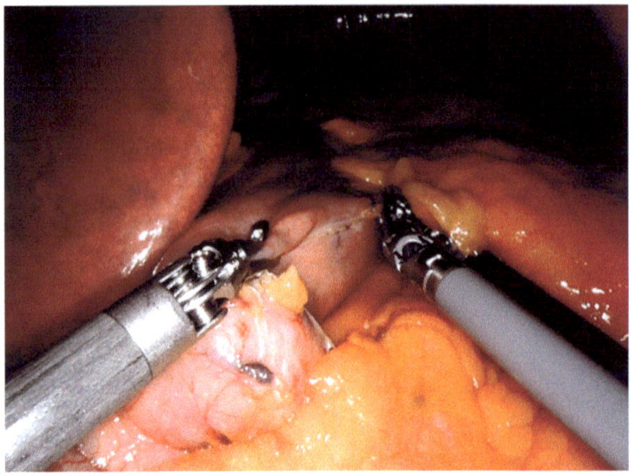

Fig. 2 Mobilization of the omentum and short gastric vessels starting approximately 5 cm from the pylorus

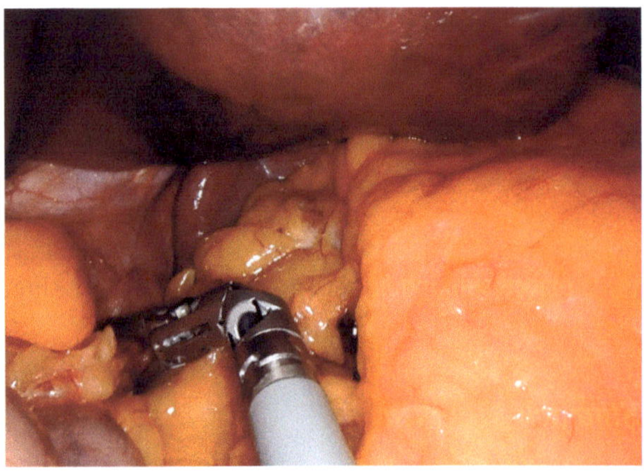

Fig. 3 Use of forth arm in the most proximal aspect of the greater curvature dissection to push the stomach medially and expose the angle of His and posterior vessels

retracting the omenum laterally to pushing the stomach medially for better exposure of the angle of His and posterior short gastric vessels (Fig. 3).

The esophageal hiatus is carefully dissected to identify any existing or potential hiatal hernias.

The left crus is completely dissected and exposed, this ultimately allows exposure of the gastroesophageal junction (GEJ). The dissection is then continued distally, mobilization the greater curvature until about 2–3 cm from the Pylorus. In some situations, posterior attachments to the stomach are released to allow full mobilization and correct placement of the stapler.

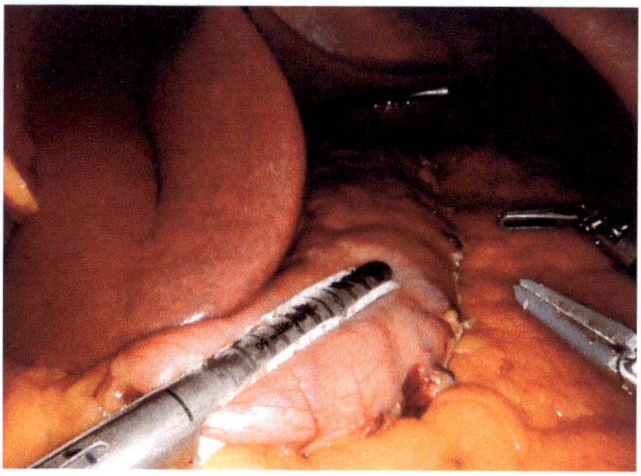

Fig. 4 Stapling of the stomach using SureForm™ 60 mm stapler

Stomach Stapling

A 36-38F bougie is orally advanced to the distal stomach to serve as a guide for the stapling step. The use or not of staple line reinforcement is generally left to the surgeon's preference and availability.

The Robotic SureForm™ 60 mm Staplers with reinforcement material is used for this step. Firing start by placing the initial green staple load approximately 5 cm proximal to the pylorus (Fig. 4). Subsequent staples are then sequentially fired along the course of the bougie. The Antrum of the stomach is stapled using green robotic loads, the body using blue stapler loads and finally the fundus is divided using white 60 mm stapler loads. The posterior aspect of fundus is retracted to facilitate optimal exposure during staple placement avoiding retained fundus (Fig. 5).

The final staple is carefully placed approximately 1 cm lateral to the gastroesophageal junction. It is of extreme importance that during the stapling portion the stomach is uniformly retracted allowing for a lateral staple line, avoiding torsion of the Sleeve. Another very important tip during the stapling of the stomach is to confirm with the anesthesia provider that no other devices are in the patient's mouth or nose, such us nasogastric tube or temperature probes, to avoid the accidental entrapment in the staple line. It is recommended to perform a time out prior to stapling to confirm every time that this is the case.

Endoscopy/Air Leak Test

Air leak is recommended in all cases. This can either be accomplished by performing an intraoperative upper endoscopic, not only allowing to perform the leak test but also visualization of the staple line and gastric mucosa. Another option is to use a flexible, single-use 36 F tube that will serve as a guide during the stapling as well as to perform an air leak test.

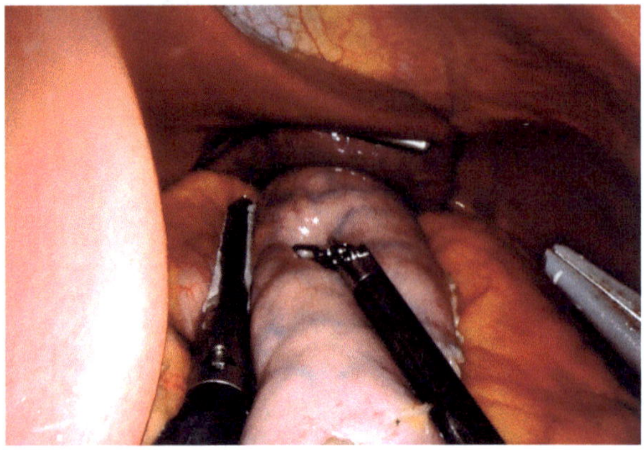

Fig. 5 Ensuring no retained fundus is left behind during the stapling of the stomach

Specimen Removal and Port Access Closure

Lastly, the specimen is removed through the 12 mm port with or without the use of an endocatch bag. The fascial defect is closed with absorbable sutures the rest of the trocars are removed, followed by standard closure of the incisions.

Conclusions

Robotic sleeve gastrectomy is increasingly favored among bariatric surgeons due to its feasibility, lower complication rates, and reduced torque on the abdominal wall, offering distinct advantages over the laparoscopic approach, particularly for patients with high BMI or super-super obesity. Robotic SG has become an excellent training model for bariatric surgeons entering the field of robotics. Mastery of the procedure's technical aspects is essential to minimize postoperative complications.

References

1. Boustani P, Sheidaei A, Mokhber S, Pazouki A. Assessment of weight change patterns following Roux en Y gastric bypass, one anastomosis gastric bypass and sleeve gastrectomy using change-point analysis. Sci Rep. 2024;14(1):17416. https://doi.org/10.1038/s41598-024-68480-x.
2. Estimate of Bariatric Surgery Numbers, 2011–2021. American Society for Metabolic and Bariatric Surgery. https://asmbs.org/resources/estimate-of-bariatric-surgery-numbers/. Accessed 2 Jan 2024.

Laparoscopic RYGB

Huy D. Hoang

Abstract This chapter explores the evolution of laparoscopic gastric bypass since its pioneering introduction in 1994 by Wittgrove and Clark. The procedure, initially a groundbreaking milestone, has gained widespread acceptance in both the medical community and the general public. Despite its complexity, the procedure stands out for its superior safety, cost-effectiveness, and patient acceptance. While the precise pathophysiology remains elusive, the positive outcomes underscore the procedure's effectiveness and enduring impact in metabolic and bariatric surgery.

Keywords Gastric bypass · Hand-sewn · Peri-gastric dissection · Ante-colic ante-gastric · Operative technique

Introduction

In 1994, Wittgrove and Clark achieved a groundbreaking milestone by conducting the inaugural laparoscopic gastric bypass. This pivotal event significantly contributed to fostering wider acceptance of metabolic and bariatric surgery within both the medical community and the general public. Over time, the laparoscopic gastric bypass has evolved into a prevalent metabolic operation, recognized for its safety and cost-effectiveness. The original technique has undergone numerous refinements, and this chapter will delve into one such variation of the operative procedures that is currently employed.

H. D. Hoang (✉)
Department of Surgery, University of Illinois at Chicago, Chicago, IL, USA
e-mail: huy.d.hoang@icloud.com

F. Schlottmann, M. A. Masrur (eds.), *Endoscopic, Laparoscopic and Robotic Techniques for Foregut Disorders*, https://doi.org/10.1007/978-3-032-00811-4_3

Procedure Description

Patient Positioning

The patient is placed in a supine position on the operating table, with consideration given to the patient's body habitus to prevent potential pressure points. Prior to the procedure, the patient receives preoperative antibiotics and venous thromboembolism prophylaxis. General endotracheal anesthesia is then administered, and sequential compression devices are placed. The abdomen is prepared and draped following standard sterile protocols.

Trocar Placement

The abdominal entry is achieved through the Optiview technique at Palmer's point, employing a 10 mm 0-degree laparoscope and a 12 mm trocar. Insufflation of the abdomen is carried out to a pressure of 15 mmHg. Subsequently, the 10 mm 0-degree laparoscope is switched to a 10 mm 30-degree one. Additional 12 mm trocars are carefully positioned under direct visualization, utilizing internal anatomy rather than external landmarks to optimize trocar placement for the operation. To aid in visualizing the hiatus, a 5 mm subxiphoid liver retractor is placed, and the patient is positioned in reverse Trendelenburg. (Fig. 1).

Fig. 1 Trocar placement

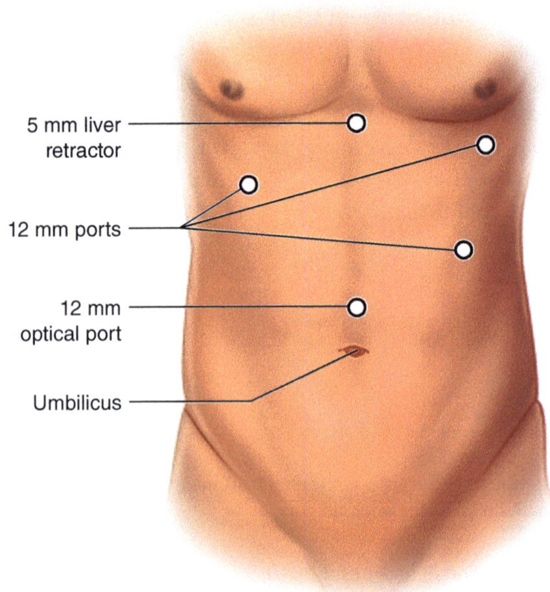

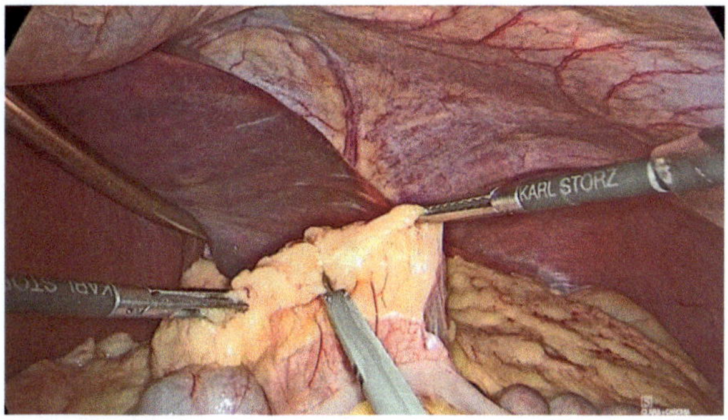

Fig. 2 Division of omentum

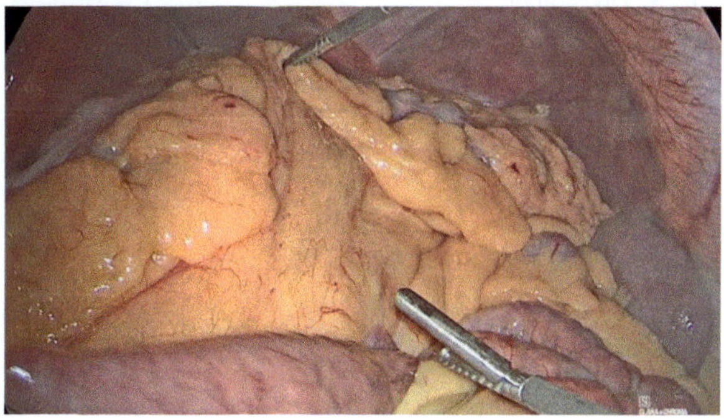

Fig. 3 Identification of ligament of Treitz

Creation of Jejunojejunostomy

The omentum is lifted cephalad and then divided using an energy device to facilitate the antecolic configuration of the Roux limb (Fig. 2). Following this, the transverse colon and its mesentery are lifted in a cephalad direction to expose the ligament of Treitz (Fig. **3**). The jejunum is measured (Fig. 4) and then transected 50 cm from the ligament of Treitz, utilizing a stapling device to create the biliopancreatic limb (Fig. 5). The mesentery of the jejunum is divided using an energy device (Fig. 6).

A measurement of a 100 cm Roux limb is performed (Fig. 7), followed by carefully created enterotomies on the common channel (Fig. 8) and the biliopancreatic limb (Fig. 9). Subsequently, a side-to-side stapled jejunojejunostomy is fashioned (Fig. 10). Special attention is emphasized to prevent any kinking or twisting of the Roux limb and to avoid inadvertently creating the notorious Roux-en-O configuration. The common enterotomy is then closed using a continuous absorbable suture (Fig. 11).

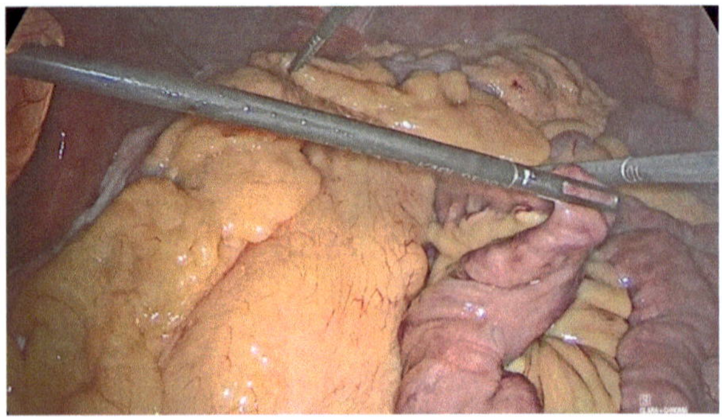

Fig. 4 Measurement of biliopancreatic limb

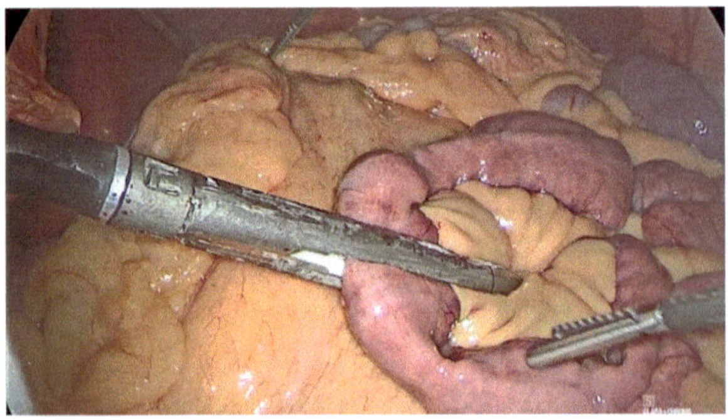

Fig. 5 Division of jejunum

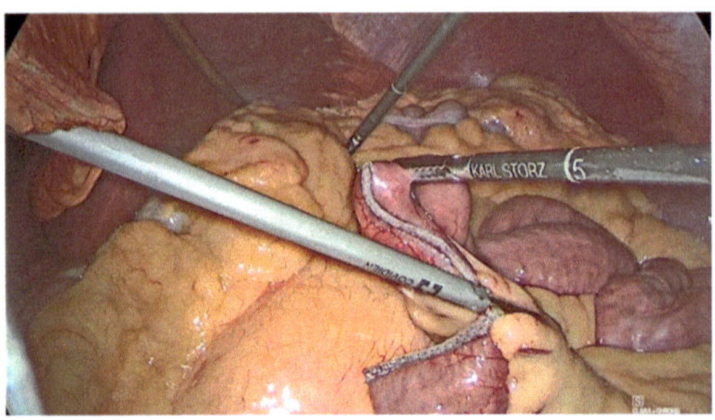

Fig. 6 Division of mesentery

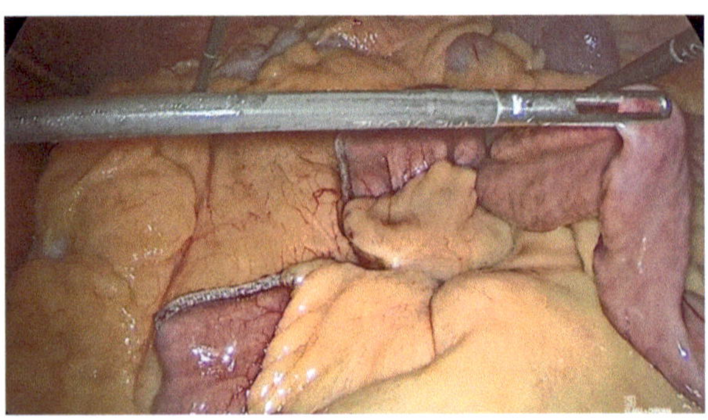

Fig. 7 Measurement of Roux limb

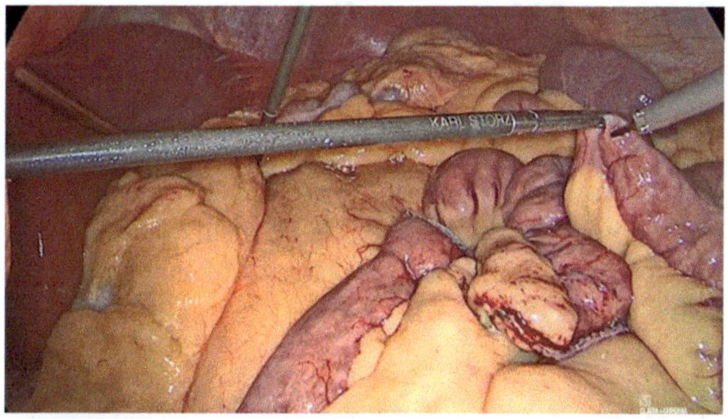

Fig. 8 Creation of jejunojejunostomy–creation of enterotomy on the common channel

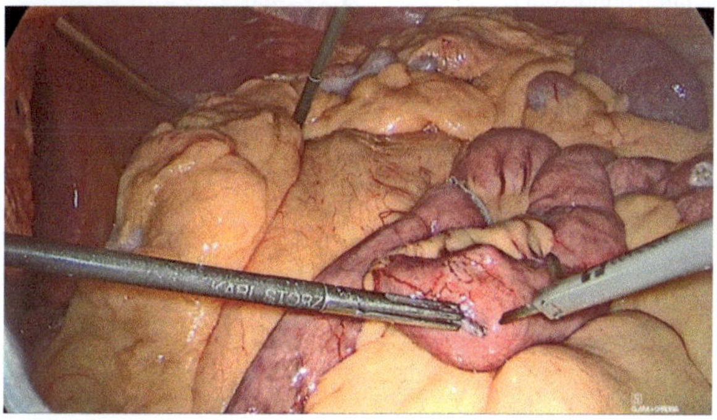

Fig. 9 Creation of jejunojejunostomy–creation of enterotomy on the biliopancreatic limb

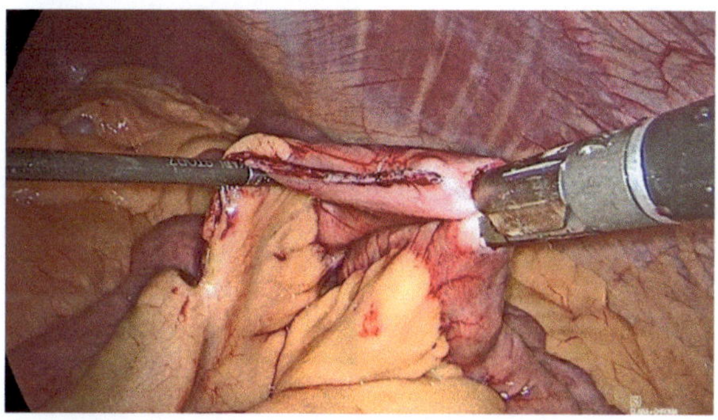

Fig. 10 Creation of jejunojejunostomy–creation of stapled side-to-side anastomosis

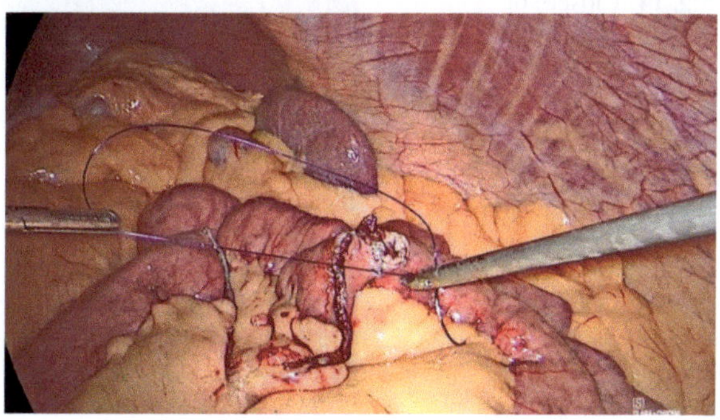

Fig. 11 Creation of jejunojejunostomy–closure of common enterotomy

Closure of Mesenteric Defects

The Roux limb is carefully elevated in a cephalad direction to ensure its optimal reach to the gastric pouch without tension. Subsequently, the mesenteric defect at the jejuno-jejunostomy is closed using a continuous non-absorbable suture (Figs. 12 and 13). Following this step, the Roux limb is gently reflected to the left of the patient, exposing the Petersen's space, and the closure of this space is executed in a similar fashion (Figs. 14 and 15).

Fig. 12 Closure of jejunojejunostomy mesenteric defect

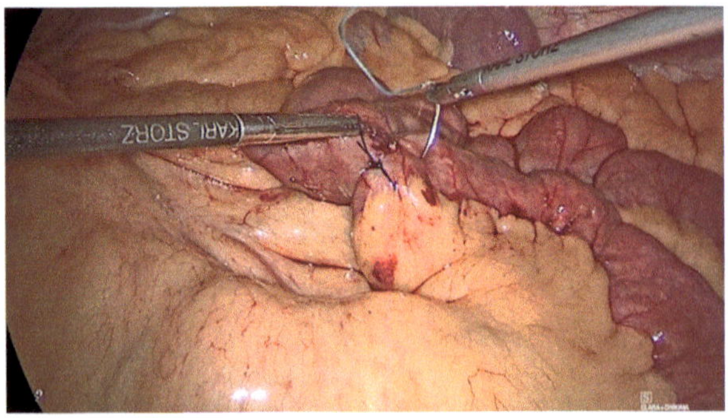

Fig. 13 Closure of jejunojejunostomy mesenteric defect

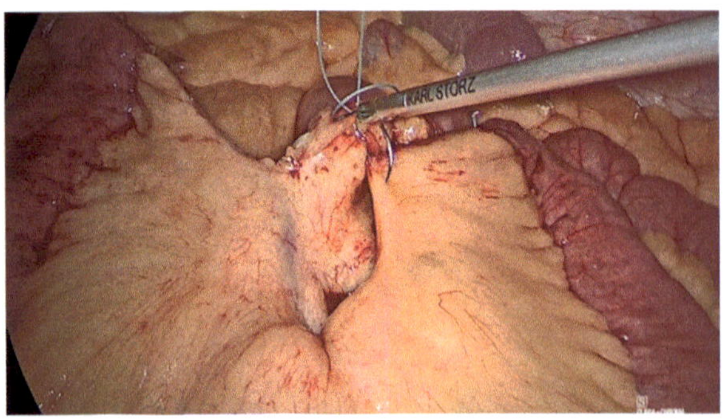

Fig. 14 Closure of Petersen's space

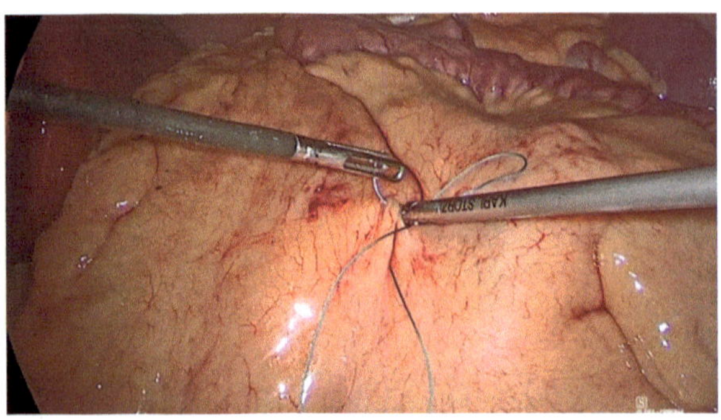

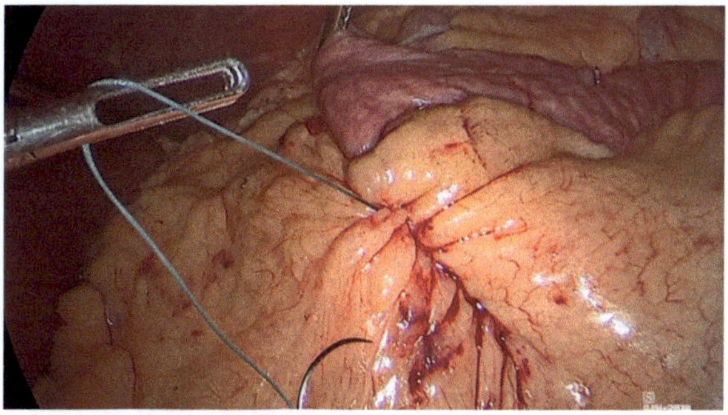

Fig. 15 Closure of Petersen's space

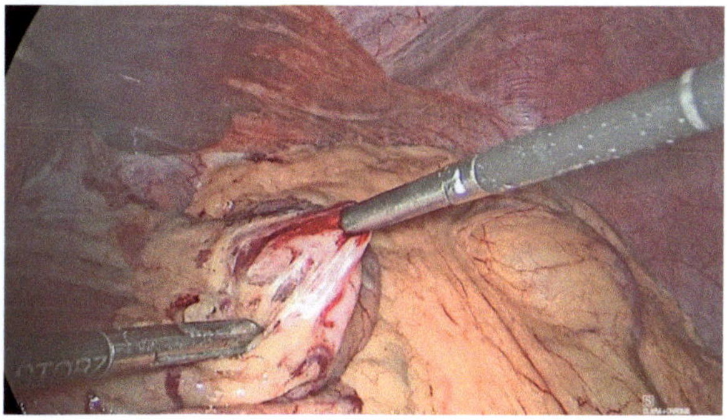

Fig. 16 Creation of gastric pouch–lesser curve dissection

Creation of Gastric Pouch

The focus then transitions to the creation of the gastric pouch, commencing with the dissection of the angel of His to expose the left crus. A perigastric dissection is carried out using an energy device approximately 5 cm distal to the gastroesophageal junction (Fig. 16). Notably, a perigastric dissection is favored over the par flaccida technique to safeguard the integrity of the vagus nerves.

The horizontal segment of the pouch is subsequently fashioned using a stapling device, with the 36 French bougie serving as a guide (Fig. 17). Following this, the posterior component of the dissection of the angle of His is performed, and the vertical segment of the pouch is created using a stapling device, once again guided by the 36 French bougie (Fig. 18). This methodical approach ensures precision and adherence to the intended dimensions of the gastric pouch.

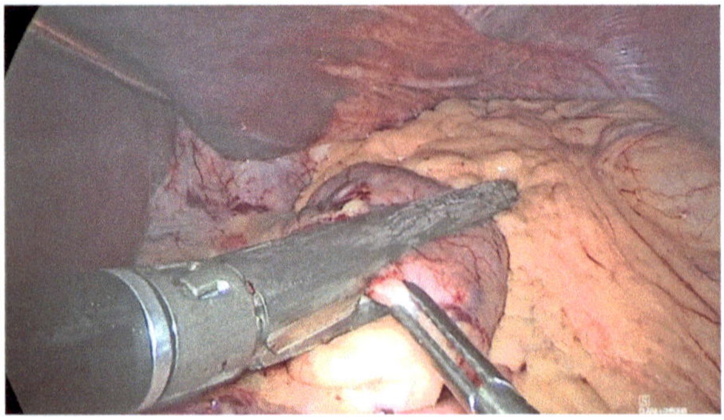

Fig. 17 Creation of gastric pouch–horizontal fire

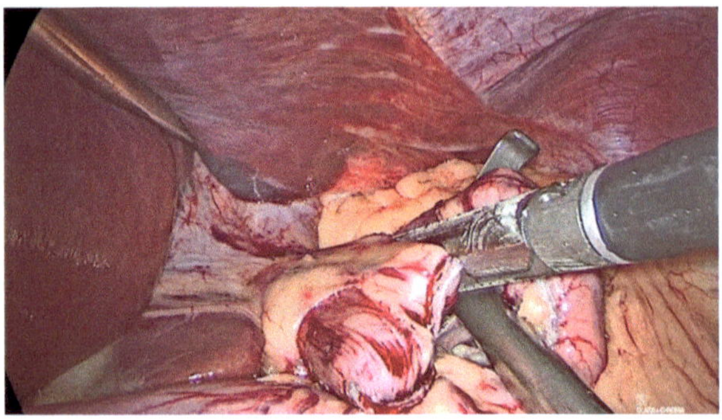

Fig. 18 Creation of gastric pouch–vertical fire

Creation of Gastrojejunostomy

The Roux limb is brought in an antecolic antegastric fashion, and a hand-sewn two-layer gastrojejunostomy is crafted using absorbable sutures. The initial layer, positioned posteriorly, is placed between the antimesenteric border of the Roux limb and the horizontal segment of the pouch (Fig. 19). Gastrotomy and enterotomy are carefully fashioned with the use of an energy device (Figs. 20 and 21). Subsequently, the posterior and anterior components of the second layer are performed (Figs. 22 and 23).

Before tying the inner layers together, the 36 French bougie is advanced through the anastomosis to prevent any inadvertent purse-string effect. The anterior component of the first layer is created in a horizontal mattress fashion and securely tied to the posterior first layer (Fig. 24). To ensure integrity, a bowel clamp is applied to the proximal Roux limb, and an air leak test is conducted (Fig. 25). This approach ensures a robust and well-constructed gastrojejunostomy (Fig. 26).

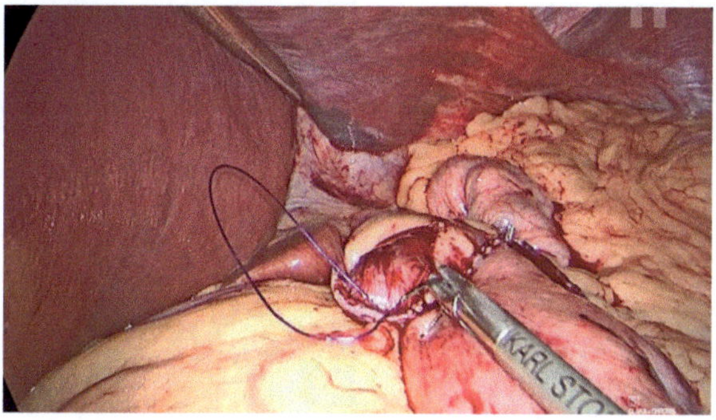

Fig. 19 Creation of gastrojejunostomy–posterior outer layer

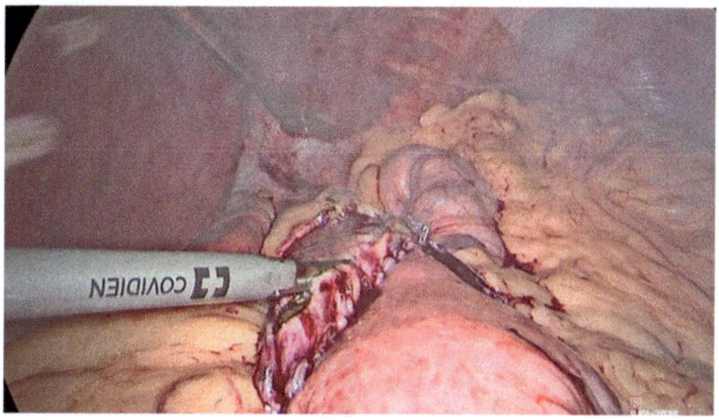

Fig. 20 Creation of gastrojejunostomy–gastrotomy

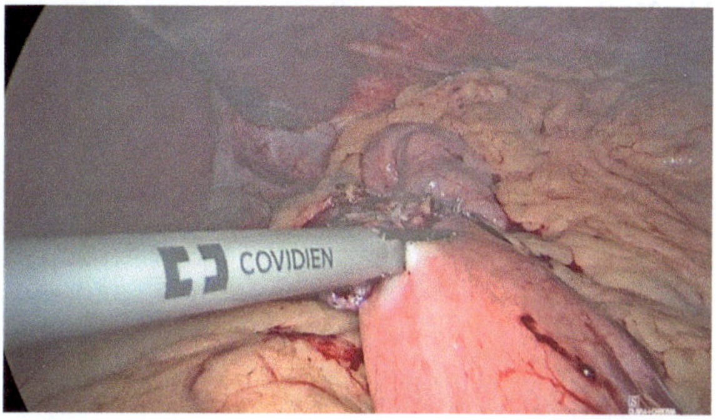

Fig. 21 Creation of gastrojejunostomy–enterotomy

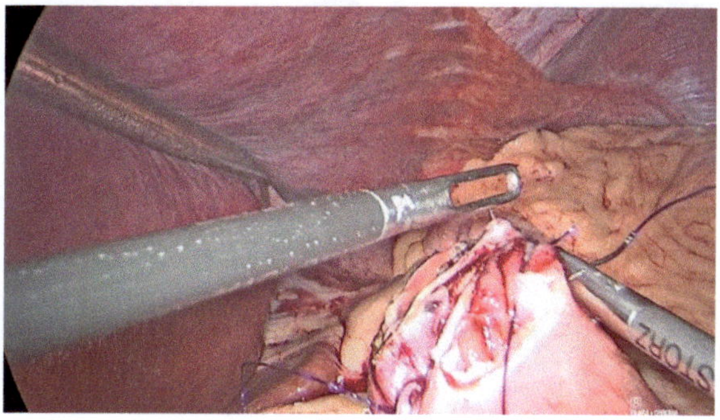

Fig. 22 Creation of gastrojejunostomy–posterior inner layer

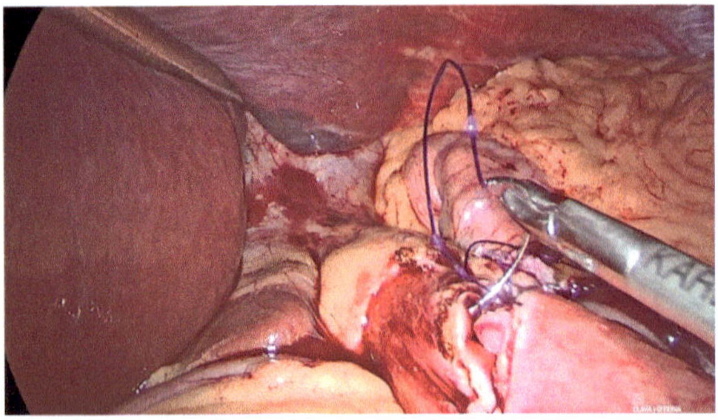

Fig. 23 Creation of gastrojejunostomy–anterior inner layer

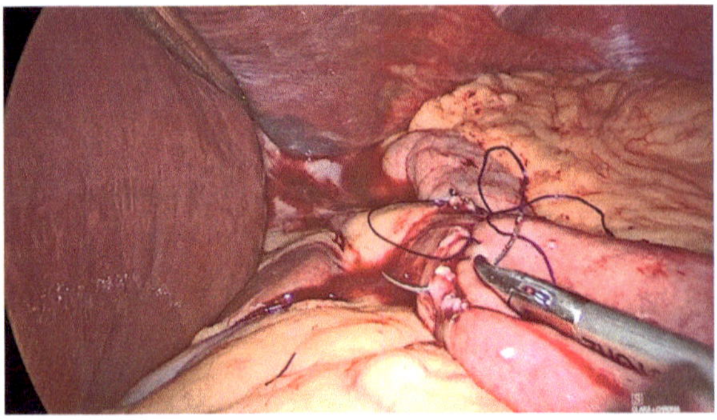

Fig. 24 Creation of gastrojejunostomy–anterior outer layer

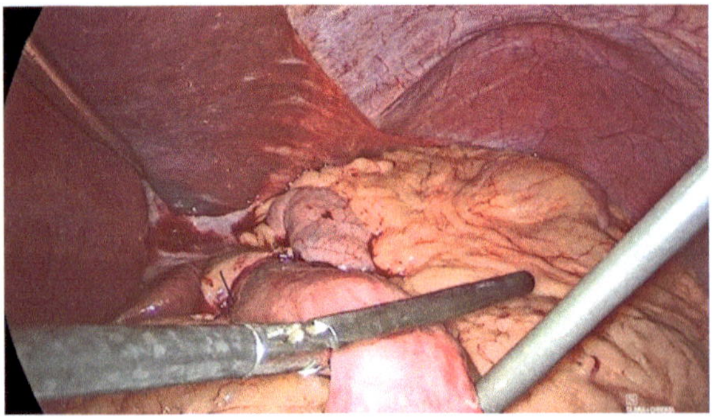

Fig. 25 Creation of gastrojejunostomy–air leak test

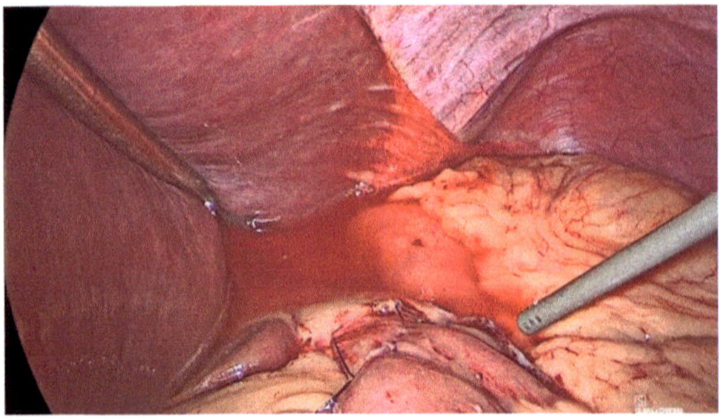

Fig. 26 Creation of gastrojejunostomy–complete anastomosis

Final Inspection

The successful completion of the gastrojejunostomy signifies the conclusion of the operation. A meticulous check for hemostasis is conducted to ensure no bleeding concerns. Subsequently, the trocars used during the procedure are carefully removed, and the skin incisions are re-approximated in the standard fashion.

Conclusions

Despite its inherent complexity and steep learning curve, the laparoscopic gastric bypass stands out as a superior choice in terms of safety, cost-effectiveness, and heightened patient acceptance. While the precise pathophysiology of the gastric bypass remains elusive, the undeniable outcomes underscore its efficacy and impact. There exists no universally acknowledged "gold-standard" for laparoscopic gastric bypass procedures. However, this chapter delineates a secure and consistently replicable variation of the operation.

Robotic RYGB

Cristina Perez Viso, Tarani Bajwa, Shinil K. Shah, and Erik B. Wilson

Abstract Obesity is a serious, common and costly chronic disease with increasing prevalence in the US and globally. Minimally invasive Roux-en-Y gastric bypass is one of the most reliable and effective operations for patients with morbid obesity. In this chapter, we describe the technique for minimally invasive Roux-en-Y gastric bypass approach with robotic assistance providing illustrations of the key intraoperative surgical steps.

Keywords Obesity · Roux-en-Y gastric bypass · Robotic surgery · Minimally invasive surgery · Surgical technique · Laparoscopic surgery

Introduction

Obesity is a serious, common and costly global disease. The CDC estimates 9.2% of Americans had severe obesity in 2017, the highest incidence ever recorded in the United States [1].

In 2023, The Center for Control of Diseases, in conjunction with the Behavioral Risk Factor Surveillance System, an ongoing state-based telephone interview survey, has reported an obesity prevalence higher than 20% in all U.S states and

C. P. Viso · T. Bajwa · E. B. Wilson (✉)
Division of Minimally Invasive and Elective General Surgery, Department of Surgery, McGovern Medical School, University of Texas Health Science Center at Houston, Houston, TX, USA

S. K. Shah
Division of Minimally Invasive and Elective General Surgery, Department of Surgery, McGovern Medical School, University of Texas Health Science Center at Houston, Houston, TX, USA

Michael E DeBakey Institute for Comparative Cardiovascular Science and Biomedical Devices, Texas A&M University, College Station, TX, USA
e-mail: shinil.k.shah@uth.tmc.edu

F. Schlottmann, M. A. Masrur (eds.), *Endoscopic, Laparoscopic and Robotic Techniques for Foregut Disorders*, https://doi.org/10.1007/978-3-032-00811-4_4

territories (more than 1 in 5 adults) Overall, the Midwest (36%) and South (34.7) had the highest prevalence of obesity, followed by the West (29%) and the Northeast (28.6%) [2].

Obesity is closely linked to chronic diseases including type 2 diabetes, heart disease, stroke and certain types of cancer. Bariatric surgery is the most effective and durable treatment for severe obesity, leading to significant weight loss and improvement, prevention or resolution of many related diseases. Roux-en-Y gastric bypass (RYGB) is one of the most reliable bariatric procedures as it allows for long lasting weight loss and effective remission of obesity-associated conditions.

Over time, the surgical technique for Roux-en-Y gastric bypass has been refined and standardized. In this chapter, we describe our technique for the minimally invasive Roux-en-Y gastric bypass approach with robotic assistance providing illustrations of the key intraoperative surgical steps.

Procedure Description

Patient Positioning

The patient is placed supine on the operative table. Appropriately chosen intravenous antibiotics and subcutaneous pharmacologic DVT prophylaxis are given within 1 hour of the incision time. Pre-operative nerve blocks can be performed before or after induction of general anesthesia, or intra-operatively by the surgeon as per surgeon and anesthesiologist preference. Once general endotracheal anesthesia is achieved, sequential compression devices are placed in both legs, arms are abducted on armboards with padding, and a footboard is positioned so that the feet lie flat (Fig. 1). Care should be taken to provide adequate padding of the midfoot and to prevent hyperflexion in a steep reverse Trendelenburg position, which may result in severe injury. A 40 Fr gastric bougie (or sizing tube of the surgeon's choice) is inserted to splint the stomach and esophagus. A Foley catheter is generally not required for the procedure, unless the surgeon anticipates the case will be longer than 3–4 h.

Pneumoperitoneum and Port Placement

The abdomen is prepped and draped in sterile fashion. The abdomen is entered under direct visualization using an optical trocar through a 5-mm incision in the right upper quadrant. If there are anticipated dense adhesions in the right upper quadrant, a left upper quadrant entry may be chosen depending on the patient's particular surgical history. Pneumoperitoneum with carbon dioxide at 12–15 mmHg is obtained. Lower insufflation pressures are encouraged if appropriate. Under direct vision a 8-mm robotic port is placed superior and left to the umbilicus, then two 8-mm robotic ports are placed on the left side of the abdomen, a 5-mm port is

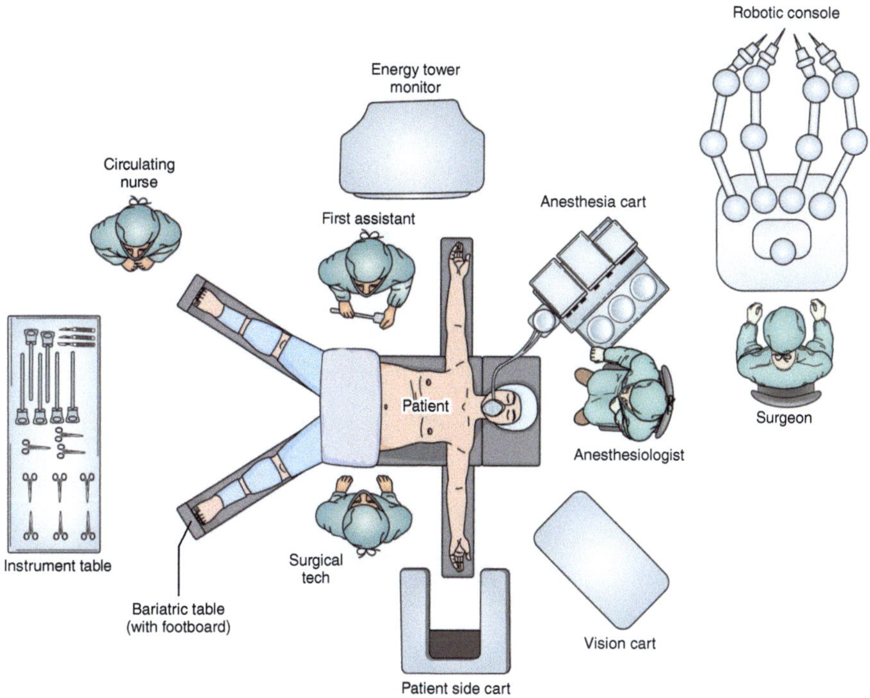

Fig. 1 Operating room set up and patient positioning

placed in the subxiphoid position (if external liver retractor is placed) and a 12–15-mm port is placed in the mid abdomen (depending on surgeon's choice of stapler). The 5-mm right upper quadrant trocar is upsized to a 8-mm robotic trocar. A Nathanson liver retractor is placed through the 5-mm subxiphoid incision. If an internal liver retractor is used (e.g., FreeHold Trio®, FreeHold Surgical, LLC, New Hope, PA), the subxiphoid incision is eliminated. The patient is placed in steep reverse Trendelenburg and the surgical robot is docked to the patient (Fig. 2).

Operative Technique

Creation of the Gastric Pouch

Using robotic assistance, the angle of His is exposed by dissecting the attachments from the stomach to the hiatus and diaphragm. We typically use a pars flaccida approach. The pars flaccida is opened widely with scissors with cautery. The left gastric artery is identified. Dissection with scissors with cautery is continued posteriorly to dissect the retroperitoneal attachments of the stomach. After the lesser sac is fully mobilized up to the left crus, the adjacent vessels are divided using a 60-mm endoscopic stapler with a vascular load and absorbable staple line reinforcement (Fig. 3).

Fig. 2 Port placement

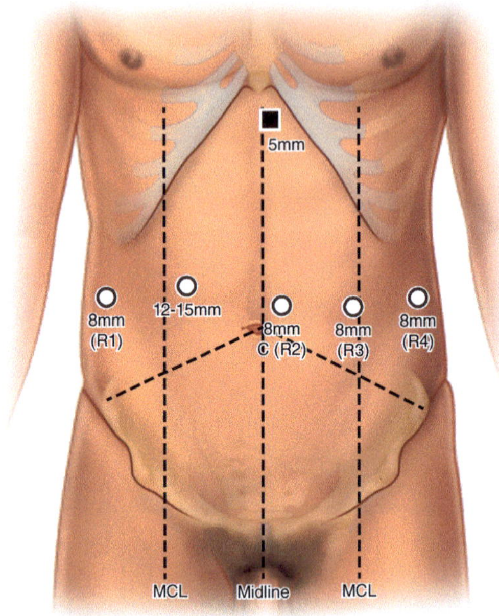

Fig. 3 Gastric pouch creation. Division of perigastric vessels

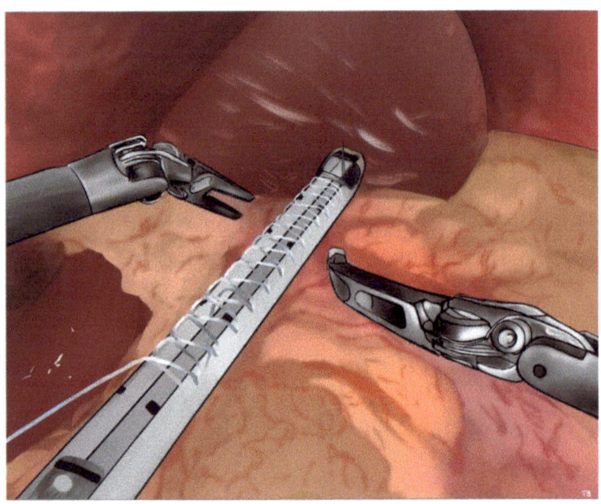

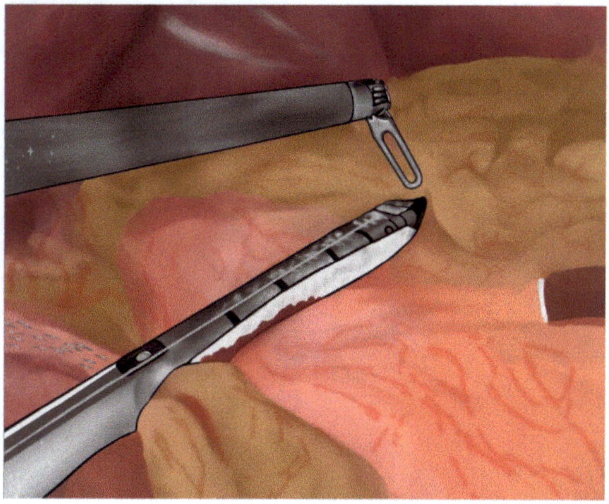

Fig. 4 Gastric pouch creation. First horizontal staple firing

In certain cases, a peri-gastric approach may obviate the need for this first staple fire. Typically, a vessel sealing device will be utilized when a perigastric approach is performed.

The upper gastric pouch is created with a single horizontal firing of the endoscopic stapler with an appropriately sized load for the proximal stomach and with absorbable staple line reinforcement (Fig. 4).

This is followed by a vertical staple fire towards the angle of His with an appropriately sized load for the proximal stomach and with absorbable staple line reinforcement. The staple fires are done around the sizing tube (Fig. 5).

An additional vertical firing of a non-reinforced 45-mm to 60-mm appropriately sized endoscopic stapler may be required to complete the pouch creation. A small 20 to 30 ml upper gastric pouch is obtained.

Creation of the Gastro-jejunostomy

In patients with a bulky greater omentum, it may be divided with a vessel sealing device to avoid tension once the alimentary limb is brought towards the gastric pouch.

The omentum and transverse colon are lifted superiorly and the ligament of Treitz is identified (Fig. 6).

The jejunum is run approximately 75–100 cm distal to the Ligament of Treitz and brought in apposition to the gastric pouch in an ante-colic position as an "omega loop". It is important the orientation is such that the biliary limb is positioned on the patient's left side (surgeon screen right) and the alimentary limb is on the patient's right side (surgeon screen left) (Fig. 7).

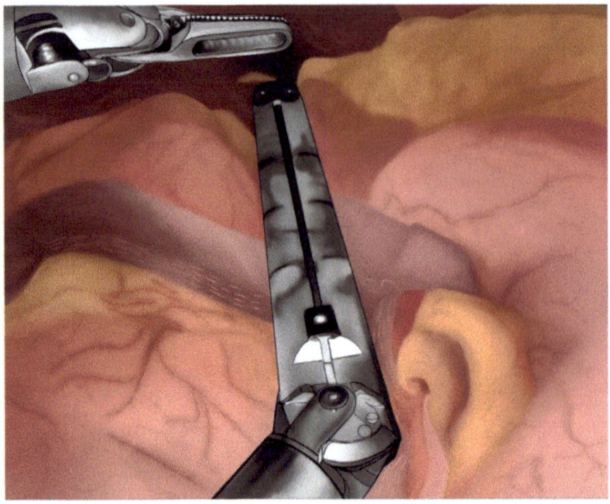

Fig. 5 Gastric pouch creation. Second vertical stapler firing

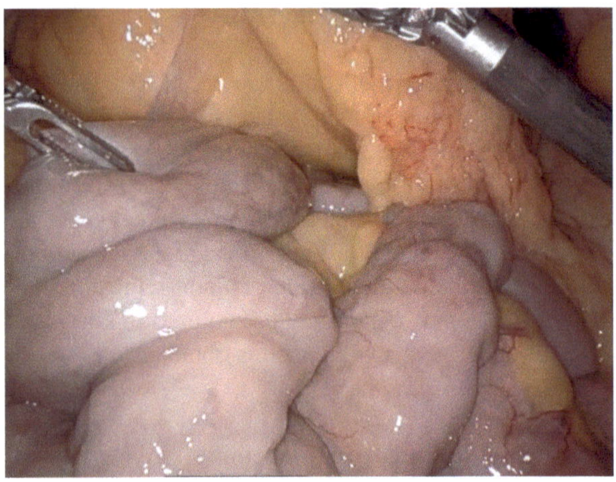

Fig. 6 Identification of the Ligament of Treitz

The gastric pouch and the jejunum are sutured together with the posterior row of the gastro-jejunostomy created with a double armed 2–0 absorbable spiral barbed suture in a running Lembert fashion (Fig. 8).

A 1.5 cm gastrotomy and enterotomy are made in the stomach and the jejunum using scissors with cautery and a 2-layer hand-sewn gastrojejunal anastomosis is performed over the previously placed 40 Fr bougie with the outer running layer of 2–0 absorbable spiral barbed suture and inner running layer of 2–0 braided Polyglactin absorbable suture. The bougie/sizing tube is removed after the gastrojejunostomy is complete (Fig. 9).

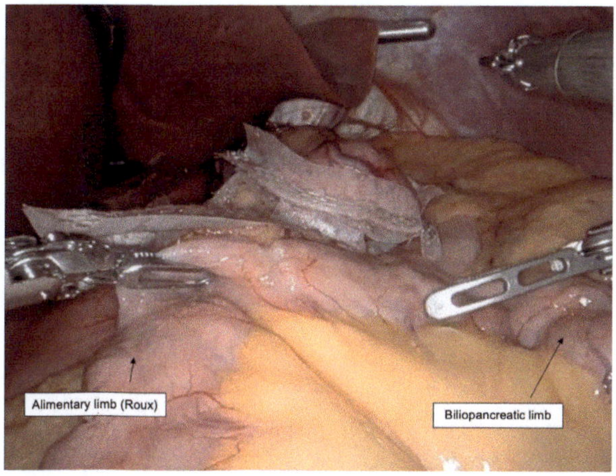

Fig. 7 Creation of "omega loop"

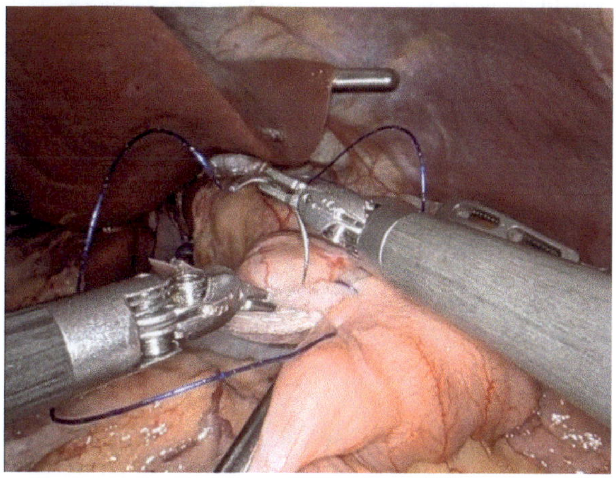

Fig. 8 Gastrojejunostomy. Posterior outer row

Division of the Jejunum and the "Omega Loop"

A defect in the jejunal mesentery just distal to the gastrojejunostomy is created and the jejunum divided using a 60-mm non-reinforced endoscopic stapler with appropriately sized load for the small intestine. This creates the biliopancreatic and and alimentary "Roux" limbs (Fig. 10).

Creation of Jejuno-jejunostomy

Once the omega loop is divided, the alimentary limb is run approximately 150 cm distal to the gastrojejunostomy and brought in apposition to the biliopancreatic limb. Both limbs are sutured with a 2–0 braided non-absorbable suture (silk).

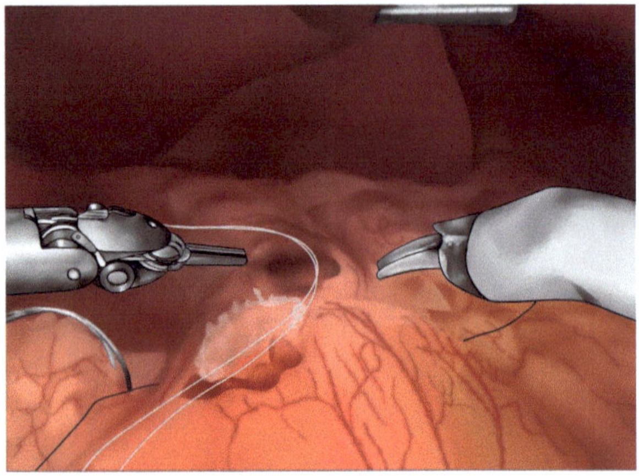

Fig. 9 Creation of gastro-jejunostomy: Posterior inner layer with running suture

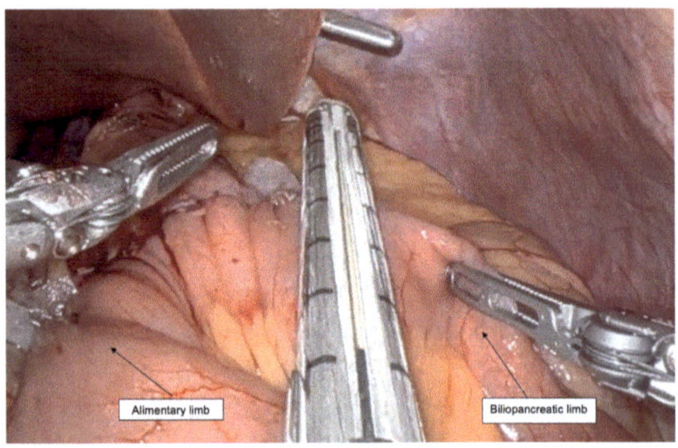

Fig. 10 Division of "omega loop"

Enterotomies are made in both segments of the bowel with scissors with cautery and an anastomosis is created using a 45–60-mm non-reinforced endoscopic stapler with an appropriately sized load for small bowel (Fig. 11).

The common enterotomy is closed using a running 2–0 braided Polyglactin absorbable suture (Fig. 12).

The mesenteric defect of the jejuno-jejunostomy is closed with a running 2–0 braided non-absorbable suture (silk) and includes a Brolin, anti-kinking suture to align the entry of the Roux limb to the jejuno-jejunostomy appropriately, and so as to prevent early post operative small bowel obstruction at this anastomosis. Care is taken not to take large bites on the Roux limb side and to appropriately advance on the biliopancreatic limb side to account for any size mismatch of the enterotomy (Fig. 13).

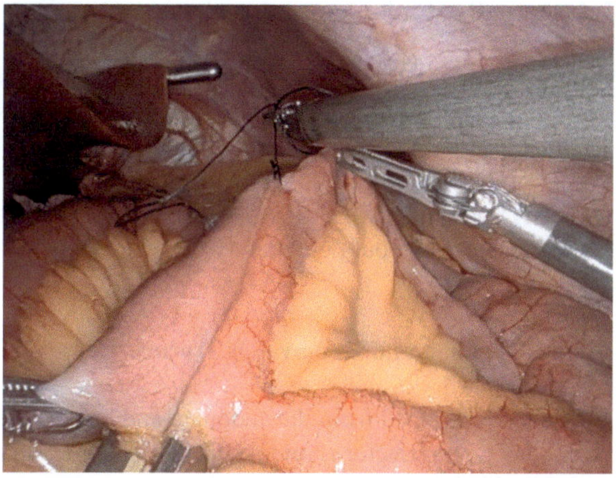

Fig. 11 Creation of jejuno-jejunostomy. Stapled common channel

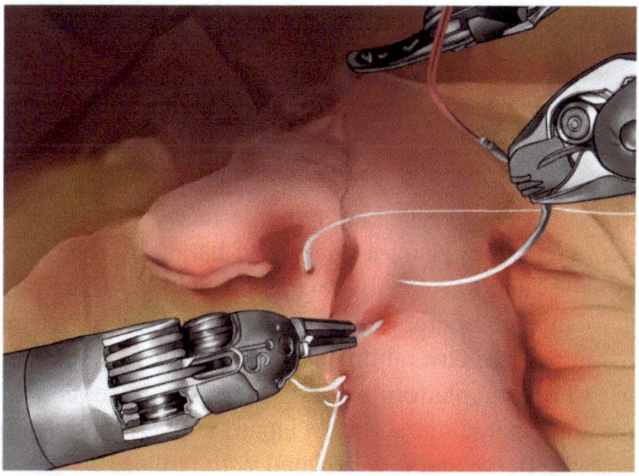

Fig. 12 Creation of jejuno-jejunostomy. Closure of enterotomy

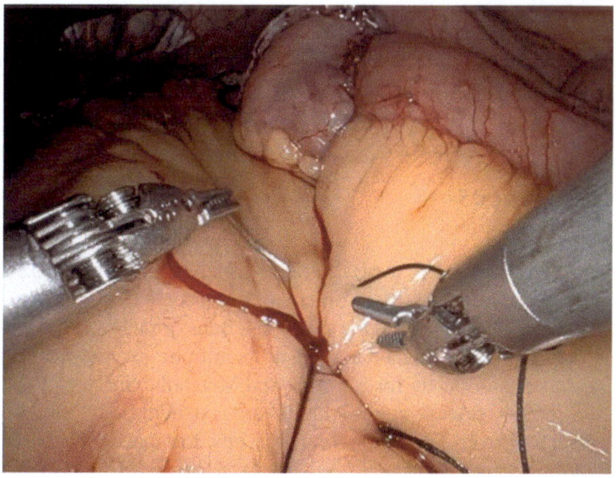

Fig. 13 Closure of mesenteric defect at the jejuno-jenunostomy

Intraoperative Endoscopy

Satisfied with our jejuno-jejunostomy, the alimentary limb is clamped distal to the anastomosis and saline solution is irrigated at the gastrojejunostomy. The endoscope is inserted through the mouth and passed down the esophagus under direct visualization into the gastric pouch. The pouch is insufflated under air pressure and leak test is performed. The scope is passed down the anastomosis to confirm patency, hemostasis and rule out potential leaks.

Final Inspection and Removal of Trocars

All fluid is suctioned from the abdomen and hemostasis is verified. The Nathanson or internal liver retractor is removed, and the 12–15-mm port fascial defect is closed with 0 braided Polyglactin absorbable sutures using a transfascial suture passer. The pneumoperitoneum is then evacuated and ports are removed under vision. Trocar sites are closed with subcuticular sutures.

Conclusions

Total robotic surgery is playing an increasing role in metabolic and bariatric surgery. With the rise in a number of bariatric procedures, surgeons are facing more complex and technically demanding surgical situations. Robotic platforms provide a solution to address these challenges. They allow for better visualization, tissue handling, maneuverability and ergonomics. Systematic reviews have revealed the use of robotic platforms lead to similar or lower complication rates in bariatric surgery, compared to traditional laparoscopy. Robotic gastric bypass requires a shorter learning curve and is associated with reduced lenghts of stay, compared to laparoscopic approaches [3].

Conflicts of Interest Erik B Wilson MD receives teaching honoraria from Intuitive Surgical, Inc. Shinil K Shah DO EdD has received prior research funding from Intuitive Surgical. There are no other relevant disclosures.

References

1. American Society for Bariatric and Metabolic Surgery 2024. ASMBS website. https://asmbs.org/resources/obesity-in-america/. Last access Oct 2024.
2. Center for Control of Diseases 2024. Behavioral Risk Factor Surveillance System. https://www.cdc.gov/obesity/data-and-statistics/adult-obesity-prevalence-maps.html. Last access Oct 2024.
3. American Society for Bariatric and Metabolic Surgery. 2024. ASMBS website. https://asmbs.org/new_releases/new-studies-suggest-benefit-of-total-robotic-metabolic-and-bariatric-surgery-over-conventional-laparoscopy. Last access Oct 2024.

Laparoscopic Duodenal Switch

Gabriela Restrepo-Rodas, Juan Cruz Lopez Meyer, Freddy Miguel Ortiz Aparicio, Suleiman Al-Baqain, and Alfredo D. Guerron

Abstract Biliopancreatic diversion is one of the oldest surgical procedures for weight loss. Over time, this technique has evolved, incorporating key features that culminated in the development of the Duodenal Switch (DS). Some properties that characterize the DS are the creation of a sleeve gastrectomy, duodenal transection with pyloric preservation, and standardized intestinal lengths. The DS is among the most effective bariatric procedures available, with a clear consensus on its benefits, particularly for those with a BMI > 50 kg/m^2 and severe type 2 diabetes.

Keywords Obesity · Bariatric surgery · Laparoscopy · Duodenal switch

Introduction and History of the Duodenal Switch

Biliopancreatic diversion (BPD) is one of the oldest surgical procedures for weight loss. Performed either as an open or laparoscopic approach, the BPD involves the resection of a portion of the stomach, followed by its anastomosis to the distal ileum [1, 2]. Over time, this technique has evolved, incorporating key features that culminated in the development of the Duodenal Switch (DS). Some properties that characterize the DS are the creation of a sleeve gastrectomy, duodenal transection with pyloric preservation, and standardized intestinal lengths [3]. Even though the technique has evolved, the goal remains the same: to offer safe metabolic surgery with favorable long-term results.

G. Restrepo-Rodas · A. D. Guerron (✉)
Department of Digestive Disease Institute, Abu Dhabi, United Arab Emirates

J. C. L. Meyer · S. Al-Baqain
Associate, Digestive Disease Institute, Abu Dhabi, United Arab Emirates

F. M. O. Aparicio
Fellowship Minimally Invasive Surgery. Universidad de los Andes–Red Salud, Santiago, Chile

F. Schlottmann, M. A. Masrur (eds.), *Endoscopic, Laparoscopic and Robotic Techniques for Foregut Disorders*, https://doi.org/10.1007/978-3-032-00811-4_5

The evolution of BPD has been challenging. In 1977, Nicola Scopinaro improved the intestinal bypass procedure by creating a bypass that excluded the duodenum and jejunum [4]. He combined this bypass with an antrectomy and a Roux-en-Y reconstruction, including a Roux limb of approximately 200 cm. Scopinaro was the first to name this procedure BPD because bile and pancreatic juices were diverted from the nutrient flow. Both juices and nutrients were mixed only within the last 50 cm before reaching the ileocecal valve. However, this procedure led to an imbalance between nutrients, pancreatic secretions, and bile, causing undesirable consequences [5, 6]. While weight loss was a positive outcome, a significant risk of protein deficit, micronutrient deficiencies, and malodorous diarrhea became evident [7]. These consequences had a profuse negative impact on the patient's quality of life [5, 7].

Between 1993 and 1998, the technique was further refined. Picard Marceau and Douglass Hess introduced four key developments [8, 9]. First, the resection of the greater gastric curvature followed by a duodenal transection distal to the pylorus. Then, the creation of a duodenal-ileal anastomosis, and finally, an ileo-ileal anastomosis 50 to 250 cm from the ileocecal valve.

In 2002, the technique advanced further. Michel Gagner and colleagues published their preliminary outcomes on the laparoscopic Biliopancreatic Diversion-Duodenal Switch (BPD-DS) [10]. To manage high-risk super-obese patients, they proposed a two-stage procedure. They observed that performing a gastric sleeve (SG) alone could result in up to 35% excess weight loss. Gagner suggested performing the SG in an initial stage while completing the Duodenal Switch (DS) or a Roux-en-Y gastric bypass (RYGB) in a second stage. Currently, the outcomes of staged BPD-DS are similar to those of the one-stage technique [11].

Laparoscopic biliary pancreatic diversion with duodenal switch (LBPD/DS) was first performed in the United States. Ren et al. described one of the first series of 40 patients who underwent a LBDP/DS, with a median BMI of 60 kg/m^2 [12]. The number of BPD/DS performed in the United States have increased over the years, with an estimated 6100 surgeries performed in 2022 [13].

Patient Selection

The DS is among the most effective bariatric procedures available, with a clear consensus on its benefits, particularly for those with a BMI > 50 kg/m^2 and severe type 2 diabetes [14]. DS offers significant advantages over BPD and distal RYGB, such as a lower ulcerogenic potential and improved food tolerance, provided by vertical gastrectomy [15]. Furthermore, the DS combines the restrictive aspects of a sleeve gastrectomy with the malabsorptive features of a distal intestinal bypass. Despite its safety, DS is not suitable for all patients. Factors such as social conditions, income, access to supplementation, and follow-up capabilities must be considered.

- **Indications**
- Patient selection for DS aligns with the criteria for other bariatric procedures [1, 16].
  - BMI > 40 kg/m^2
  - BMI > 35 kg/m^2 with obesity-related comorbidities
  - Failed non-operative weight loss treatments
- **Special Considerations**
  - Super-obese patients (SOP) are typically ideal candidates for hypoabsorptive procedures.
  - Patients with metabolic disorders, specially type two diabetes, as remission rates at one year are far superior than with other bariatric techniques [14, 17].
  - DS is also considered for patients with binge eating behaviors.
- **Contraindications**
- The primary contraindications for DS are related to its potential side effects and include:
  - Pregnancy
  - Patient-related contraindications for surgery (e.g., cardiovascular or anesthetic risks)
  - Substance misuse (e.g., alcoholism)
  - Severe coagulopathies
  - Eating disorders
  - Lack of mental health clearance
  - Severe psychiatric illness

Other contraindications are related to the techniques involved in DS [1, 18]:

- Gastrectomy
  - Severe reflux (esophagitis with Los Angeles grade greater than B or giant hiatal hernias)
- Hypo-absorptive conditions
  - Inflammatory bowel disease
  - Immunosuppressant therapies
  - Hypo-absorptive syndromes
  - Familial polyposis colonic disease
  - Colonic resections
  - Fecal incontinence

Preoperative Evaluation

Preoperative examinations for DS do not differ significantly from those required for other metabolic bariatric surgery (MBS) techniques [3]. There has yet to be a consensus on the imaging modalities to be obtained before bariatric procedures. Some studies have evaluated the use of abdominal ultrasounds to assess liver pathology, size, and cholelithiasis [19, 20]. However, they have shown that imaging does not change patient outcomes and offers no benefit to the procedure [20].

Clinical guidelines, such as those from the International Federation for the Surgery of Obesity and Metabolic Disorders (IFSO), recommend EGD for all patients with upper gastrointestinal symptoms and those undergoing bariatric surgery [21, 22]. EGD is also recommended routinely for populations at high risk of esophageal and gastric diseases and as a postoperative follow-up one year after sleeve gastrectomy (SG) or one-anastomosis gastric bypass (OAGB) [21].

Strengths and Limitations of the Laparoscopic Approach

The development of minimally invasive surgery techniques has significantly contributed to the success of bariatric surgery. The laparoscopic approach reduces morbidity, shortens hospital stays, and minimizes intraoperative blood loss, among other well-documented benefits [2]. However, laparoscopic surgery presents challenges, such as operating in multiple quadrants, requiring a skilled assistant, and longer learning curves [4, 23]. Similarly, the learning curve for laparoscopic duodenal switch is around thirty cases, after which complications decrease [24].

Procedure Description

1. **Anesthesia, Positioning, and Docking**

   Patients should be positioned supine with outstretched arms [4]. After the induction of general anesthesia, appropriate padding of all pressure points and a foot board to support the lower extremities is necessary. SCIP measures are followed, including deep vein thrombosis (DVT) prophylaxis, antibiotic prophylaxis. An orogastric tube may be inserted to decompress the stomach. Securing the patient to the operating table is imperative as many maneuvers in the surgery require changes in table position to facilitate optimal execution of the steps.

   Pitfall: *Ensure the patient has appropriate padding and is well secured to the operating table. Changing the table position from Trendelenburg to reverse Trendelenburg and right side up are needed for adequate execution of surgical maneuvers.*

2. **Access and Exposure**

The operation is performed with the surgeon working from the patient's right side and the assistant standing on the left. Some surgeons prefer to perform the operation from the patient's left arguing better triangulation and access to crucial structures.

Pneumoperitoneum is established using a Veress needle at Palmer's point. Once pneumoperitoneum is successfully achieved endoscopic access begins by using an Optiview trocar in the periumbilical position. Four accessory trocars are placed in a "lazy U" disposition to allow free movement of instruments (Fig. 1). It is our preference to use two 5 mm trocars, one 12 mm trocar for the right hand of the assistant and to perform aa triple stapler technique for the ileo-ileostomy and finally a 15 mm port to construct the distal portion of the sleeve gastrectomy. An extra thick reload with triple stapler technology is used (Medtronic, Inc). Several methods to retract the liver are available. The Nathanson retractor is placed in the subxiphoid position that displaces the left lobe of the liver and exposes the hiatus, angle of His and greater curvature.

For instruments, atraumatic graspers with or without a preexisting 10 cm measurement are preferred (for bowel limb counting), needle driver or end-ostitch, a monopolar cautery for enterotomies and a bipolar energy device for advance coagulation.

Ensure proper placement of trocars to avoid instrument collision and provide adequate exposure. The right left sided ports might need to be placed at a lower

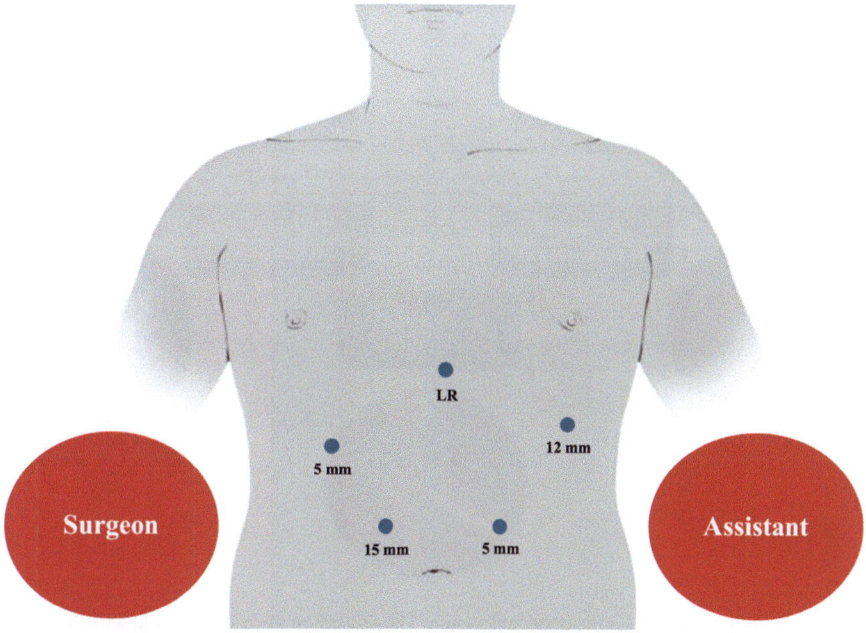

Fig. 1 Port Placement. LR: Liver Retractor, Mm: millimeters

level to ensure adequate access to the distal bowel and appropriate angles for the construction of the duodeno-ileostomy anastomosis.

The technique uses a step-up approach that enables the surgeon the option to retrieve in case problems are encountered. A clockwise approach is used starting with bowel identification, assessment and counting, duodenal dissection, sleeve construction, duodenal dissection, duodeno-ileal anastomosis creation and ileo-ileal anastomosis construction (Fig. 2). During all steps, there is an option to retrieve if problems are encountered and complete a sleeve only if needed.

3. **Small Bowel Assessment**

The surgical table is placed in Trendelenburg with slight right side up. The ileocecal valve is identified following the Tinea colis or by identifying the fold of Treves (Fig. 3). The bowel is ran sequentially from distal to proximal ensuring

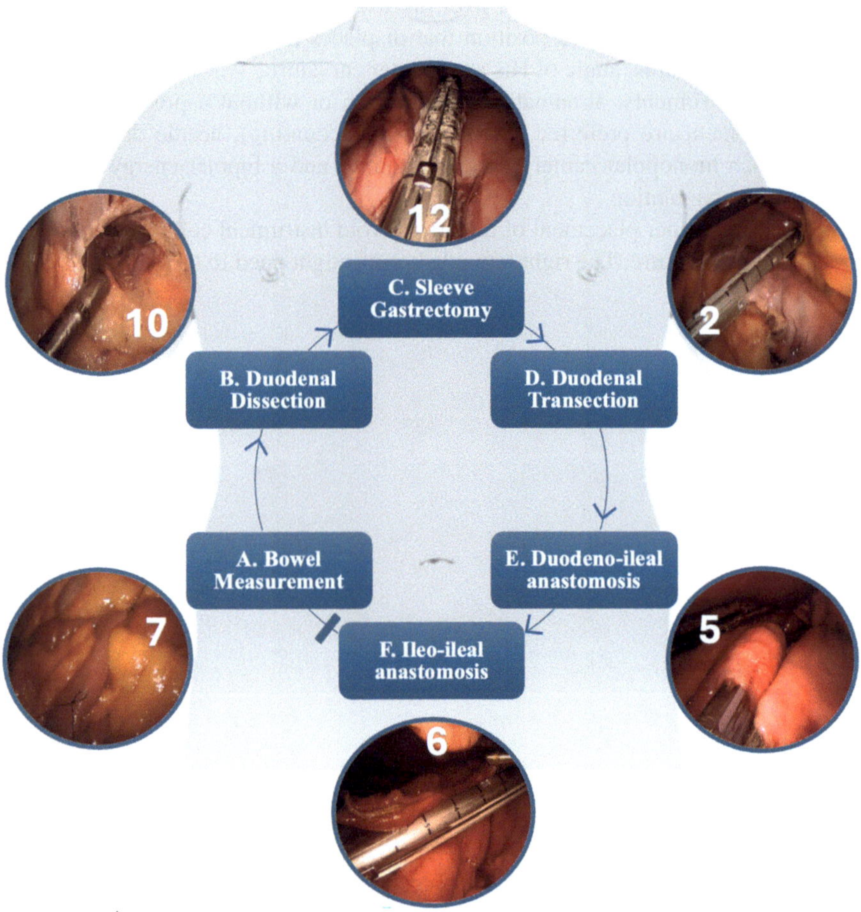

Fig. 2 Step-up approach for the duodenal switch: The procedure starts at 7 o clock, with the bowel measurement, and continues in a clock-wise form according to the approximate anatomical location of the organ involved in the next step (A-F)

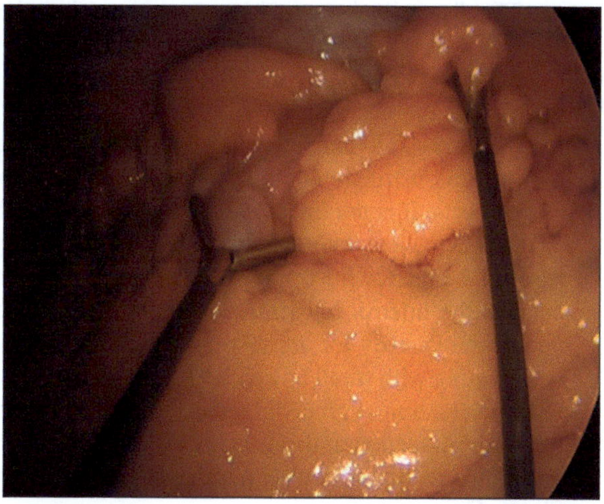

Fig. 3 Bowel Identification. A: Cecum, B: Fold of Treves (ileocecal valve)

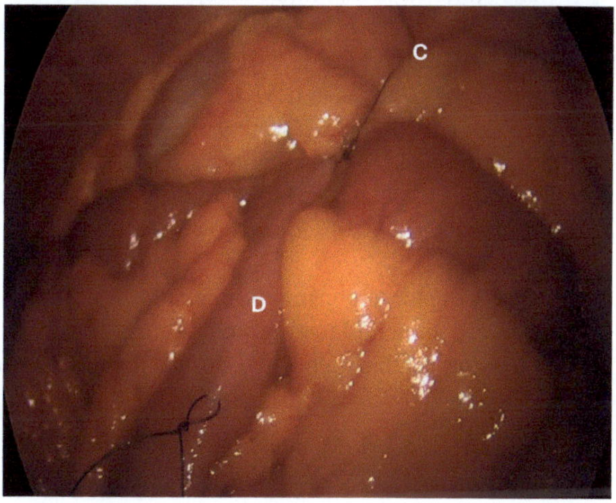

Fig. 4 Bowel Identification. C: marking suture, D: Orientation suture

adequate orientation at all time. The small bowel is measured at 5 cm intervals proximally. We routinely anchored the bowel at 250–300 cm from the ileocecal valve, securing it to the periduodenal fat using absorbable braided suture (purple color). Simultaneously, an interrupted stitch is placed proximally few cm to the anchoring suture to mark on the bowel and keep the bowel orientation and to use as a handle for subsequent duodeno-ileal construction (Fig. 4).

It is important to maintain a proper orientation of the bowel. Marking the proximal loop helps avoid re-running the bowel. A purple-colored suture is used, as the 'P' in purple indicates the proximal side.

4. **Mobilization of Stomach and Duodenum**

The gastrocolic ligament is opened to access the greater curvature of the stomach. Dissection then proceeds along the lesser curvature towards the pylorus. The dissection is carried past the pylorus into the duodenum. Approximately 3 cm into the first portion of the duodenum, a retroduodenal tunnel is created. Then, the duodenum is carefully dissected from its posterior attachments until visualizing the gastroduodenal artery (Fig. 5). The right gastric artery is routinely preserved to enhance duodenal blood flow; however, it may be sacrificed during the construction of the duodeno-ileal anastomosis if there is tension at the anastomosis. It is not uncommon to encounter bleeding at this area due to presence of the pancreatoduondal arcade. Bipolar energy is useful as is gentle pressure. The superior border of the first portion of the duodenum is dissected to connect the inferior border and retroduondeal tunnel (Fig. 6). At this point the duodenum is ready for transection.

Initiating with small bowel assessment and duodenal dissection allows for the initial evaluation of procedural feasibility. The gastroduodenal artery is the landmark for dissection and subsequent transection. A clear dissection of retroduodenal tunnel allows for easy placement of the stapler.

5. **Sleeve Gastrectomy**

The stomach is mobilized along its greater curvature, dividing the short gastric vessels to release the fundus and facilitating posterior dissection until the left crus of the diaphragm is visualized for complete mobilization. A 40-French bougie-sized calibration device is inserted and guided towards the antrum. The sleeve is created closely around the 40-French bougie using laparoscopic staplers positioned from the patient's right trocar (Fig. 7). Tri-stapler technology (Medtronic, Inc) is preferred, using reinforced 60 mm extra thick "black" loads for the first staple, subsequently we switch to reinforced 60 mm medium thick "purple" loads.

A proper sleeve construction avoiding twist and stenosis is advisable. Some authors recommend larger sized bougies. As well as routinely performed a cholecystectomy at this point advocating a potential reduction of the risk of choledocholithiasis and difficult access to endoscopic treatment due to altered anatomy.

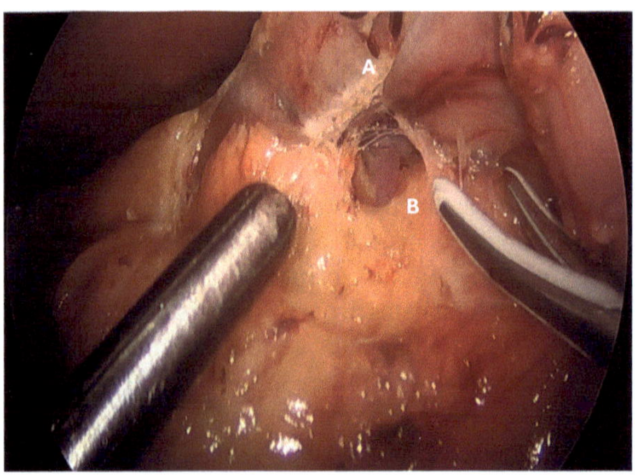

Fig. 5 Duodenal dissection and creation of retroduodenal tunnel. A: Duodenum. B: Gastroduodenal artery (GDA)

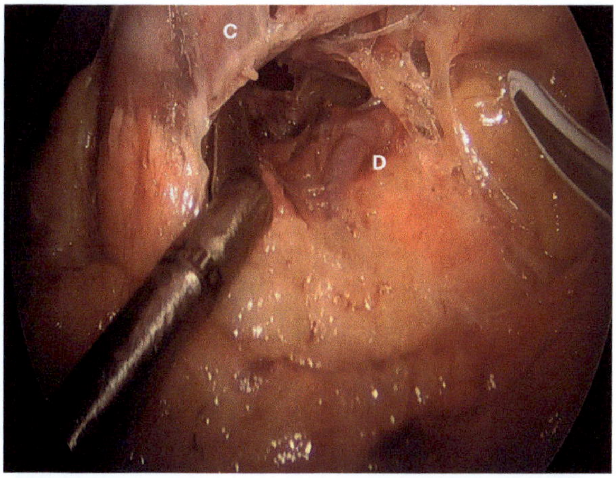

Fig. 6 Duodenal dissection and creation of retroduodenal tunnel. C: Duodenum, D: Gastroduodenal artery (GDA)

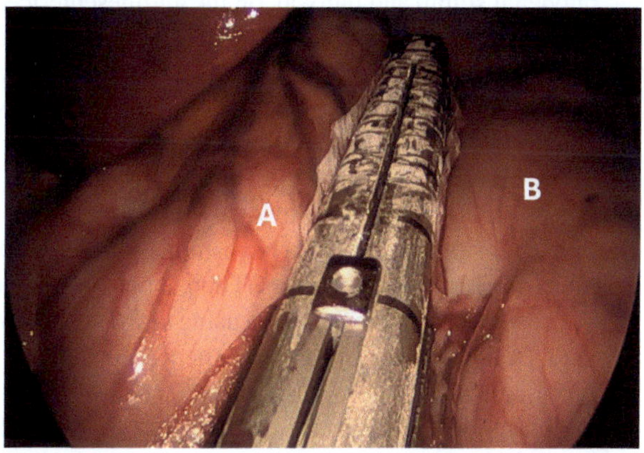

Fig. 7 Sleeve Gastrectomy. A: Sleeve, B: Specimen

We do not advocate for this practice as the risk of biliary obstruction is similar in non-DS population [25, 26].

6. **Duodenum Division**

The duodenal division is performed using a 45 mm tan non reinforced tri stapler tan load. (Fig. 8). Careful introduction of the stapler in the retroduodenal space is mandatory due to the proximity to several major structures such as the pancreatic head, the gastroduodenal artery and the common bile duct. Close observation of the tips of the stapler is needed to avoid iatrogenic injuries.

It is crucial to ensure a perpendicular position at a 90-degree angle to the axis of the duodenum during stapling to avoid forming ischemic dog ears at the edges.

7. **Duodenoileal Anastomosis**

(a) **Hand sewn technique**

The previously anchored loop of bowel is approximated to the duodenal stump. A handsewn anastomosis is performed using slow absorbing 3.0 barbed

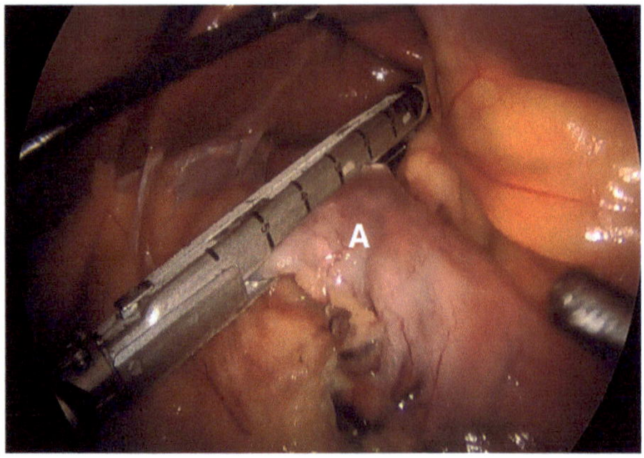

Fig. 8 Duodenal Division. A: Duodenum

sutures. A posterior outer wall is performed, incorporating the staple line of the duodenal stump and halfway on the antimesenteric side of the ileum. This suture line aligns the ileum and duodenum in preparation for the anastomosis and provides and additional layer to prevent tension prior to the construction of our duodenal ileal anastomosis. Matching enterotomies are made with monopolar electrocautery. A duodenotomy is performed 0.5 cm from the staple line that compromises almost the entire width of the duodenal stump to ensure a wide and patent anastomosis. As previously mentioned, it is important to obtain a 3 cm duodenal stump in order to have enough room to construct the anastomosis and avoid working on the pylorus. Then, a two-layered anastomosis is completed on the posterior and anterior walls using a slow-absorbing 3.0 barbed suture. Connel stitches are performed at the corners to invaginate the tissue and secure leak-proof corners.

In case of experiencing tension, the selective ligation of the right gastric artery is performed as a second technical step, allowing for duodenal straightening and tension-free anastomosis. Some surgeons advocate for routine division of the right gastric pedicle and surrounding attachments to maximize exposure and decrease tension.

(b) **Stapler technique**

As previously described, the anchored loop of bowel is apposed to the duodenal stump avoiding unnecessary tension. A duodenotomy using monopolar electrocautery is executed at the inferior border of the duodenal stump. A matching enterotomy at anti-mesenteric border of the ileum is performed using monopolar cautery. A 30 mm medium thick purple stapler is introduced and a anastomosis is created (Fig. 9). The common enterotomy is closed using absorbable barbed or braided suture (Fig. 10). A stay suture is placed at the inferior border of the common enterotomy to aid with retraction.

It is important to note that the duodenal section may take on a purple hue due to venous congestion, which does not justify changing the surgical strategy.

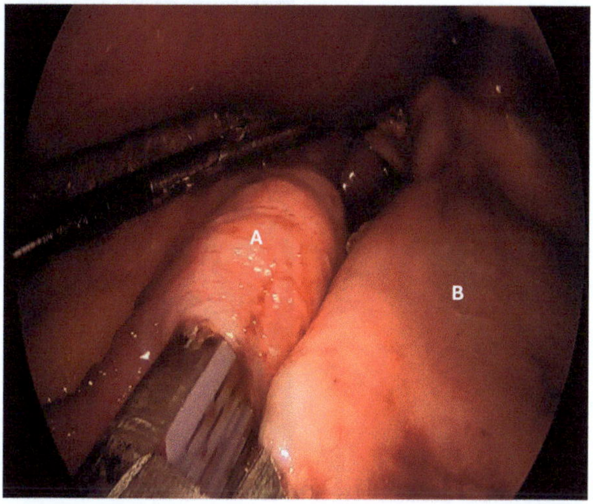

Fig. 9 Stapled Duodeno-ileal anastomosis. A: Ileum, B: Duodenum

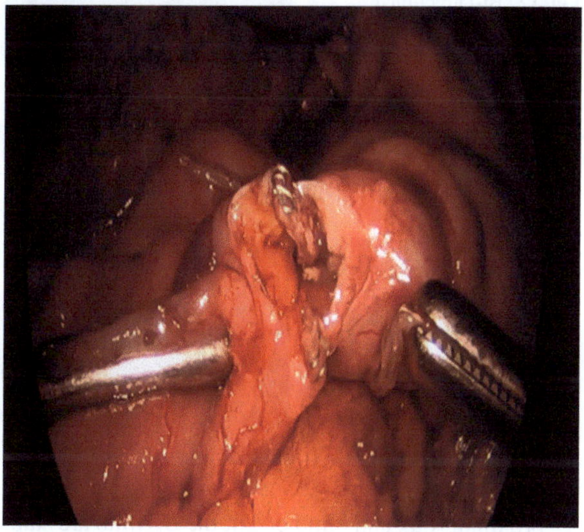

Fig. 10 Closure of enterotomies Duodeno-ileal anastomosis

8. **Ileal Division and Ileoileal Anastomosis**

   Carefully identify the correct bowel loop using the reference barbed suture point. A tan load stapler is used to section the BP limb just proximal to the previously formed DI anastomosis. A Roux limb of 150–200 cm is carefully counted starting from the DI towards the ileocecal valve. A common channel of 120 to 150 cm is confectioned. The ilieoileal anastomosis is constructed using a bidirectional tri stapler technique (Fig. 11). Enterotomies are made with monopolar electrocautery in the common channel and the biliary limb leaving approximately 5 cm from the enterotomy to the blind of on the stapler. A 45 mm medium thick tan stapler is introduced through the 15 mm port on the right side and the

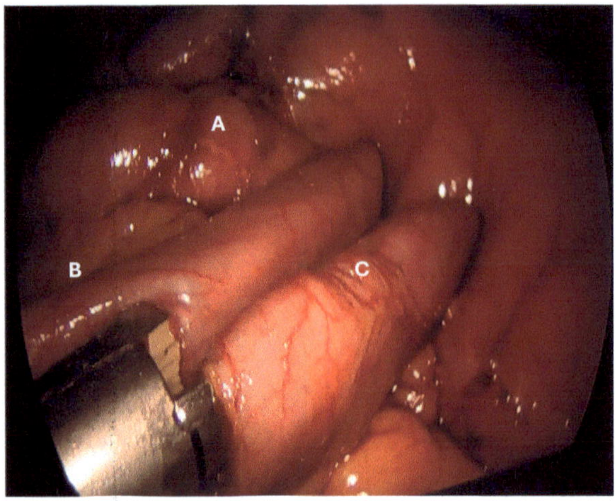

Fig. 11 Bi-Directional Stapled Ileo-ileal anastomosis. A: Proximal limb (roux), B: Distal limb (common channel), C: Biliopancreatic limb

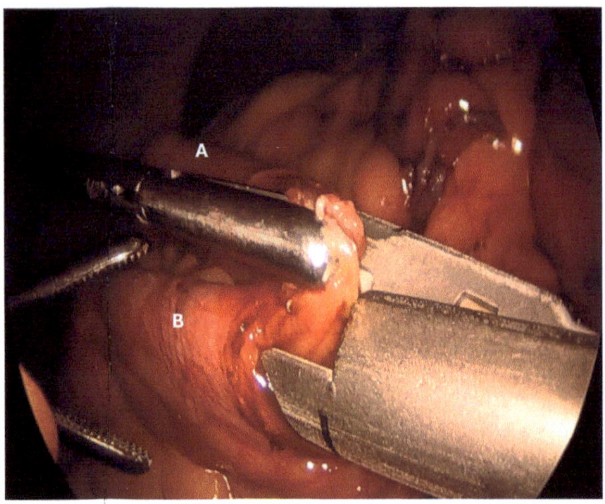

Fig. 12 Bi-Directional Stapled Ileo-ileal anastomosis. A: Proximal limb (roux), B: Distal limb (common channel)

proximal roux and blind end of the BP limb are stapled. Next, the common channel and roux are aligned, and a 45 mm medium thick tan stapler is introduced through the 12 mm subcostal port aiming towards the RLQ. The stapler is introduced into the Roux/common channel and proximal end of the BP limb (Fig. 12). The common enterotomy is closed with a 60 mm medium thick purple stapler (Fig. 13).

Exercise great caution when handling the ileum; its thin muscular wall and rough manipulation without direct vision can cause injuries. Ensure the serosa of the common enterotomy is visible prior to fire the stapler.

9. **Mesenteric Closure and Testing**

A non-absorbable 3.0 barbed suture is recommended to close the mesenteric defect as it facilitates continuous and rapid closure. Similarly, the pseudopetersen space is closed using non-absorbable barbed suture 3.0. Finally, a routine intra-

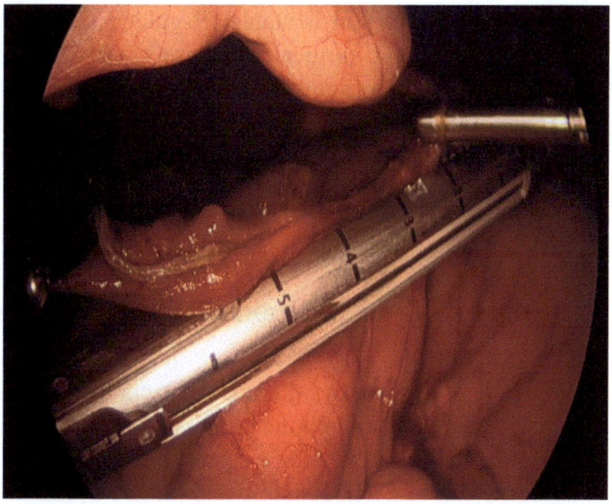

Fig. 13 Bi-Directional Stapled Ileo-ileal anastomosis. Common enterotomy closure

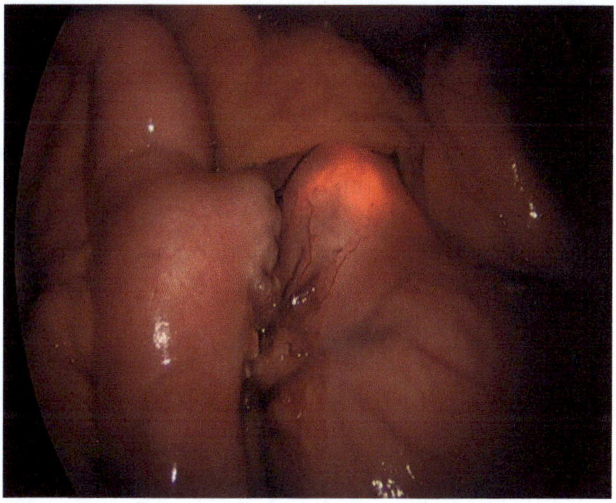

Fig. 14 Endoscopic evaluation of Duodeno-ileal anastomosis

operative endoscopic examination is conducted (Fig. 14). This allows adequate hydro-pneumatic leak testing and bleeding detection along the suture line. It also provides training for surgeons in post-surgical endoscopic anatomy.

Complications and Management Strategies

The management of postoperative complications in laparoscopic surgery is similar to other techniques [27]. It is essential to consider that the procedure includes creating a gastric sleeve and two anastomoses; thus, associated complications must also be considered. If leaks are detected early, it is imperative to avoid or try to control the sepsis. If the patient is stable IR-guided drains can be used. If the patient is unstable laparoscopic surgical resolution should be attempted. In addition, patients should receive appropriate antibiotic therapy and nutritional support [1]. Similarly, endoscopic interventions can be used in selected cases [28]. As aforementioned, careful handling of the distal bowel is imperative to avoid inadvertent enterotomies, serosal tears and overall damage to the bowel.

Future Directions in Duodenal Switch Surgery

Although less common now, the DS has contributed valuable insights into managing malabsorption and complications, which have been applied to newer, less invasive techniques like the Single Anastomosis Sleeve-Ileal Bypass (SASI) and the Single Anastomosis Duodenal Switch (SADI-S) [29]. Nonetheless, the DS may still play a role in specific cases, such as severe obesity (BMI > 50 kg/m^2) or previous bariatric surgery failures [30]. Long-term studies are needed to further understand the outcomes of duodenal switch compared to newer procedures.

Additionally, robotic surgery opens up the future for the DS, offering greater precision and reduced complications, which could renew interest in the technique for complex cases [27, 31, 32]. Similarly, advances in nutritional management and post-operative follow-up could make the procedure more sustainable. While its frequency has diminished, there is still potential for adaptation and selective use, especially with the integration of robotic technology.

References

1. Teixeira A, Jawad MA, Galvão Neto MDP, Torres A, Biertho L, Marchesini JC, Wilson E, editors. Duodenal switch and its derivatives in bariatric and metabolic surgery: a comprehensive clinical guide. Cham: Springer International Publishing; 2023.
2. Al-Mazrou AM, Bellorin O, Dhar V, Dakin G, Afaneh C. Minimally invasive versus open duodenal switch: a nationwide retrospective analysis. Surg Endosc. 2022;36:7000–7.
3. Biertho L, Bouvet-Bouchard L, Vourtzoumis P. Laparoscopic biliopancreatic diversion with duodenal switch: surgical technique. In: Teixeira A, Jawad MA, Galvão Neto M d P, Torres A, Biertho L, Marchesini JC, Wilson E, editors. Duodenal switch and its derivatives in bariatric and metabolic surgery: a comprehensive clinical guide. Cham: Springer International Publishing; 2023. p. 235–46.
4. Scopinaro N, Marinari GM, Camerini G. Laparoscopic standard biliopancreatic diversion: technique and preliminary results. Obes Surg. 2002;12:362–5.
5. Addeo P, Cesaretti M, Anty R, Iannelli A. Liver transplantation for bariatric surgery-related liver failure: a systematic review of a rare condition. Surg Obes Relat Dis. 2019;15:1394–401.
6. Gagner M. For whom the bell tolls? It is time to retire the classic BPD (bilio-pancreatic diversion) operation. Surg Obes Relat Dis. 2019;15:1029–31.
7. Iannelli A, Petrucciani N, Schiavo L, Anty R. Severe protein malnutrition after bariatric surgery and liver failure: a dangerous sequence. Obes Surg. 2021;31:3860–1.

8. Marceau P, Hould F-S, Simard S, Lebel S, Bourque R-A, Potvin M, Biron S. Biliopancreatic diversion with duodenal switch. World J Surg. 1998;22:947–54.
9. Hess DS, Hess DW. Biliopancreatic diversion with a duodenal switch. Obes Surg. 1998;8:267–82.
10. Gagner M, Matteotti R. Laparoscopic biliopancreatic diversion with duodenal switch. Surg Clin North Am. 2005;85:141–9.
11. Biertho L, Thériault C, Bouvet L, Marceau S, Hould F-S, Lebel S, Julien F, Tchernof A. Second-stage duodenal switch for sleeve gastrectomy failure: a matched controlled trial. Surg Obes Relat Dis. 2018;14:1570–9.
12. Ren CJ, Patterson E, Gagner M. Early results of laparoscopic biliopancreatic diversion with duodenal switch: a case series of 40 consecutive patients. Obes Surg. 2000;10:514–23.
13. Clapp B, Ponce J, Corbett J, Ghanem OM, Kurian M, Rogers AM, Peterson RM, LaMasters T, English WJ. American Society for Metabolic and Bariatric Surgery 2022 estimate of metabolic and bariatric procedures performed in the United States. Surg Obes Relat Dis. 2024;20:425–31.
14. Guerron AD, Perez JE, Risoli T, Lee H-J, Portenier D, Corsino L. Performance and improvement of the DiaRem score in diabetes remission prediction: a study with diverse procedure types. Surg Obes Relat Dis Off J Am Soc Bariatr Surg. 2020;16:1531–42.
15. Kerrigan DD, Almerie Q, Leuratti L, Khwaja HA, Harper CE. Laparoscopic biliopancreatic diversion with duodenal switch (BPD-DS) surgery. In: Agrawal S, editor. Obesity, bariatric and metabolic surgery: a practical guide. Cham: Springer International Publishing; 2023. p. 787–805.
16. Eisenberg D, Shikora SA, Aarts E, et al. 2022 American Society for Metabolic and Bariatric Surgery (ASMBS) and International Federation for the Surgery of Obesity and Metabolic Disorders (IFSO): indications for metabolic and bariatric surgery. Surg Obes Relat Dis. 2022;18:1345–56.
17. Chumakova-Orin M, Vanetta C, Moris DP, Guerron AD. Diabetes remission after bariatric surgery. World J Diabetes. 2021;12:1093–101.
18. Conner J, Nottingham JM. Biliopancreatic diversion with duodenal switch. StatPearls; 2024.
19. Nagarajan B, Gupta K, Nasta A, Gayatri A, Goel R. Usefulness of preoperative trans-abdominal ultrasound prior to bariatric surgery. SN Compr Clin Med. 2020;2:11–5.
20. Abou Hussein BM, Khammas A, Makki M, Makki M, Al Bastaki U, Al Mazrouei A, Badri FS. Role of routine abdominal ultrasound before bariatric surgery: review of 937 patients. Obes Surg. 2018;28:2696–9.
21. Brown WA, Johari Halim Shah Y, Balalis G, et al. IFSO position statement on the role of esophago-gastro-duodenal endoscopy prior to and after bariatric and metabolic surgery procedures. Obes Surg. 2020;30:3135–53.
22. Quake SYL, Mohammadi-Zaniani G, Musbahi A, Old O, Courtney M, Small P. Routine use of esophago-gastro-duodenoscopy (EGD) in bariatric surgery—an international survey of our current practice. Obes Surg. 2022;32:3627–34.
23. Sorribas M, Casajoana A, Sobrino L, Admella V, Osorio J, Pujol-Gebellí J. Experience in biliopancreatic diversion with duodenal switch: results at 2, 5 and 10 years. Cirugia Espanola. 2022;100:202–8.
24. Topart PA, Vandenbroucke F, Ferrand L, Lozac'h P (2005) Laparoscopic biliopancreatic diversion with duodenal switch (LBPD-DS): how long is the learning curve? Surg Obes Relat Dis 1:247.
25. Clapp B, Janik M, Corbett J, Vahibe A, Ul Hassan O, Husain F, Pullat R, Ghanem OM. Duodenal switch without versus with laparoscopic cholecystectomy: a perioperative risk comparative analysis of the MBSAQIP database (2015-2019). Surg Endosc. 2023;37:219–24.
26. Sucandy I, Abulfaraj M, Naglak M, Antanavicius G. Risk of biliary events after selective cholecystectomy during biliopancreatic diversion with duodenal switch. Obes Surg. 2016;26:531–7.
27. Al-Mazrou AM, Cruz MV, Dakin G, Bellorin-Marin OE, Pomp A, Afaneh C. Robotic duodenal switch is associated with outcomes comparable to those of laparoscopic approach. Obes Surg. 2021;31:2019–29.

28. Boules M, Chang J, Haskins IN, Sharma G, Froylich D, El-Hayek K, Rodriguez J, Kroh M. Endoscopic management of post-bariatric surgery complications. World J Gastrointest Endosc. 2016;8:591–9.
29. Gebellí JP, Lazzara C, de Gordejuela AGR, Nora M, Pereira AM, Sánchez-Pernaute A, Osorio J, Sobrino L, García AJT. Duodenal switch vs. single-anastomosis duodenal switch (SADI-S) for the treatment of grade IV obesity: 5-year outcomes of a multicenter prospective cohort comparative study. Obes Surg. 2022;32:3839–46.
30. DeCicco JP, Barajas-Gamboa JS, Dang JT, et al. Bariatric surgery outcomes in patients with severe obesity compared to patients with non-severe obesity at a new institution in The United Arab Emirates. J Clin Med. 2024;13:1907.
31. Antanavicius G, Katsichtis T, Alswealmeen W, Assali M. Three hundred four robotically assisted biliopancreatic diversion with duodenal switch operations with gradual robotic approach implementation: short-term outcomes, complication profile, and lessons learned. Obes Surg. 2020;30:3961–7.
32. Teixeira A, Jawad M, Ghanem M, Sanchez A, Inchausti C, Mogollon I, Lind R. Robot-assisted duodenal switch with DaVinci xi: surgical technique and analysis of a single-institution experience of 661 cases. J Robot Surg. 2022;17:923–31.

Robotic Duodenal Switch

Rebecca C. Dirks and Ranjan Sudan

Abstract As the problem of obesity evolves and grows, so too does the role of the duodenal switch. The duodenal switch is the most effective bariatric surgery currently performed for weight loss and treatment of diabetes type 2. As obesity becomes more prevalent and more severe, the value of the duodenal switch increases. Additionally, this procedure is an excellent conversion operation for weight regain after sleeve gastrectomy. The technical difficulty of the duodenal switch can be ameliorated by the current robotic platform available. In this chapter, we present the steps to the duodenal switch using the current daVinci Robot platform.

Keywords Obesity · Morbid obesity · Duodenal switch · Biliopancreatic diversion · Bariatric surgery · Robotic surgery

Introduction

Obesity has become more pervasive and severe in the United States. The CDC reports the prevalence of obesity (BMI $\geq$ 30) at approximately 40% and severe obesity (BMI $\geq$ 40) at approximately 9%, with the ratio of severe obesity to overall obesity increasing as well in recent decades [1]. The duodenal switch is the most effective bariatric surgery at achieving weight loss [2, 3]. As more patients present with severe, or class III, obesity, the value of the duodenal switch increases. This procedure also presents an excellent option for revision in patients who have already undergone sleeve gastrectomy and require greater weight loss.

Although the original biliopancreatic diversion with duodenal switch (BPD-DS) was described in the 1990s, the modern minimally invasive duodenal switch (BPD/DS) was not performed until 2000 with the laparoscopic and robotic approaches

R. C. Dirks · R. Sudan (✉)
Department of Surgery, Duke University, Durham, NC, USA
e-mail: ranjan.sudan@duke.edu

F. Schlottmann, M. A. Masrur (eds.), *Endoscopic, Laparoscopic and Robotic Techniques for Foregut Disorders*, https://doi.org/10.1007/978-3-032-00811-4_6

[4–6]. Its popularity has been tempered in part by technical difficulty and by lack of training or demand, which can be ameliorated by the current robotic platform and additional surgeon and patient education, respectively. Prior research has shown that both operative time and complications associated with the duodenal switch can improve with surgeon experience on the robotic platform [7]. In this chapter, we present the steps to the duodenal switch using the da Vinci Robot Xi platform.

Procedure Description

Patient Positioning

The patient is placed in the supine position. Bilateral SCD's are placed, and 40 mg of subcutaneous Enoxaparin Sodium is given for VTE prophylaxis before induction of anesthesia. Preoperative antibiotics are given within an hour of incision. Typically, three grams of Ancef and 500 mg of Metronidazole are used and the selection is adjusted based on patient allergies. The patient's arms are placed on arm boards and partially abducted. A pillow is placed under the knees, and then a footboard is placed so the feet lie flush against the board. Appropriate padding and straps are needed to prevent pressure injuries. A 32 French gastric calibration tube is placed to decompress the stomach; and proper placement confirmed with the anesthetist. An orogastric tube can be used as an alternative, but we use the calibration tube for decompression, shaping our sleeve, and a leak test using dye or air. For primary duodenal switches, a foley catheter is not routinely placed. While draping, we use an additional half sheet to cover the arms so the arm board near the robot can be moved next to the bed in a sterile fashion after port placement. As an alternative, the arm on the side with the robot can be tucked during initial positioning taking care to protect any intravenous lines.

Pneumoperitoneum and Port Placement

We use a STEP® needle at Palmer's point to establish pneumoperitoneum after using sterile water and syringe to perform a "drop test." An 8 mm robotic optical port and a 0-degree laparoscope is used to enter the abdomen in a supraumbilical position under visualization. The site of the STEP® needle and trocar are checked for any injuries, then additional ports are placed under direct visualization (Fig. 1). An 8 mm robotic port is placed in the left subcostal and right subcostal positions, a 15 mm port in the right hemiabdomen, and a 12 mm laparoscopic assistant port in the left lateral abdomen. We also place a Nathanson liver retractor in the subxiphoid area. All port sites are preinjected with a local anesthetic (0.25% Bupivacaine or long acting lipoidal bupivacaine). A transverses abdominis plane block may also be utilized for optimal pain control.

Fig. 1 Port placement

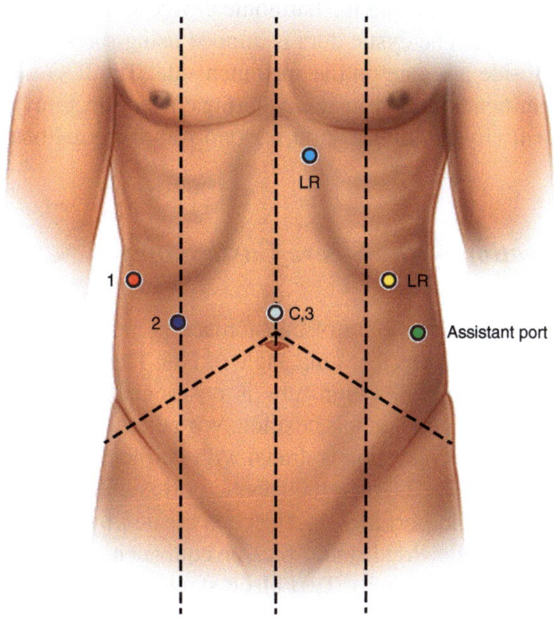

Measuring the Bowel

We measure our small bowel laparoscopically before docking the robot. This allows a single dock procedure, which has previously been described [8]. Starting at the ileocecal valve, 100 cm is measured, and the small bowel marked with two sutures, the distal stitch is longer than the other to maintain orientation. An additional marking suture is placed at 250 cm from the ileocecal valve, and then the bowel at this point is secured to the abdominal wall with an additional suture. This marks our future common channel at 100 cm and total alimentary limb at 250 cm. These limb lengths can be adjusted if performing the single anastomosis version of the duodenal switch. Care is taken to anchor the bowel between the two right sided ports, to ensure it will not be in the way of our stapler while making the sleeve. We then position the patient in reverse Trendelenburg, elevate the left lobe of the liver with the Nathanson retractor, and dock the robot. Two of the robotic arms are placed to the left of the Nathanson retractor, and two are placed to the right of the retractor.

Cholecystectomy

If cholecystectomy is performed in conjunction with the duodenal switch, it is performed prior to the sleeve and switch portions of the case. Intravenous indocyanine green (ICG) is administered at the start of the case. The gallbladder is dissected from its fossa using the harmonic device and the cystic artery is also taken with the harmonic. The cystic duct is clipped using robotic hemolok clips, with two on the stay side and one on the specimen side. The ICG view on the robot enables clear identification of the anatomy during cholecystectomy and demonstrates with greater sensitivity any bile leak during removal of the gallbladder.

Creation of the Sleeve Gastrectomy

The greater curvature of the stomach is mobilized starting at approximately 5 cm from the pylorus up to the angle of His. This is performed with a robotic harmonic scalpel. The calibration tube is positioned along the lesser curve and suction is applied to keep it in this position. With the stomach in a neutral position, an approximate line of resection is drawn with purple marker. The stomach before stapling is shown in Fig. 2. Next, the robotic port is undocked and removed from the 15 mm laparoscopic port and the sleeve is created by a series of 45 mm staple black and purple loads (Medtronic, Inc) or equivalent with staple line reinforcement using Seamguards (Gore®). Two black staple loads are used at the antrum followed by purple staple loads more proximally.

Creation of the Duodeno-Ileostomy

Mobilization from the sleeve is continued distally until a tunnel underneath the first portion of the duodenum can be created (Fig. 3). A tan 60 mm load of the staple is used to divide the duodenum at this point. A stay stitch with Vicryl® suture is placed

Fig. 2 Mobilized stomach with calibration tube and approximate line of resection

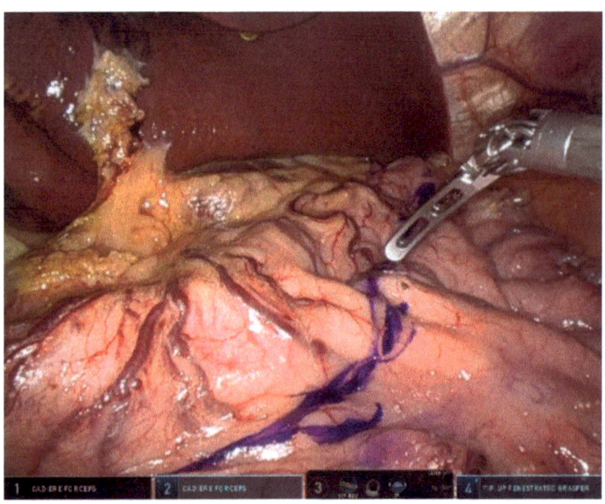

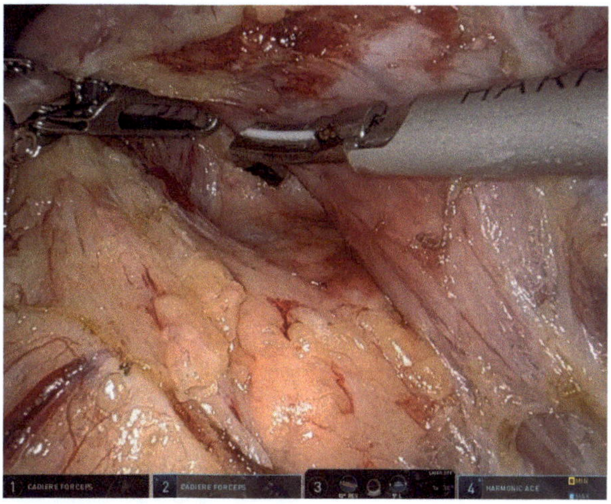

Fig. 3 Retroduodenal dissection

at the lateral corner of the duodenal staple line for retraction. The small bowel marked at 250 cm from the ileocecal valve is detached from the abdominal wall, maintaining correct orientation of the bowel during creation of the duodeno-ileal anastomosis (D-I). A two-layer handsewn anastomosis is created by suturing the bowel to the duodenal staple line with a six-inch running absorbable 3 zero V-loc® suture for the posterior layer of the D-I anastomosis (Fig. 4). Enterotomies are started with a hook cautery, then extended with the *harmonic* scalpel (Fig. 5). A second full thickness posterior layer of the D-I anastomosis is created with a new running absorbable V-loc® (Fig. 6), which is continued around the corner and then used for an anterior layer (Fig. 7). The original V-loc® from the first seromuscular posterior layer is then used to create a second partial thickness anterior layer with running seromuscular bites (Fig. 8).

Creation of the Ileo-Ileostomy

The bowel distal to the D-I is then run until the prior marking stitch at 100 cm is found. An enterotomy with the harmonic is created on the antimesenteric side of the bowel. This is done adjacent to the suture to keep the orientation of the bowel while creating the ileo-ileal anastomosis (I-I). An enterotomy on the antimesenteric side of the bowel is also created at the biliary limb approximately 10 cm proximal to the D-I anastomosis. Bi-directional firing of the stapler is then used to create the anastomosis. The left upper port is undocked, and a low profile 45 mm white staple load used to create the first side of the anastomosis, then the assistant port in the left subcostal area is used to introduce the second staple load for the I-I anastomosis (Figs. 9, 10, and 11). The common enterotomy is closed with a 45 mm tan load transversely from the assistant port to complete the I-I anastomosis (Fig. 12).

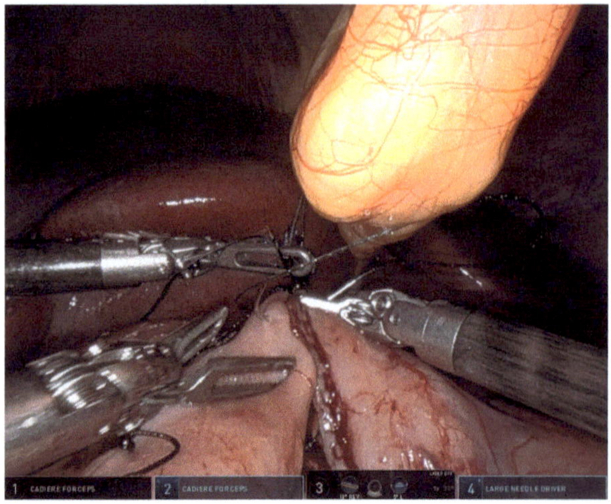

Fig. 4 Posterior layer of the duodeno-Ileostomy

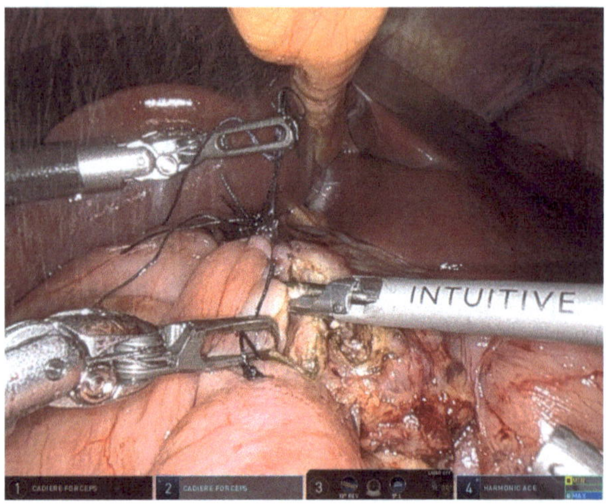

Fig. 5 Duodeno-Ileostomy enterotomies

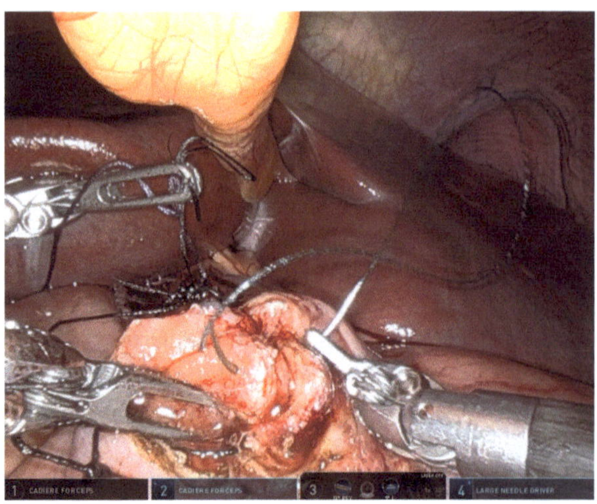

Fig. 6 Second posterior layer of the duodeno-Ileostomy

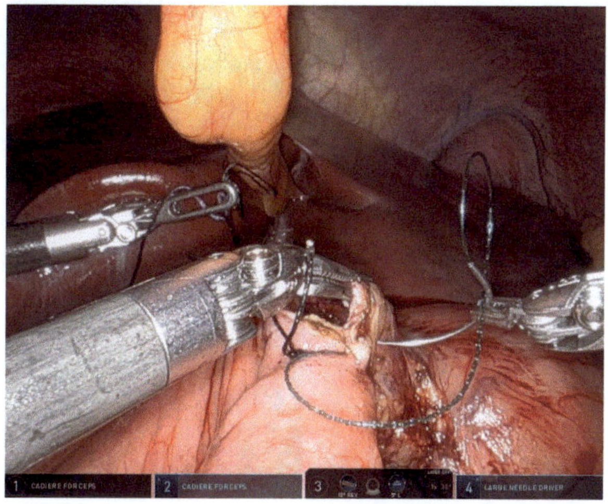

Fig. 7 Anterior layer of the duodeno-Ileostomy

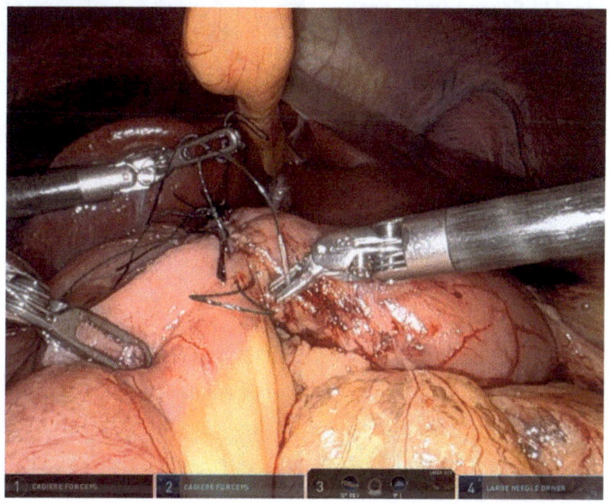

Fig. 8 Second anterior layer of the duodeno-Ileostomy

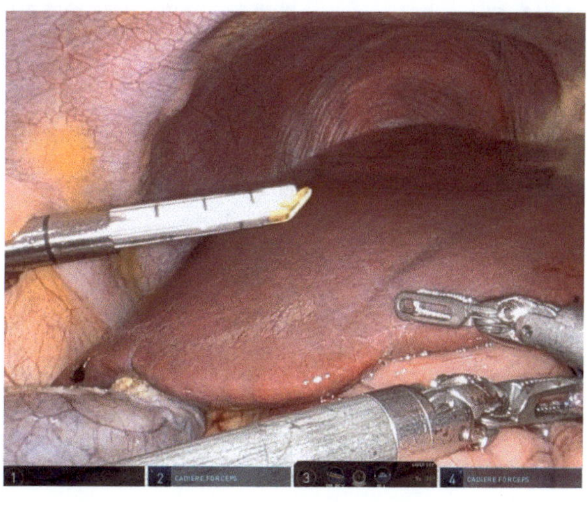

Fig. 9 Port and staple load for first fire of the bi-directional ileo-ileostomy

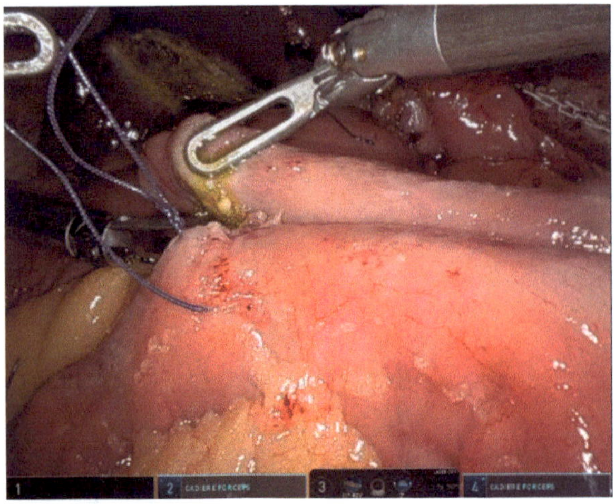

Fig. 10 First staple fire of the ileo-ileostomy

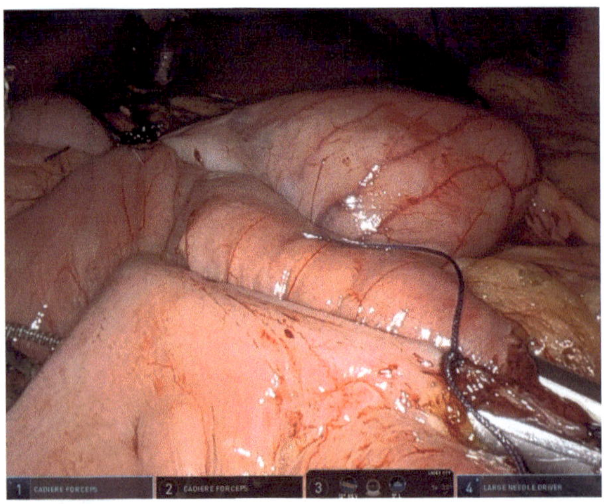

Fig. 11 Second staple fire of the ileo-ileostomy

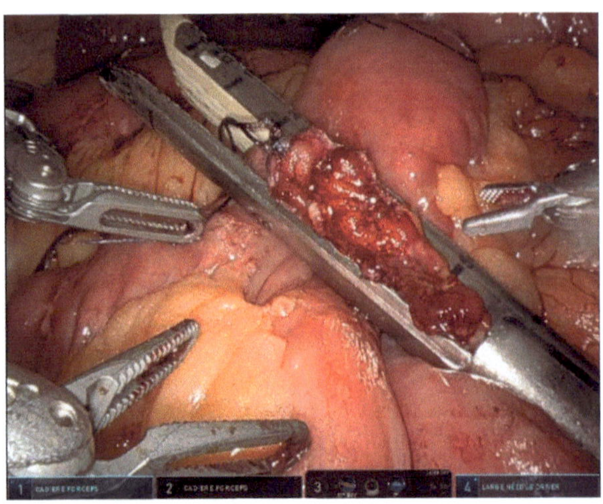

Fig. 12 Closure of ileo-ileostomy common enterotomy

Closure of the Mesenteric Defect and Separation of the Biliopancreatic Limb

The mesenteric defect of the ileo-ileostomy is first closed with a running non-absorbable V-loc 3 zero suture (Medtronic®) (Fig. 13). Next, the biliopancreatic limb is divided from the D-I anastomosis and alimentary limb. A hole in the mesentery next to the D-I is created with a harmonic, then a 60 mm tan staple load is used to divide the biliopancreatic limb from the D-I anastomosis (Fig. 14). Next, the space between the transverse mesocolon and the newly separated roux limb, Peterson's space, is also closed with running six inch non-absorbable 3 zero V-loc suture (Fig. 15).

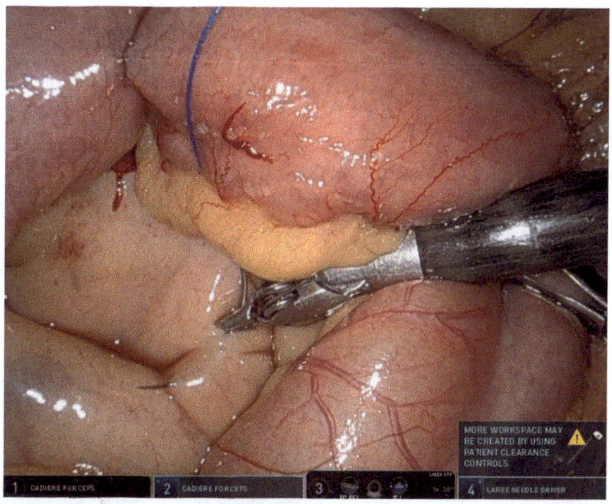

Fig. 13 Beginning of the closure of the ileo-ileostomy mesenteric defect

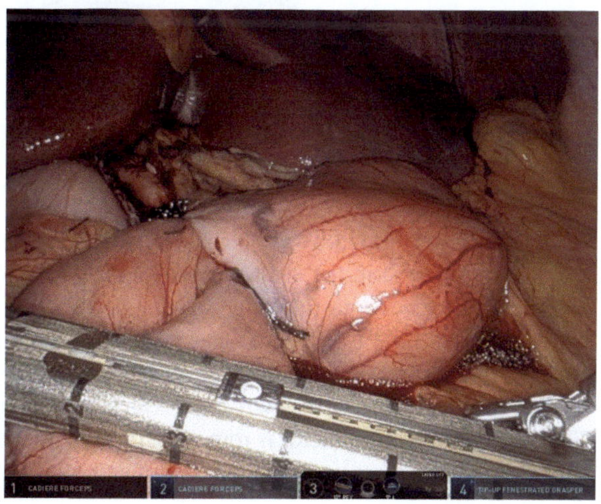

Fig. 14 Separation of biliopancreatic limb from duodeno-ileostomy

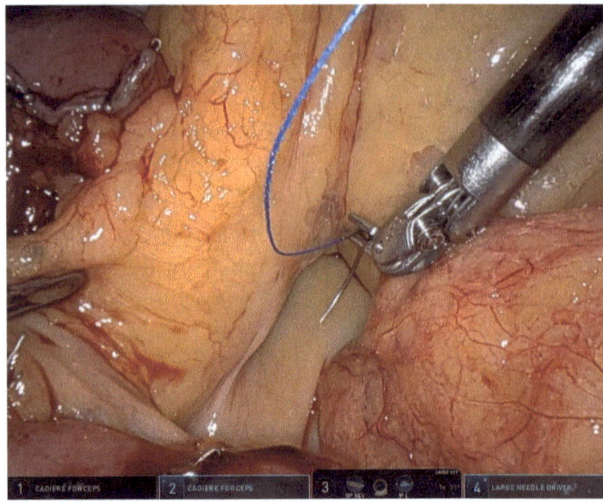

Fig. 15 Beginning of the closure of Peterson's space

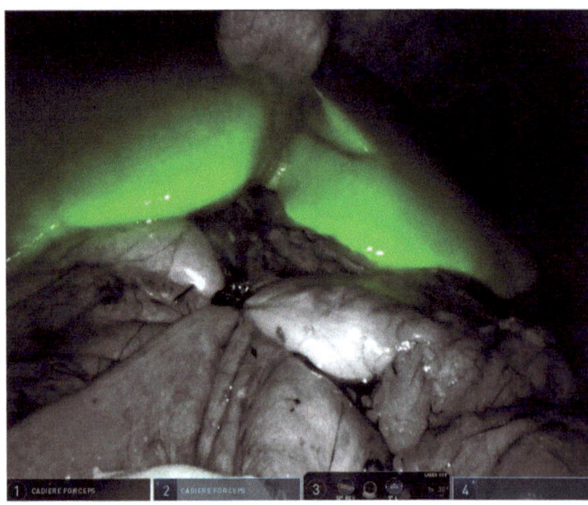

Fig. 16 Leak test with ICG

Leak Test and Closure

A leak test is performed by administering intraluminal ICG or methylene blue into the calibration tube in the sleeve lumen to check for leaks at the D-I anastomosis and along the sleeve gastrectomy staple line (Fig. 16). Alternatively, insufflation with air can be used to check for gas leak. After negative leak tests, hemostasis is confirmed, and the specimen(s) are removed via the 15 mm port. The fascia of the 15 mm port is closed with interrupted Vicryl® suture using a port closure device. The Nathanson liver retractor is removed, the pneumoperitoneum evacuated, and all skin closed with subcuticular vicryl suture and surgical glue.

Conclusions

The duodenal switch is a made more accessible by the robotic platform. We present a combined laparoscopic and robotic approach, utilizing the robot's magnification and increased articulation to facilitate the duodeno-ileal anastomosis in particular. By using bedside stapling, this technique can also be easily used in newer robot platforms without staplers available. In the current daVinci platform, robotic staplers can be used depending on individual surgeon practice. Regardless of preferred technique, as obesity increases in severity and prevalence, the robot can help bring the duodenal switch into the armamentarium of more bariatric surgeons.

References

1. Hales CM, Carroll MD, Fryar CD, Ogden CL. Prevalence of obesity and severe obesity among adults: United States, 2017–2018. NCHS Data Brief. 2020;360:1–8.
2. Gulinac M, Miteva DG, Peshevska-Sekulovska M, Novakov IP, Antovic S, Peruhova M, et al. Long-term effectiveness, outcomes and complications of bariatric surgery. World J Clin Cases. 2023;11(19):4504–12. https://doi.org/10.12998/wjcc.v11.i19.4504.
3. Prachand VN, Davee RT, Alverdy JC. Duodenal switch provides superior weight loss in the super-obese (BMI > or =50 kg/m2) compared with gastric bypass. Ann Surg. 2006;244(4):611–9. https://doi.org/10.1097/01.sla.0000239086.30518.2a.
4. Ren CJ, Patterson E, Gagner M. Early results of laparoscopic biliopancreatic diversion with duodenal switch: a case series of 40 consecutive patients. Obes Surg 2000;10(6):514–23; discussion 24. doi: https://doi.org/10.1381/096089200321593715.
5. Sudan R, Puri V, Sudan D. Robotically assisted biliary pancreatic diversion with a duodenal switch: a new technique. Surg Endosc. 2007;21(5):729–33. https://doi.org/10.1007/s00464-006-9171-y.
6. Hess DS, Hess DW. Biliopancreatic diversion with a duodenal switch. Obes Surg. 1998;8(3):267–82. https://doi.org/10.1381/096089298765554476.
7. Sudan R, Bennett KM, Jacobs DO, Sudan DL. Multifactorial analysis of the learning curve for robot-assisted laparoscopic biliopancreatic diversion with duodenal switch. Ann Surg. 2012;255(5):940–5. https://doi.org/10.1097/SLA.0b013e31824c1d06.
8. Sudan R, Podolsky E. Totally robot-assisted biliary pancreatic diversion with duodenal switch: single dock technique and technical outcomes. Surg Endosc. 2015;29(1):55–60. https://doi.org/10.1007/s00464-014-3653-0.

Laparoscopic SADI-S

Antonio J. Torres, Jose L. Romera, Adriana Ruano, and Andrés Sánchez-Pernaute

Abstract Single-anastomosis duodeno-ileal bypass with sleeve (SADI-S) was first described in 2007 as a simplified version of the biliopancreatic diversion with duodenal switch. SADI-S has achieved satisfactory short and long-term results for the treatment of both morbid obesity and its metabolic comorbidities. SADI-S is a safe, reproducible and effective bariatric procedure that offers excellent weight loss and metabolic outcomes as a malabsorptive technique. In this chapter, the procedure is described step by step, including representative intraoperative images.

Keywords SADI-S · Obesity surgery · Metabolic surgery · Biliopancreatic diversion · Single anastomosis · Duodeno-ileal bypass · Duodenal switch

Introduction

Laparoscopic single anastomosis duodenal switch with sleeve or SADI-S (single-anastomosis duodeno-ileal bypass) was first described in 2007 with the intention of simplifying a complex surgical technique, the biliopancreatic diversion with duodenal switch (BPD-DS), whilst maintaining its metabolic principles. SADI-S was initially designed by associating a SG resulting in a single-anastomosis duodeno-ileal bypass with sleeve gastrectomy (SADI-S). This was achieved by practising a vertical gastrectomy as a restrictive procedure with pyloric preservation, followed by an end-to-side duodeno-ileal anastomosis in the first duodenal portion, beyond the pylorus (Fig. 1).

A. J. Torres (✉) · J. L. Romera · A. Ruano · A. Sánchez-Pernaute
General and Digestive Surgery Service, Hospital Clínico San Carlos, Madrid, Spain

Department of Surgery, Complutense University Medical School, Universidad Complutense de Madrid (UCM), Madrid, Spain

IdISSC, Madrid, Spain

F. Schlottmann, M. A. Masrur (eds.), *Endoscopic, Laparoscopic and Robotic Techniques for Foregut Disorders*, https://doi.org/10.1007/978-3-032-00811-4_7

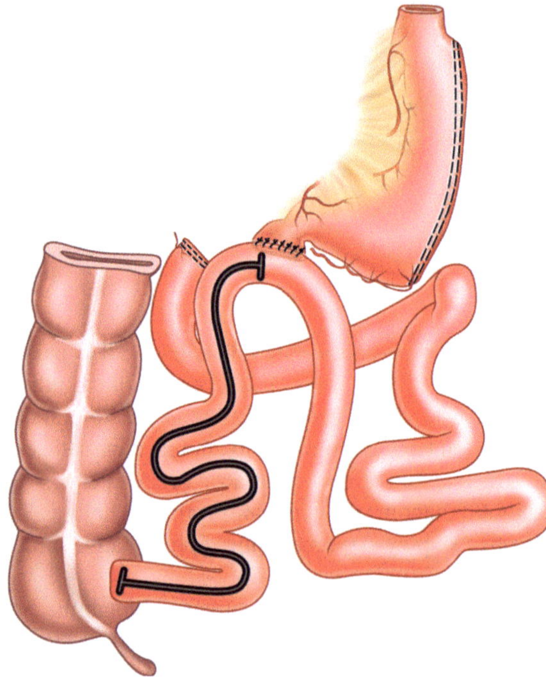

Fig. 1 SADI-S configuration

Reducing the procedure to a single anastomosis diminishes surgical time and postoperative risk of leakage. Moreover, it avoids the opening of the mesentery, normally preventing complications derived from other bariatric procedures such as Roux-en-Y gastric by-pass. Favorable outcomes have been clearly demonstrated over the years. However, as in all surgical procedures, setbacks have been encountered, although these side effects have been well tolerated and postoperative complications have appeared to be minimal. Initially, the procedure was performed with a 200 cm common limb. The initial series of 50 patients achieved excellent weight loss results after 3 years of follow-up. However, nearly 5% of the patients had to be submitted to reoperation for persistent diarrhea or malabsorption, and so the length of the common limb was increased to 250 cm. In certain situations, such as aged patients, liver or bowel disease disorders, 300 cm is the preferred length of the common limb to avoid severe nutritional complications [1–6].

In this chapter, each surgical step of minimally invasive SADI-S is thoroughly described along with representative surgical images.

Procedure Description

Position of the Patient and the Surgical Team

The operation is performed as a two-step technique, starting with a sleeve gastrectomy and continuing with a one-loop duodeno-ileostomy. In this chapter we will concentrate on the latter. The initial part of the procedure is performed with the operating table under forced anti-Trendelenburg position. The surgeon is positioned between the legs of the patient, the first assistant on the patient's left side, holding the camera, and the second assistant on the patient's right side, holding the liver retractor (Fig. 2). For the second part of the surgery, the duodeno-ileal bypass, the position is changed. The patient is placed horizontally, and the surgeon now moves from the initial position between the legs towards the left side of the patient, as well

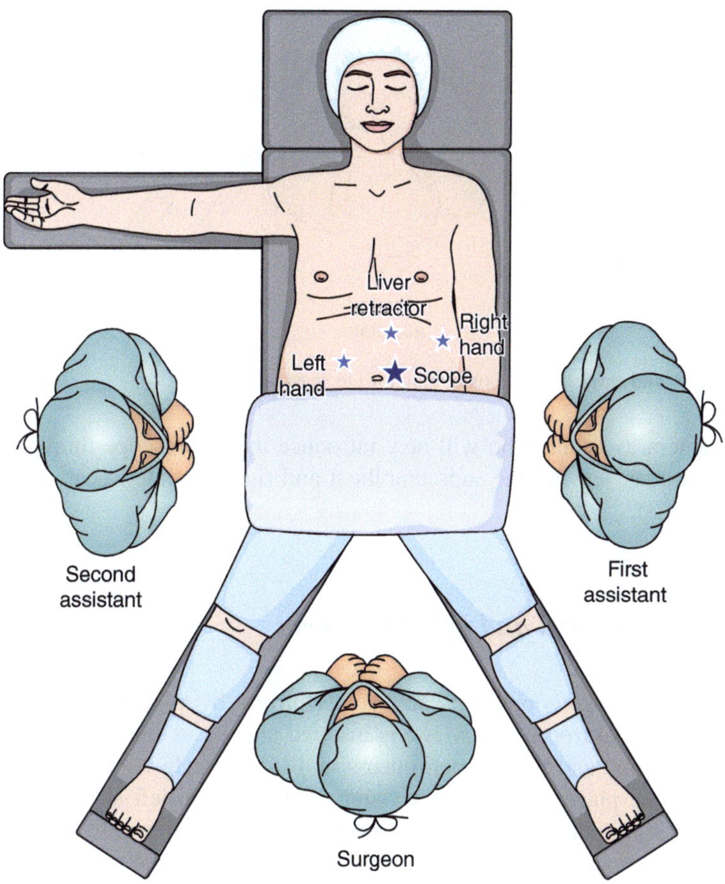

Fig. 2 Initial trocar and surgical team positioning

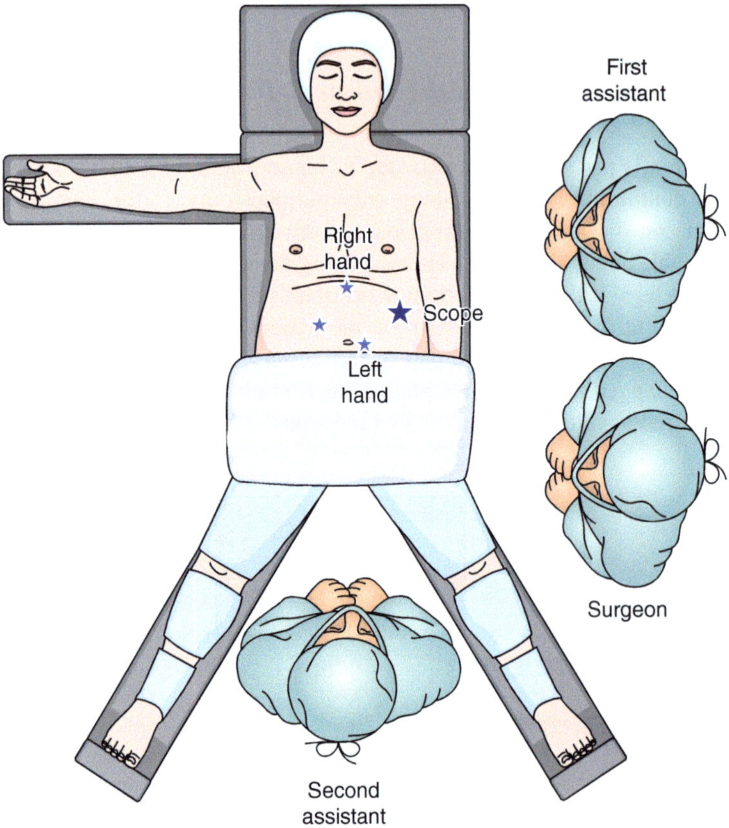

Fig. 3 Trocar and surgical team positioning for the anastomosis

as the camera assistant, who will now introduce the laparoscope through the left subcostal trocar, leaving the supraumbilical and right midline trocars as working trocars (Fig. 3).

Pneumoperitoneum and Port Placement

The standard laparoscopic approach is performed by placing four trocars. A 10–12 mm optical trocar (Optiview) is inserted above the umbilicus, slightly left from the midline, and pneumoperitoneum at 14–15 mmHg is created. All subsequent ports are placed under direct vision. A 10–12 mm left subcostal trocar is introduced for the surgeon's right hand and for the introduction of the stapler for the duodenal section during the second step. A 5 mm trocar for the surgeon's left hand initially, and subsequently for the hepatic retractor, is placed in a subxiphoid position. Finally, a 10–12 mm trocar is placed right from the midline position for the surgeon's left hand and to introduce the stapler during the sleeve gastrectomy.

Duodenal Dissection

The first step begins with a standard sleeve gastrectomy. Afterwards, by applying gentle traction of the posterior gastric wall, the antrum is raised leaving the duodenum in a vertical position. The duodenum is dissected proximally, taking care not to injure the right gastric artery. The peritoneum overlying the hepatoduodenal ligament is slightly opened and a vessel loop is passed posteriorly. A precise and complete circumferential dissection of the first duodenal portion is performed, up until 3–4 cm from the pylorus (Fig. 4). The aim of this step is to facilitate its mobilization and perform an easy and safe anastomosis. If this is not possible, division of the right gastric artery should be done at its origin. The peritoneum overlying the hepatoduodenal ligament is slightly opened and a vessel loop is passed posteriorly surrounding the duodenum to facilitate its section afterwards (Fig. 5). Dissection of the duodenum from the pancreatic surface is carried out until the pancreatoduodenal groove is reached and the gastroduodenal artery is identified (Fig. 6). The duodenum is then sectioned with a linear stapler as distal as possible from the pylorus, introducing the stapler through the left subcostal trocar (Fig. 7).

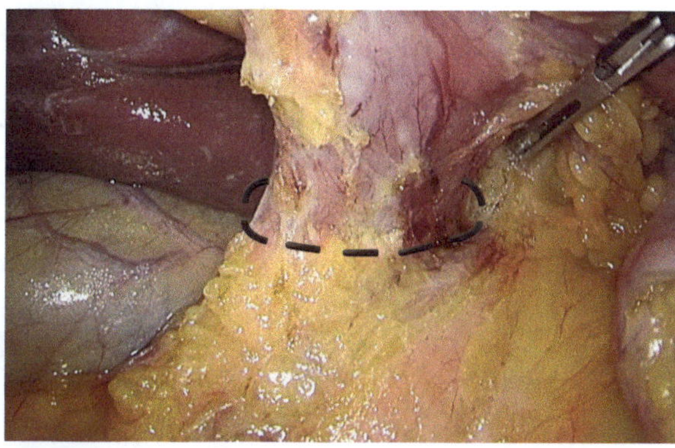

Fig. 4 Verticalization of the duodenum and complete circumferential dissection of its first portion

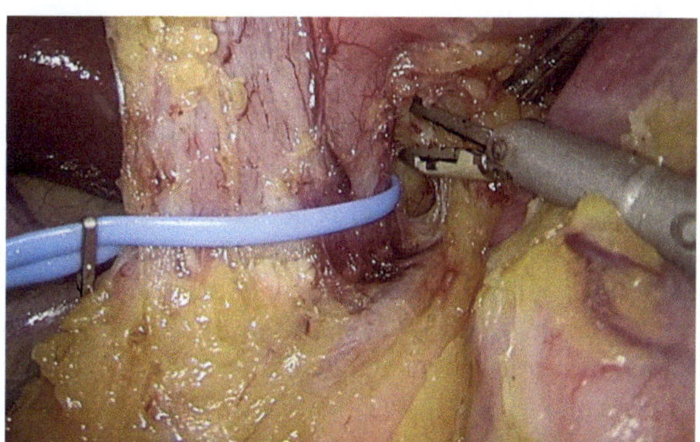

Fig. 5 The peritoneum overlying the hepatoduodenal ligament is opened and a vessel loop is passed posteriorly

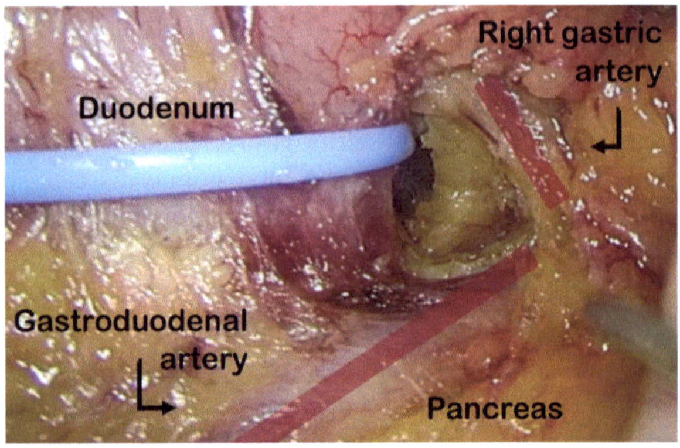

Fig. 6 Gastroduodenal and right gastric arteries

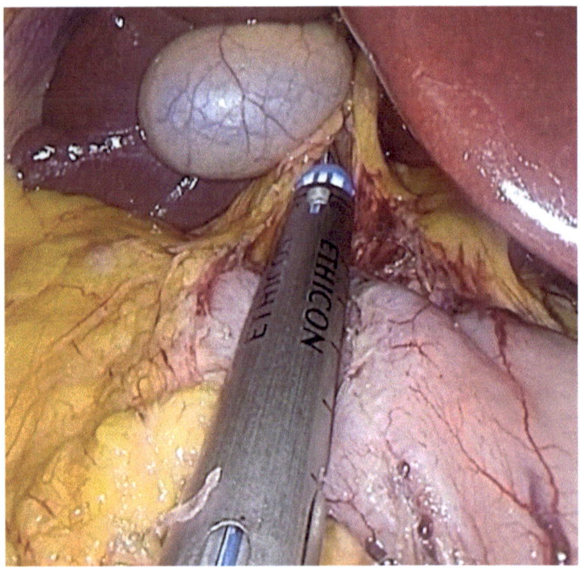

Fig. 7 Duodenal section with a linear stapler as distal as possible from the pylorus

Duodeno-Ileal Bypass

The patient is placed horizontally, and the surgical team moves to the second position. The ileo-cecal junction is identified and 250–300 cm are measured upwards. Measurement of the bowel is performed at 10 cm intervals after infusion of hyoscine butylbromide to completely relax the bowel wall and obtain the maximum possible length. The measurement of the common limb should be precise, as a short limb will predispose to malnutrition. A less effective weight loss technique is preferred over a severe malnourishment. The selected loop is ascended in an antecolic fashion and an end-to-side, two-layer, hand-sewn anastomosis to the proximal duodenal stump is carried out with running and single 3/0 polydioxanone absorbable sutures (Fig. 8).

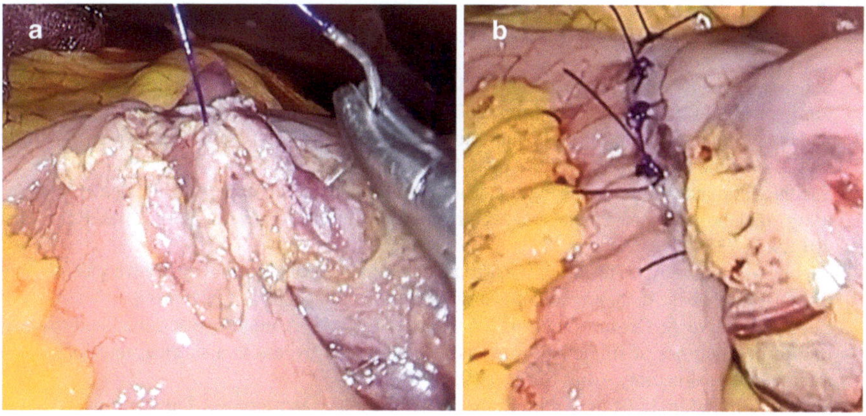

Fig. 8 An end-to-side, two-layer, hand-sewn duodeno-ileal anastomosis with running (**a**) and interrupted 3/0 polydioxanone absorbable sutures for both layers (**b**)

Final Inspection and Removal of Trocars

Once the anastomosis is done, methylene blue is routinely used to rule out any leaks at the duodeno-ileal anastomosis. Hemostasis is confirmed and the operation is then completed with the placement of a vacuum drain. The pneumoperitoneum is then evacuated, and all ports are removed under direct vision.

Conclusions

SADI-S offers better weight loss as a malabsorptive operation and better metabolic results when compared to other bariatric techniques. Pyloric preservation is more physiologic and avoids biliary reflux. This reproducible technique is relatively easy to dismantle in case of complications. No mesenteric defects are created, and so no internal hernias are normally expected. Side effects are well tolerated, and the postoperative complications are minimal. Technical pitfalls may be insufficient circumferential dissection of the first duodenal portion (by confirming up to 3–4 cm from the pylorus), duodenal devascularisation which may affect the anastomosis, errors measuring the common limb and technical difficulties concerning the anastomosis.

Conflict of Interest Authors declare that they have no conflicts of interest.

References

1. Sanchez-Pernaute A, et al. Proximal duodenal-ileal end-to-side bypass with sleeve gastrectomy: proposed technique. Obes Surg. 2007;17(12):1614–8.
2. Sanchez-Pernaute A, et al. Single anastomosis duodeno–ileal bypass with sleeve gastrectomy (SADI-S). One to three-year follow-up. Obes Surg. 2010;20:1720–6.
3. Sanchez-Pernaute A, et al. Single-anastomosis duodenoileal bypass with sleeve gastrectomy: metabolic improvement and weight loss in first 100 patients. Surg Obes Relat Dis. 2013;9(5):731–5.
4. Sanchez-Pernaute A, et al. Single-anastomosis duodenoileal bypass with sleeve gastrectomy (SADI-S) for obese diabetic patients. Surg Obes Relat Dis. 2015;11(5):1092–8.
5. Zaveri H, Surve A, Cottam D, Ng PC, Enochs P, Billy H. A multi-institutional study on the mid-term outcomes of single anastomosis Duodeno-ileal bypass as a surgical revision option after sleeve gastrectomy. Obes Surg. 2019;29(10):3165–73.
6. Shoar S, Poliakin L, Rubenstein R, Saber AA. Single anastomosis Duodeno-ileal switch (SADIS): a systematic review of efficacy and safety. Obes Surg. 2018 Jan;28(1):104–13.

Robotic SADI

Emiliano G. Manueli Laos, Beatriz Figueroa, Alvaro Ducas, and Mario A. Masrur

Abstract Single Anastomosis Duodeno-Ileal Gastric Bypass (SADI) has emerged as a popular bariatric and metabolic surgery procedure, particularly following its endorsement by the American Society for Metabolic and Bariatric Surgery (ASMBS) in 2021. While traditionally performed laparoscopically, the robotic approach offers several advantages, including enhanced visualization, precision, and dexterity. This chapter provides a detailed technical description of the robotic SADI procedure, emphasizing key steps such as duodenal dissection, window creation, stapling, and anastomosis. The importance of Indocyanine Green (ICG) fluorescence imaging for real-time assessment of duodenal perfusion is highlighted. By mastering the robotic SADI technique, bariatric surgeons can offer patients a safe and effective treatment option for weight loss and metabolic disease.

Keywords Single anastomosis duodeno-ileal bypass · Bariatric and metabolic surgery · Obesity surgery · Robitc SADI

Introduction

Single anastomosis duodeno-ileal gastric bypass (SADI) was described in 2009 as a novel procedure in the bariatric and metabolic surgery field [1]. It has gained significant popularity in US since its endorsement by ASMBS in 2021. It proposes similar weight loss outcomes as duodenal switch (DS), with lower complication rates [2]. SADI can be performed both as a revisional after a Sleeve Gastrectomy (SG) or as

E. G. Manueli Laos · B. Figueroa · A. Ducas · M. A. Masrur (✉)
Department of Surgery, University of Illinois Chicago, Chicago, IL, USA
e-mail: mmasrur@uic.edu

F. Schlottmann, M. A. Masrur (eds.), *Endoscopic, Laparoscopic and Robotic Techniques for Foregut Disorders*, https://doi.org/10.1007/978-3-032-00811-4_8

a primary procedure with a simultaneous SG (SADI-S). In this chapter, a detailed description of the technical aspects of the robotic approach for SADI will be discussed.

Procedure Description

Patient Preparation

Once the patient is placed supine on the operative table, three grams of cefazolin are administered intravenously, continued by 5000-7500 units of subcutaneous heparin for thrombosis prophylaxis. Afterwards, general anesthesia is achieved, pneumatic compression devices are placed in both legs, as well as a footboard for feet to lie flat. Arms are placed on boards with padding, at 90° abduction.

Pneumoperitoneum and Port Placement

The abdomen is prepped and draped with antiseptic and aseptic standards to guarantee sterility. To create pneumoperitoneum, a Veress needle is placed in the left upper quadrant mid-clavicular line (Plamer's point) and insufflation begins until 15 mmHg of intraabdominal pressure achieved.

Port placement starts with a 5 mm trocar placed in the left upper quadrant using Optiview technology. A diagnostic laparoscopy is then performed through this 5 mm port. The rest of the robotic 8 mm trocars are positioned under direct vision in the left upper quadrant, left flank (replacing the 5 mm port) and periumbilical area, above the umbilicus. A 12 mm robotic trocar is then placed on the right flank. Lastly, a Nathanson liver retractor is introduced in the epigastrium through a 5 mm incision (Fig. 1). The patient is then positioned in 30 degrees reverse Trendelenburg and the surgical robot is docked from the patient's lateral.

Operative Technique

Diagnostic Laparoscopy and Anatomy Identification

The procedure starts with identifying the ileocecal valve (Fig. 2). About 300 cm of bowel are run proximally from this point. This area of the anastomosis is fixed near the Duodenum with interrupted stitches marking the proximal and distal segment as can be observed in Fig. 3.

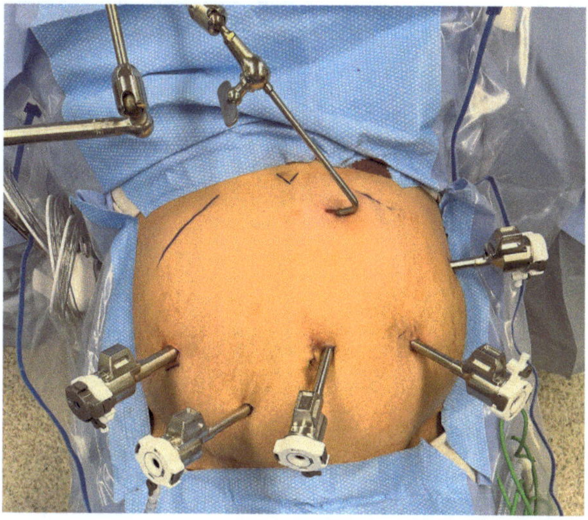

Fig. 1 Patient positioning and port placement

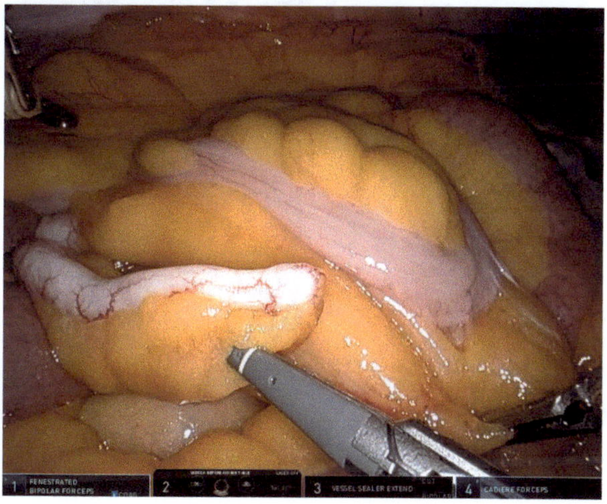

Fig. 2 Identification of the ileocecal valve

Dissection and Transection of the Duodenum

Dissection begins in the inferior aspect of the first portion of the duodenum using robotic vessels sealer (Fig. 4). To guarantee proper perfusion of the duodenal stumps, the surgeon needs to maintain the integrity of the vasculature as much as

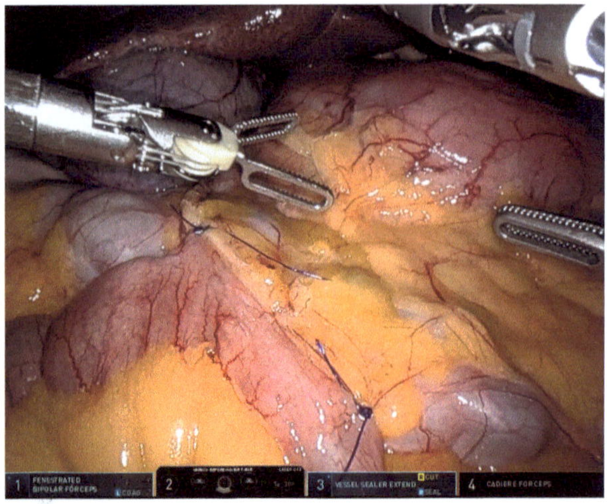

Fig. 3 Temporal fixation of the ileum

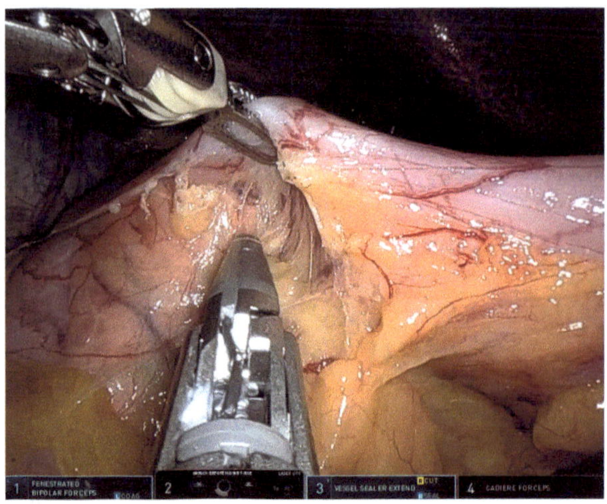

Fig. 4 Dissection of the inferior aspect of the first segment of the duodenum

possible. Caution needs to be taken, given the proximity of delicate structures such as the head of the pancreas and the gastroduodenal artery. The superior foramina of the window is created by dissecting the lesser omentum over the superior margin of the first portion of the Duodenum. Once the window is created (Fig. 5), a 60 mm White Load Robotic Stapler is used to seal and transect the duodenum (Figs. 6 and

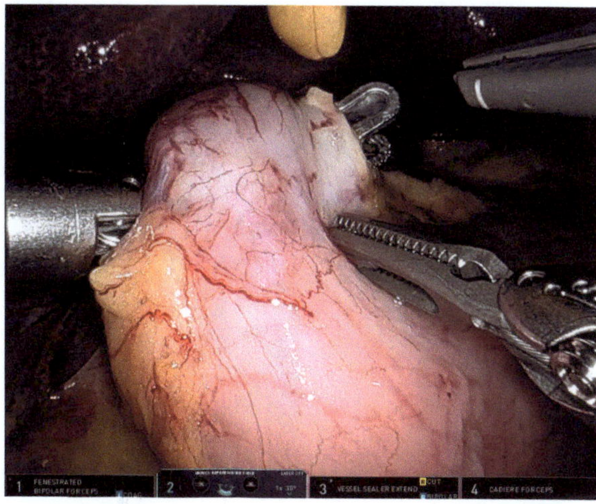

Fig. 5 Retro-duodenal window

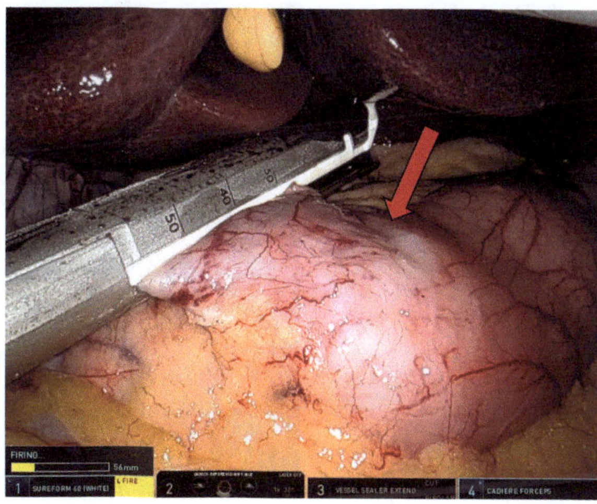

Fig. 6 Stapler positioning. (*red arrow marking the pylorus)

7). Before proceeding with the anastomosis, the patient is given an infusion of Indocyanine Green dye (ICG). Using the robotic Firefly™ mode (Intuitive Surgical, Sunnyvale California), perfusion of both distal and proximal duodenal stumps is assessed (Fig. 8). Lastly, interrupted stitches of Polydioxanone 3/0 are placed to reinforce the distal Duodenal stump (Fig. 9).

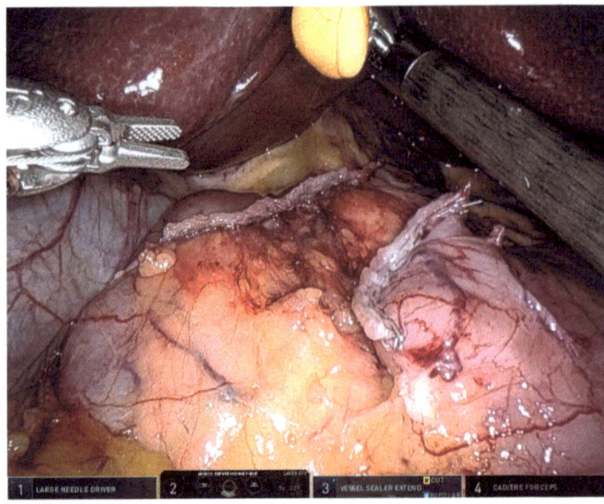

Fig. 7 Duodenal stumps after stapling

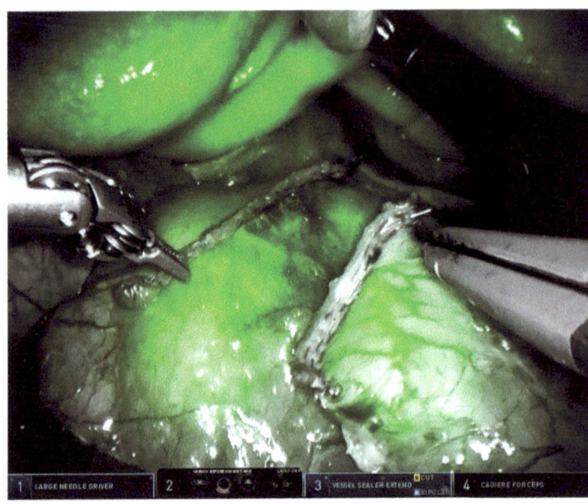

Fig. 8 Duodenal Perfusion assessment using ICG

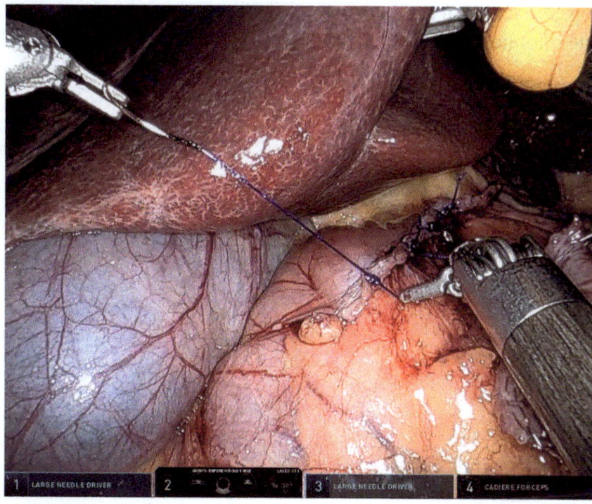

Fig. 9 Reinforcement of the Duodenal stump

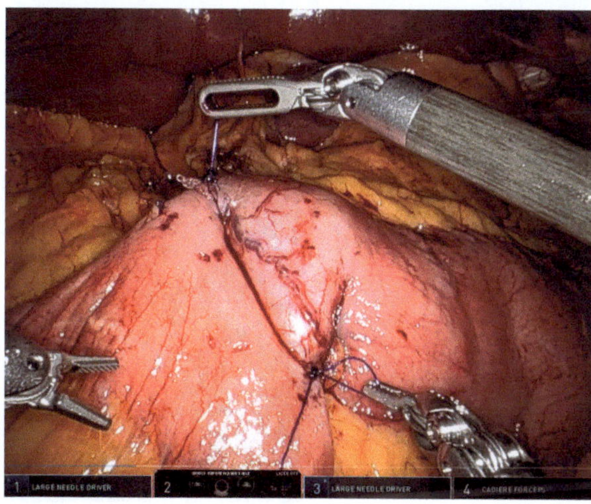

Fig. 10 External posterior layer of the anastomosis

Duodeno-Ileal Anastomosis

The duodeno-ileal anastomosis is done in a double-layer fashion. The technique begins with the creation of the external posterior layer using a running suture of Polydioxanone 3/0 in a termino-lateral fashion (Fig. 10). Using a monopolar hook, enterotomies of 1.5 cm long incision are made in both proximal duodenum and ileal loop (Fig. 11). The internal posterior layer of the anastomosis is performed with a running 3/0 Polydioxanone suture starting from the superior corner (Fig. 12).

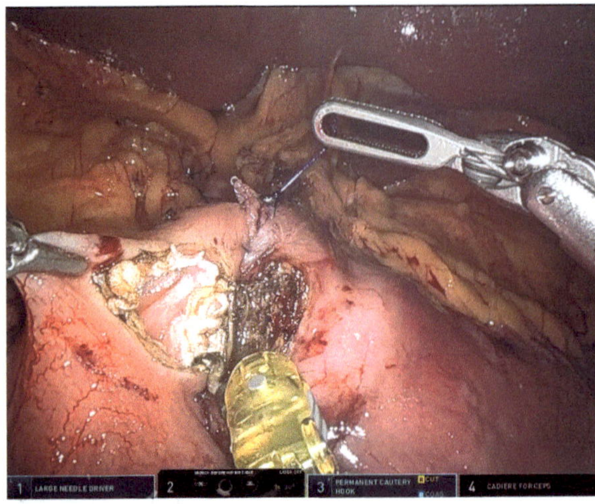

Fig. 11 Creation of the enterotomies

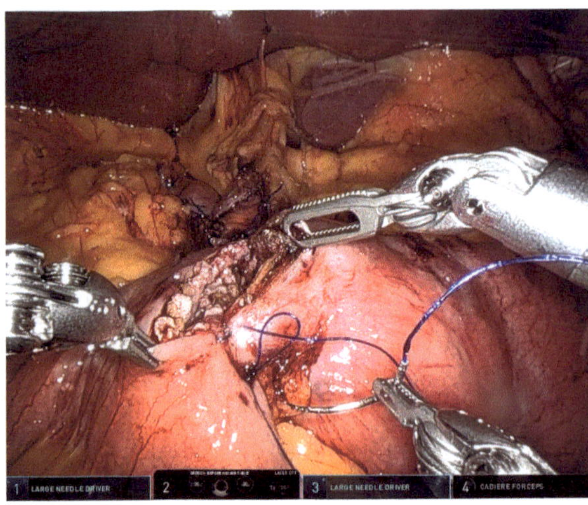

Fig. 12 Closure of the posterior inner layer

Similarly, a running suture is utilized to close the internal and external anterior layers (Fig. 13). Surgeons should perform the technique in a way that prevents mucosal prolapses or stenosis. The ileal loop is then fixated proximally and distally to the anastomosis with two interrupted stitches. This maneuver is performed to avoid potential twisting of the anastomosis (Fig. 14). Mesenteric gaps are not close as no mesenteric defects are created in this technique.

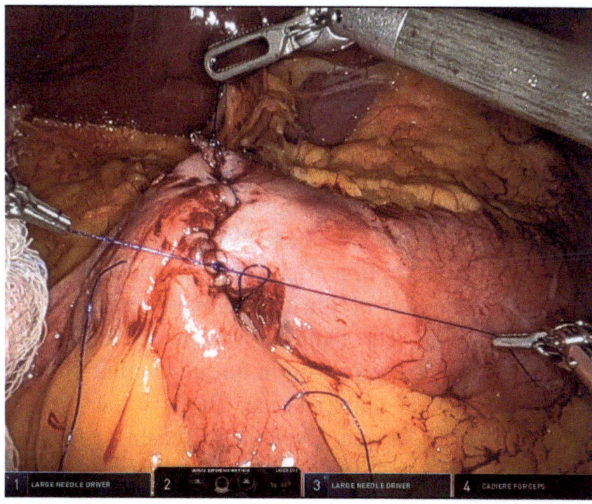

Fig. 13 Closure of the anterior inner layer

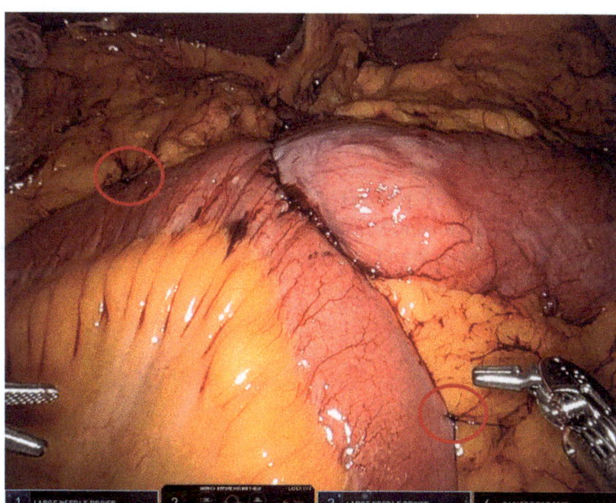

Fig. 14 Closure of the external anterior layer. (*red circles mark the fixating sutures)

Final Evaluation and Trocar Removal

An esophago-gastro-duodenoscopy (EGD) is performed intraoperatively to check the integrity of the anastomosis, assessment of leaks or intraluminal bleeding. The liver retractor is removed, and the fascia of the 12 mm port is closed using #0 Polyglactin sutures. Lastly, after a final inspection of the abdomen, the trocars are removed, and pneumoperitoneum is evacuated. Skin incisions are closed with subcutaneous sutures.

Conclusions

SADI has been increasing applicability in the US since its endorsement by ASMBS in 2021. Although is a well establish primary procedure, it has become more popular as a revisional option after weight regain post SG. The Robotic assistance facilitates the execution of intricate procedures in otherwise high-risk patients with enhanced safety. The main advantages include application of ICG of perfusion evaluation and the reduction in torque exerted by the abdominal wall translates to smoother surgical manipulation. Bariatric surgeons must be well-versed in this approach and technique, given the increasing prevalence of SADI procedures. They are likely to encounter patients who may benefit from or require such interventions.

References

1. Sánchez-Pernaute A, Rubio Herrera MA, Pérez-Aguirre E, et al. Proximal duodenal-ileal end-to-side bypass with sleeve gastrectomy: proposed technique. Obes Surg. 2007;17(12):1614–8. https://doi.org/10.1007/s11695-007-9287-8.
2. Verhoeff K, Mocanu V, Zalasky A, et al. Evaluation of metabolic outcomes following SADI-S: a systematic review and meta-analysis. Obes Surg. 2022;32(4):1049–63. https://doi.org/10.1007/s11695-021-05824-w.

Laparoscopic OAGB

Luciano Deluca and Ezequiel Fernandez

Abstract Bariatric surgery continues to be the most effective treatment for patients with obesity. Laparoscopic one-anastomosis gastric bypass (OAGB) is currently the third most performed bariatric surgery worldwide and has experienced the greatest growth in the last 10 years. In this chapter, we will describe the surgical technique step by step with representative images of the procedure.

Keywords OAGB · One anastomosis gastric bypass · Minigastric bypass

Introduction

Bariatric surgery is the most effective treatment for patients with obesity and laparoscopic one-anastomosis gastric bypass (OAGB) is currently the third most performed bariatric surgery worldwide with the greatest growth in the last 10 years.

There is controversy regarding potential adverse effects such as bile reflux or protein malnutrition [1]; however, current evidence shows that it is a safe and effective surgery in well-selected patients [2–5]. Also, when compared to Roux-en-Y gastric bypass (RYGB), OAGB has shown to be a shorter and simpler technique to perform, with a lower incidence of postoperative complications [6–8].

In this chapter, we will describe the surgical technique step by step with representative images of the procedure.

L. Deluca (✉)
Complejo Médico Policial Churruca, Buenos Aires, Argentina

Centro de Rehabilitación Quirúrgica de la Obesidad, Buenos Aires, Argentina

E. Fernandez
Complejo Médico Policial Churruca, Buenos Aires, Argentina

F. Schlottmann, M. A. Masrur (eds.), *Endoscopic, Laparoscopic and Robotic Techniques for Foregut Disorders*, https://doi.org/10.1007/978-3-032-00811-4_9

Procedure Description

Patient Positioning

The patient is placed in a supine position with abducted arms and intermitent pneumatic boot compression. The screen is positioned over the patient's head. The surgeon stands on the patient's right side, while the first and second assistant are placed on the left (Fig. 1). After trocars are placed, position is then set to Fowler.

Orogastric 27 Fr tube is used for gastric decompression and ulterior calibration. Placement of any other kind of tube is avoided to prevent inadvertent stapling incidents. Antibiotic prophylaxis with 1 g of intravenous cephalothin is usually performed.

Pneumoperitoneum and Port Placement

We perform skin, fascia and preperitoneal infiltration with bupivacaine. Pneumoperitoneum with a Veress needle is perform subcostal to achieve an intraperitoneal pressure of 12-14 mmHg depending on surgical exposure. In patients with a history of abdominal surgery, the midclavicular line just below the costal margin is the preferred access for Veress needle puncture before trocar placement.

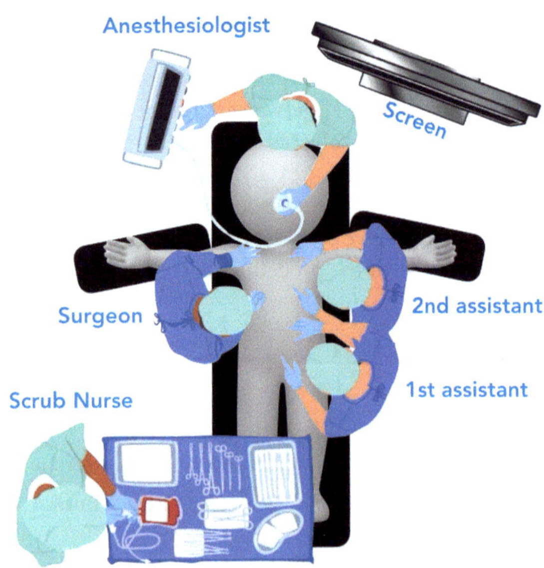

Fig. 1 Patient positioning

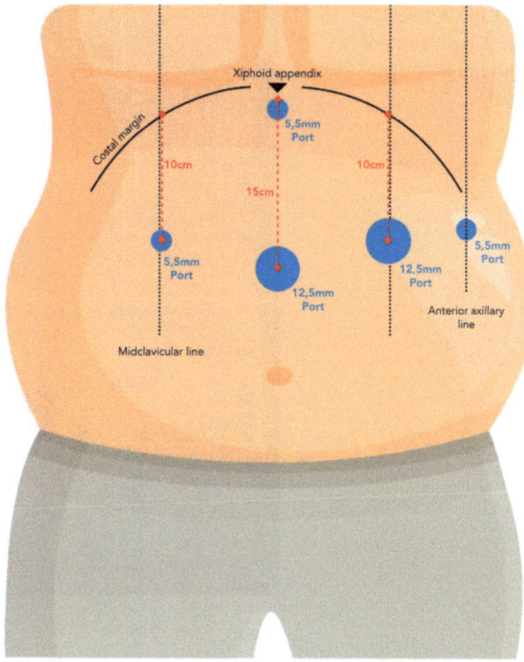

Fig. 2 Port placement

Once pneumoperitoneum is set, the ports are placed under direct vision. A 12.5 mm port is placed left midclavicular line 10 cm subcostal, the second 12.5 mm trocar is placed 15 cm below the xyphoid in the midline. Three 5.5 mm ports are placed following, one on the right flank symmetrical to the second port; one on the midaxillary line at the left costal margin, and one subxiphoid to retract the liver during the procedure (Fig. 2).

Liver Retraction and Greater Omentum Transection

Liver retraction is usually achieved with a 5 mm fan liver retractor. In some cases, a polypropylene stitch is passed through the right crus and retrieved through the epigastrium, as published previously [9] (Fig. 3).

Subsequently, the Treitz angle and the presence of any adhesions that could hindered the OAGB are identified. Then, the greater omentum is split with an unltrasonic scalpel until reaching the transverse colon. This is critical to reduce tension at the anastomosis (Fig. 4).

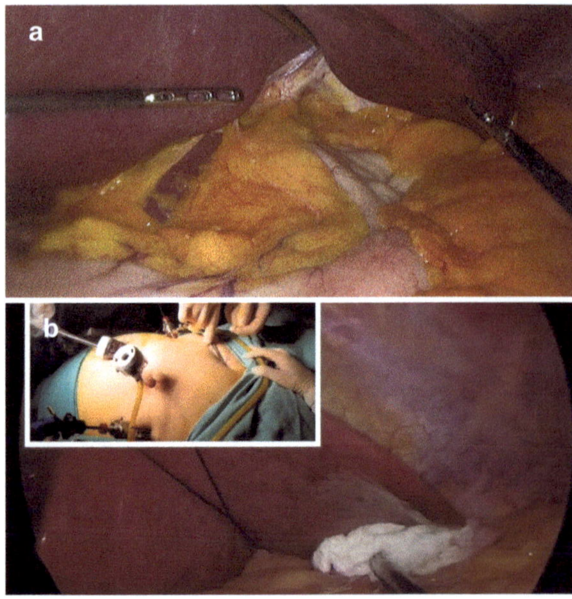

Fig. 3 Liver retraction with fan Liver retractor (**a**) and with polipropilene stitch (**b**)

Creation of Gastric Pouch

The His angle is dissected and the periesophageal fat pad is resected to facilitate stapling. The incisura angularis is identified and dissection is started 2 cm below this landmark using ultrasonic scalpel until the lesser sac is accesed. Then, the stomach is transected calibrated with the 28fr tube. The first transversal stapling is performed with a green or gold (Echelon GST 60 or Ezisurg™ R45G or L45C) or purple reload (Endo GIA Tri Staple™) (Fig. 5), followed by vertical stapling with gold or blue (Echelon GST 60 or Ezisurg™ L45C or R45C) or purple (Endo GIA Tri Staple™) reloads following the calibrating tube as a guide.

The objective is to create a thin pouch of at least 18–20 cm long. It is important to dissect all adhesions on the posterior wall of the stomach in order to perform a homogeneous pouch. The last staple is placed 1–2 cm away from the angle of His to avoid stapling the lower esophageal sphincter (Fig. 6). The calibrating bougie is moved back and forth with every staple to confirm adequate placement. If a hiatal hernia is found, dissection is done until a 2–3 cm long intra-abdominal esophagus is achieved and a hiatoplasty with interrupted 2–0 polyester or silk figure-of-eight stitches.

Finally, reinforcement is performed over the gastric remnant staple line with a 2–0 polypropylene transfixing running suture. The gastric pouch stapler line is reinforced as well, then anchored to the jejunum side using the same stitch material (Fig. 7).

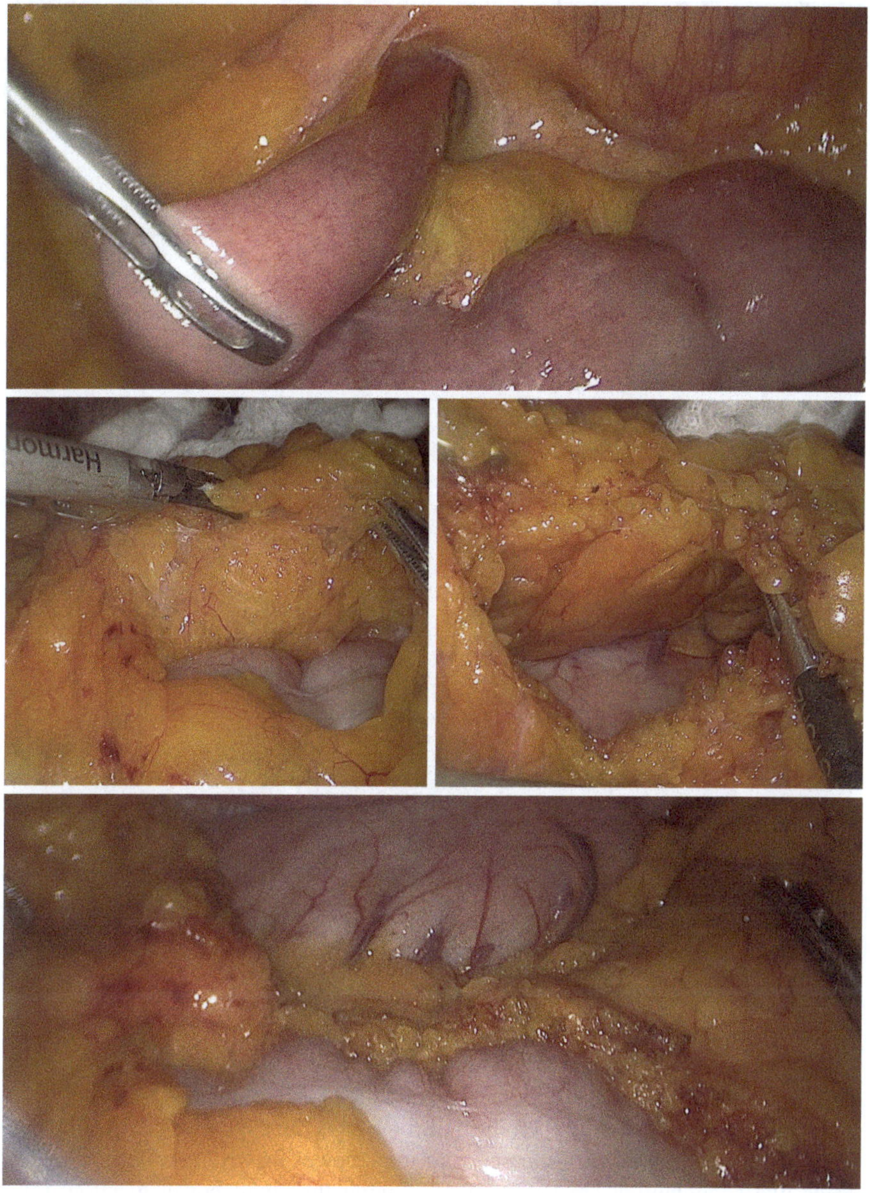

Fig. 4 Treitz identification and greater omentum section

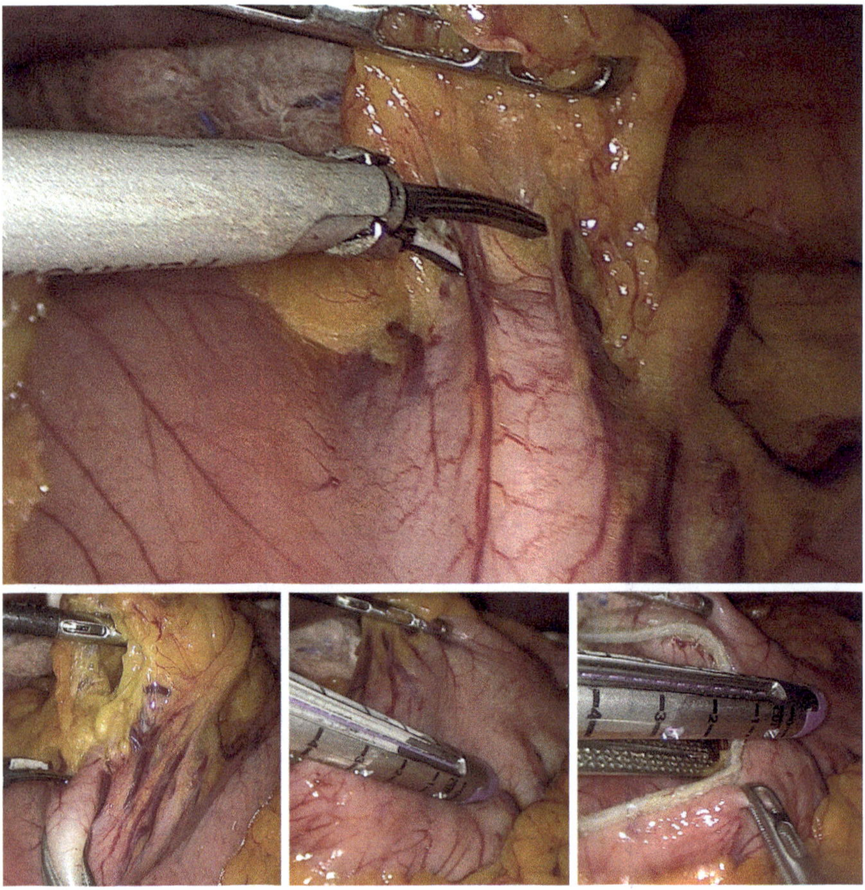

Fig. 5 Gastric transection

Gastrojejunal Anastomosis

The Treitz angle is identified once again and 200 cm of jejunum are run distally, assuring that there are at least 250 cm of jejunum distal to this point. Although rare, if the small bowel is shorter, then the anastomosis is done at at least 250 cm proximal to the ileocecal valve to secure enough small bowel absortion. Antiespasmodical drugs like scopolamine are used before running the small bowel to allow for a smoother manuever.

Once the length is established, a side-to-side running suture 10 cm long is placed between the anti-mesenteric side of the jejunum and the gastric pouch staple line using the same polyproplylene suture of the pouch reinforcement. The jejunal limb

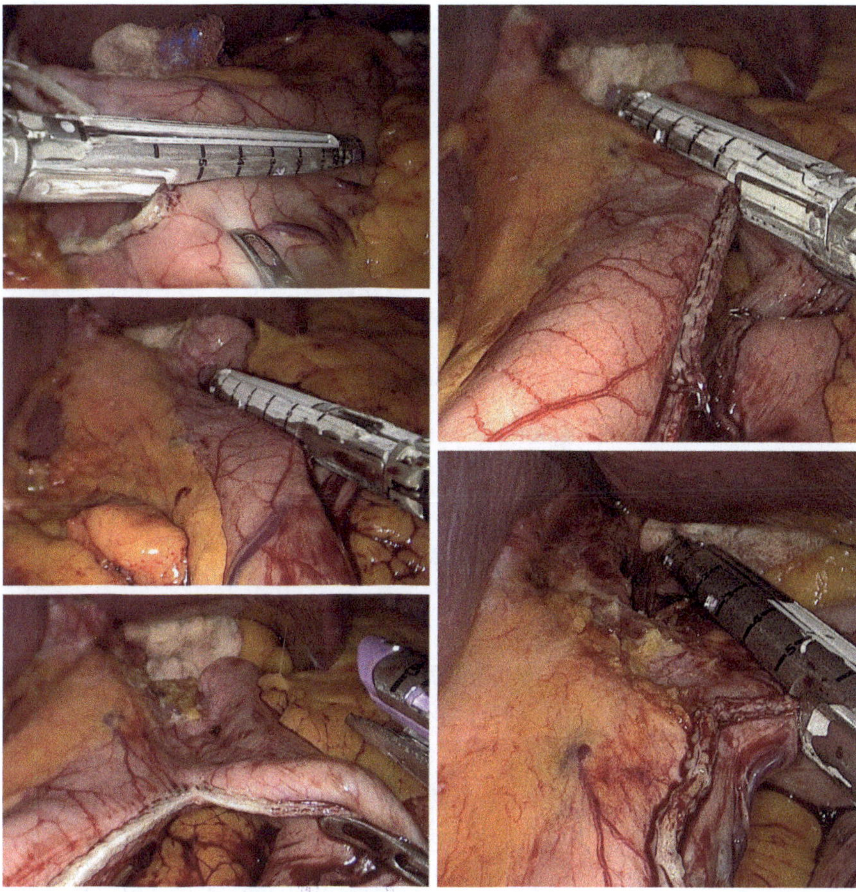

Fig. 6 Gastric pouch confection

is placed on an isoperistaltic fashion in relation to the anastomosis. This also works as an anti-reflux mechanism, as it favors gravitational bile drainage [5] (Fig. 8).

Lastly, a 1 cm enterotomy and gastrotomy are done using ultrasonic scalpel to perform a 3 cm long side-to-side gastro-jejunal anastomosis with a linear-stapled (blue load Echelon GST 60 or Ezisurg ™ R45C or purple Endo GIA Tri Staple™). The bougie is advanced through the anastomosis and the gastroenterotomy is closed with a seromuscular 2-0 polidioxanone running suture (Fig. 9).

A methylene blue leak test is performed through the 28 Fr tube after clamping the afferent and efferent limbs placing a gauze in the back of the gastroyeyunostomy to identify leaks of methylene blue posteriorly (Fig. 10).

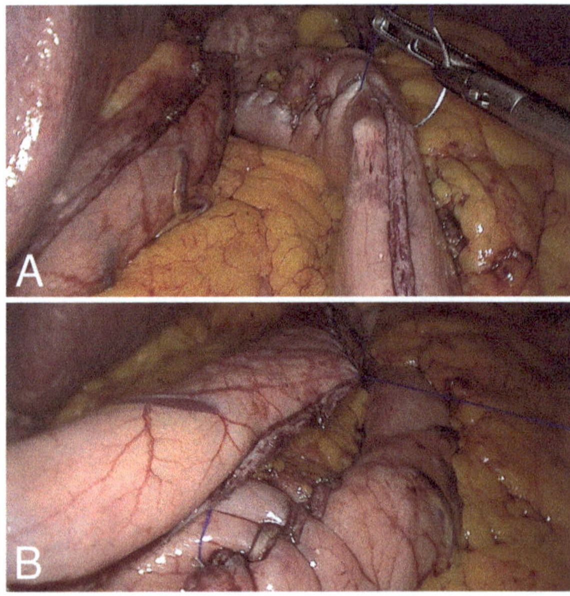

Fig. 7 Gastric remanent (**a**) and gastric pouch (**b**) reinforcement

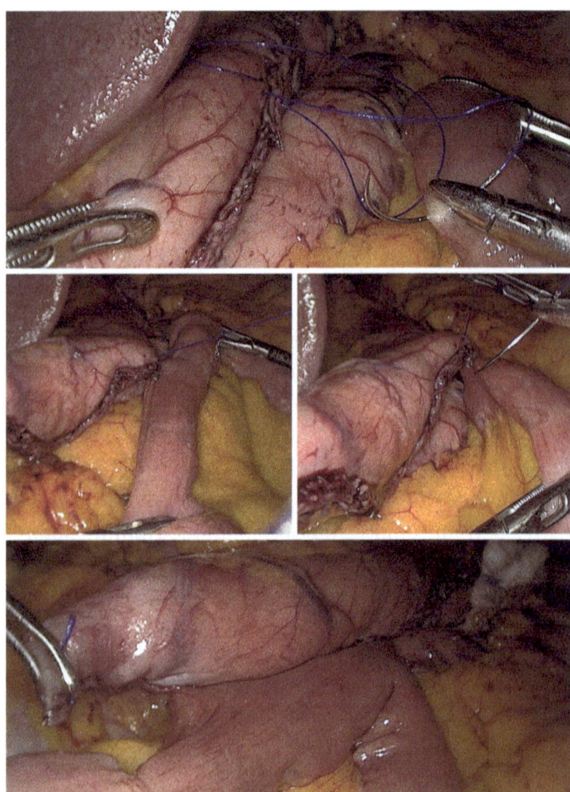

Fig. 8 Anti-reflux mechanism confection

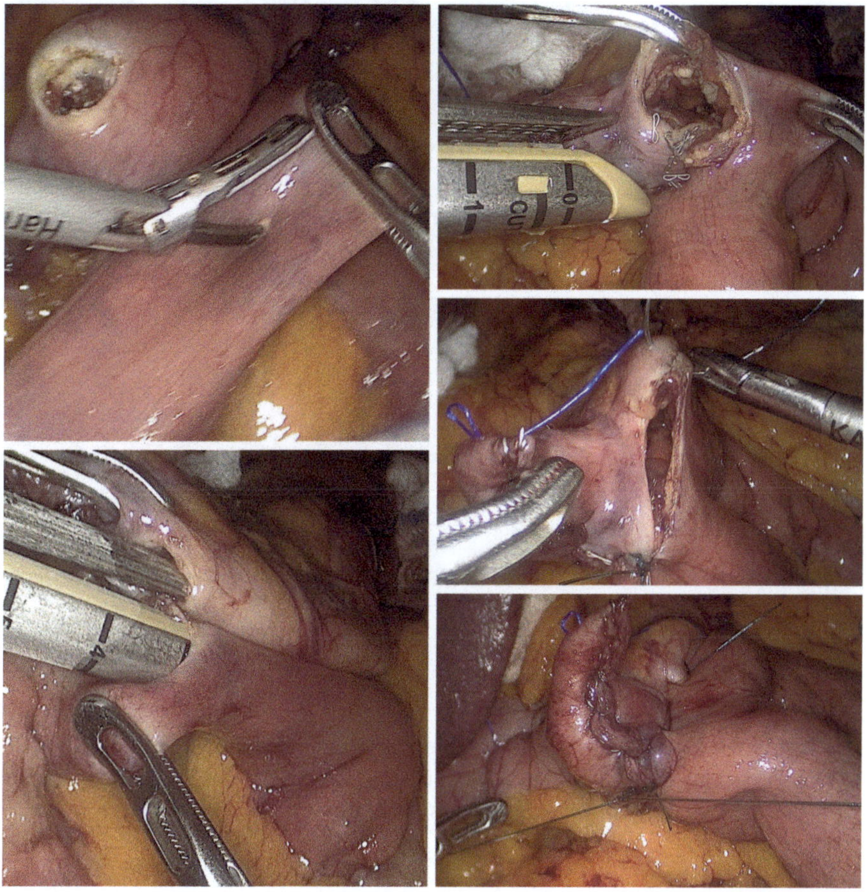

Fig. 9 Gastrojejunal anastomosis confection

Hemostasis Control and Final Inspection

Exhaustive hemostasis control is performed. The use of routine drainage is not adopted, except in selected cases based on surgical team's consideration. Twenty milliliters of 0.5% bupivacaine are instilled into the left subphrenic space and between the liver and de gastric pouch to minimize postoperative pain [10]. All ports are retrieved under direct vision. Before the last port is extracted, the abdominal cavity is deflated fully. Skin is closed with absorbable suture.

Fig. 10 Methylene blue leak test

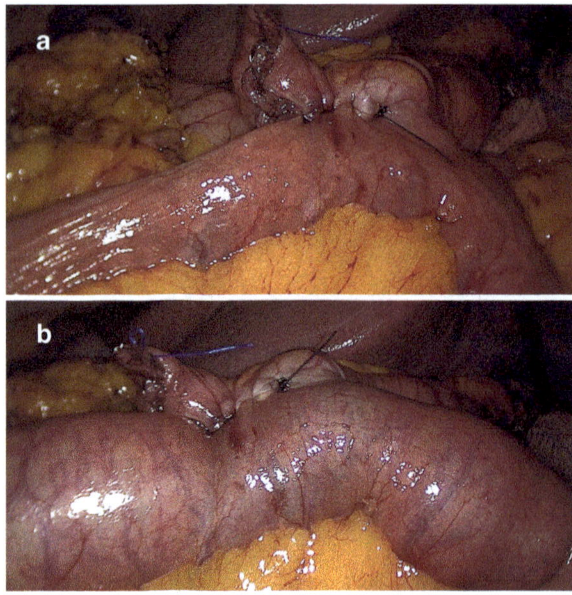

Conclusions

One-anastomosis gastric bypass is a more reproducible technique with fewer post-operative complications compared to Roux-en-Y gastric bypass. As the technique with the greatest growth in recent years, it is important to systematize it for its proper execution.

References

1. Mahawar KK, Carr WRJ, Balupuri S, Small PK. Controversy surrounding "mini" gastric bypass. Obes Surg. 2013;24(2):324–33.
2. Carbajo MA, Luque-de-León E, Jiménez JM, et al. Laparoscopic one-anastomosis gastric bypass: technique, results, and long-term follow-up in 1200 patients. Obes Surg. 2017;27:1153–67.
3. Chevallier JM, Arman GA, Guenzi M, et al. One thousand single anastomosis (omega loop) gastric bypasses to treat morbid obesity in a 7-year period: outcomes show few complications and good efficacy. Obes Surg. 2015;25:951–8.
4. Chiappetta S, Weiner R. Evidence of the mini-/one-anastomosis-gastric-bypass for being a standard procedure in obesity and metabolic surgery. Chirurg. 2018;89:589–96.
5. García-Caballero M, Carbajo M. One anastomosis gastric bypass: a simple, safe and efficient surgical procedure for treating morbid obesity. Nutr Hosp. 2004;19:372–5.
6. Lee W-J, Yu P-J, Wang W, Chen T-C, Wei P-L, Huang M-T. Laparoscopic roux-en-Y versus mini-gastric bypass for the treatment of morbid obesity. Ann Surg. 2005;242(1):20–8.

7. Jung JJ, Park AK, Witkowski ER, Hutter MM. Comparison of short-term safety of one anastomosis gastric bypass to roux-en-Y gastric bypass and sleeve gastrectomy in the United States: 341 cases from MBSAQIP-accredited Centers. Surg Obes Relat Dis. 2022;18(3):326–34.
8. Robert M, Espalieu P, Pelascini E, Caiazzo R, Sterkers A, Khamphommala L, et al. Efficacy and safety of one anastomosis gastric bypass versus roux-en-Y gastric bypass for obesity (YOMEGA): a multicentre, randomised, open-label, non-inferiority trial. Lancet. 2019;393(10178):1299–309.
9. Cal P, Deluca L, Jakob T, Parasporo L, Lonardi D, Fernández E. Low-cost incisionless liver retraction for laparoscopic sleeve gastrectomy: a prospective controlled trial. J Laparoendosc Adv Surg Tech. 2019;29(12):1556–60.
10. Omar I, Abualsel A. Efficacy of intraperitoneal instillation of bupivacaine after bariatric surgery: randomized controlled trial. Obes Surg. 2019;29(6):1735–41. https://doi.org/10.1007/s11695-019-03775-x.

Suturing Endoscopic Primary Bariatric Procedures

Ravishankar Asokkumar, Gontrand Lopez-Nava, and Natan Zundel

Abstract Endoscopic suturing and gastroplasties represent an important evolution in obesity management, offering a less invasive, effective alternative to traditional weight loss surgery. These procedures reduce the gastric volume or alter its shape, promoting early satiety and limiting food intake. Endoscopic gastroplasties have the advantage of being incisionless, having quick recovery, and having fewer complications, making them an attractive option to patients who may not be suitable candidates or are unwilling to undergo surgery. Several endoscopic gastroplasty options are currently available, along with other newer techniques in development. However, a learning curve exists to gain proficiency with different endoscopic gastroplasty procedures. In this chapter, we describe the method of performing endoscopic gastroplasty using the available suturing platforms and discuss evidence on their efficacy and safety.

Keywords Overstitch · Endoscopic sleeve Gastroplasty · Obesity · Bariatric endoscopy · POSE · Endozip · Automated suturing

R. Asokkumar
Department of Gastroenterology and Hepatology, Singapore General Hospital, Singapore, Singapore

DUKE-NUS, Graduate Medical School, Singapore, Singapore

Bariatric Endoscopy Unit, HM Sanchinarro University Hospital, Madrid, Spain

G. Lopez-Nava
DUKE-NUS, Graduate Medical School, Singapore, Singapore

N. Zundel (✉)
Department of Surgery, University at Buffalo, Buffalo, NY, USA

Florida International University, Miami, FL, USA

F. Schlottmann, M. A. Masrur (eds.), *Endoscopic, Laparoscopic and Robotic Techniques for Foregut Disorders*, https://doi.org/10.1007/978-3-032-00811-4_10

Introduction

Obesity has become a global health concern and is an established risk factor for diabetes mellitus, hypertension, metabolic-associated liver steatosis disease, cardiovascular disease, and increased all-cause mortality. In 2022, according to the WHO report, one in 8 people in the world were living with obesity, and 2.5 billion adults were overweight [1]. For long, the treatment of obesity has been limited to diet and lifestyle intervention, pharmacotherapy, and surgery. However, the proportion of patients achieving significant weight loss with lifestyle intervention alone is modest. Likewise, the number of patients opting for surgery as a treatment option for obesity has consistently remained low, thus creating a massive need for patient-preferred interventions [2]. Newer pharmacotherapeutic agents have created excitement in obesity treatment with better weight loss results [3]. However, lack of widespread availability, higher cost, need for long-term use, and increased gastrointestinal symptoms have restricted their wider use.

In the last few decades, several innovations and advancements have occurred in interventional endoscopy, expanding the horizon for minimally invasive treatment. In particular, the ability to perform full-thickness suturing and approximate tissue through natural orifice without incision has expanded the field of endo-bariatrics to address both obesity and accompanying metabolic conditions using reversible approaches [4]. Since its introduction, several devices, suturing techniques, and modifications in treatment have been described. They are used both for primary weight loss treatment and to manage weight regain and complications following bariatric surgery. Broadly, endoscopic bariatric and metabolic therapies can be classified into those targeting the stomach for primary weight loss and metabolic improvements and those targeting the small bowel for metabolic alterations alone.

In this chapter, we describe the technique and outcomes of endoscopic gastroplasty and gastric volume reduction using the widely available suturing device and provide guidance for successful clinical outcomes.

Choosing Patients for Endoscopic Gastroplasty

The American Society for Gastrointestinal Endoscopy–European Society of Gastrointestinal Endoscopy guideline [5] and the NICE recommendations [6] consider that endoscopic suturing and gastric volume reduction as a treatment option for obesity would be beneficial to

(a) Patients with BMI >30 kg/m^2 for whom non-surgical weight loss treatments had not worked. (In South Asian, Chinese, other Asian, Middle Eastern, Black African, or African-Caribbean ethnicity, BMI >27.5 kg/m^2 is recommended as the threshold).
(b) Patients with obesity Class III, for whom invasive surgery is considered as high risk.

(c) Patients who decline bariatric surgery because of associated risks and complications.
(d) Patients with a BMI of 27.0 to 29.9 kg/m^2 with at least one obesity-related comorbidity to prevent the progression of obesity and associated comorbidities.

Careful patient selection is crucial for successful technical outcomes. It is advisable to avoid endoscopic gastroplasty in patients with (a) active gastric ulcer in the fundus and body of the stomach, (b) large esophageal or gastric varices, (c) moderated to severe portal hypertensive gastropathy, (d) gastric polyposis syndrome, (e) malignant and pre-malignant gastric lesions, (f) strictures or stenosis in the upper GI tract, and (g) uncontrolled psychiatric disorders.

Endoscopic Suturing Platforms

Multiple endoscopic gastroplasty methods to induce gastric restriction are available (Fig. 1). These include the Endoscopic sleeve gastroplasty using the Overstitch second generation and the Overstitch Sx platform (Boston Scientific, Texas, USA), primary obesity surgery endoluminal (POSE) procedure using the incisionless operating platform (USGI, San Clemente, CA), and the robotic automated endoscopic suturing using the Endozip system (Nitinotes, Israel).

Procedure	Manufacturer	Device	Technique
Endoscopic Sleeve Gastroplasty (ESG)	Overstitch, Boston Scientific, USA	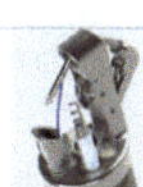	Full thickness continuous suturing
Endoscopic Sleeve Gastroplasty (ESG)	Overstitch Sx, Boston Scientific, USA	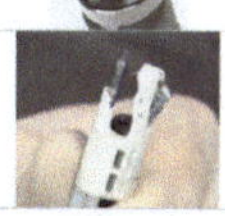	Full thickness continuous suturing
Primary Obesity Surgery Endoluminal (POSE)	USGI Medical, USA	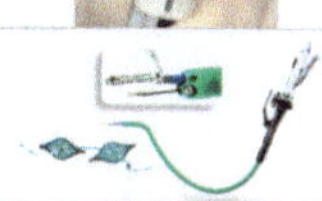	Tissue plication using snowshoe suture anchors
Endozip	Nitinotes Surgical, Israel	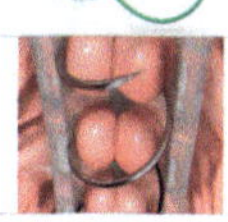	Automated full thickness suturing

Fig. 1 Endoscopic gastroplasty techniques and devices available for endoscopic suturing

Endoscopic Sleeve Gastroplasty (ESG)

Overstitch Suturing Device

The suture system comprises the needle driver assembly, anchor exchange device, 2.0 polypropylene sutures, and accessories such as the tissue helix and suture cinch. The second-generation suturing device (Overstitch, Boston Scientific, Austin, Texas) is compatible only with dual channel endoscopes (Olympus GIF-2TH180, GIF-2 T160, and Fujifilm EI740 D/S). The needle driver assembly is fitted to the larger channel at the distal end of the scope, and the handle is seated next to the working channel. Squeezing the handle locks the needle body, and using the anchor exchange catheter, the suture can be engaged and retrieved from the needle body to perform continuous suturing. As dual-channel scopes are not widely available, to overcome this limitation, a single-channel suturing platform has been made available (Fig. 2).

The single channel Overstitch Sx and NXT device (Overstitch Sx, Boston Scientific, Austin, Texas) can be mounted easily on most commercially available endoscopes (diameter: 8.8–9.8 mm). It has two separate working channels on the external sheath independent of the scope channel and can be used to advance the accessories and perform suturing. The side mounting of the external sheath does not interfere with the view. The additional channel allows better suctioning of the clots and debris during the procedure. However, some training is required to become familiar with the mounting technique and to achieve the correct distal endcap orientation.

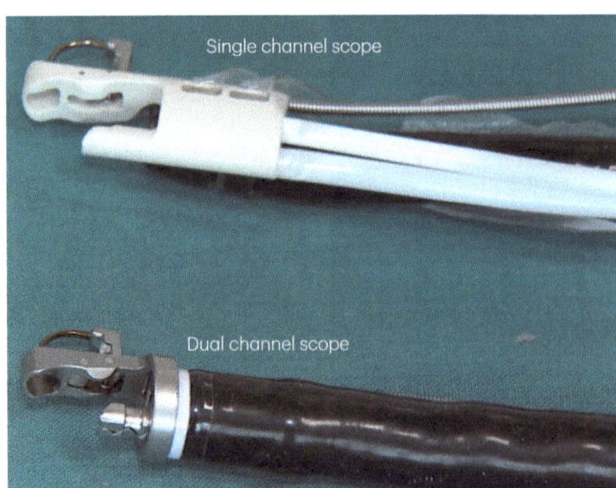

Fig. 2 Overstitch and Overstitch Sx device mounted on a dual and single channel endoscope

Procedure Description

ESG- Technical Description

ESG procedure is performed in the operating room or ambulatory center with monitored anesthesia care. The patient is placed in the left lateral position and administer antibiotics before the procedure. An upper endoscopy is performed to evaluate the stomach for any contraindications. If none, an overtube is introduced when using a dual channel device to allow easy advancement of the device and to maintain adequate gastric distention during the procedure. For the Overstitch Sx system, the use of overtube is not recommended. CO2 use for insufflation and water jet function is routinely used. Argon plasma coagulation is not used to mark the location of suturing.

Suturing starts at the distal body slightly above the incisura at the anterior wall and follow a "U" shaped suture pattern [7]. The suture is run continuously with no loop formation or tangling when moving from the anterior to the posterior wall and back to the anterior wall. Six to eight full-thickness bites are taken per row of sutures maintaining a distance of approximately 1–2 cm between each bite. Approximately 5–7 rows of suturing are performed to reduce the gastric volume and achieve a sleeve configuration (Fig. 3). The gastric fundus is spared to minimize the risk of esophageal reflux after the procedure. The gastric volume is reduced by 75–80%.

The technical success of the ESG procedure is dependent on the ability to perform full full-thickness suturing consistently. To achieve that, enough tissue is captured using the tissue helix and place it perpendicular to the needle driver assembly so that when the handle is squeezed, the needle always drives through the serosa to achieve a full-thickness bite (Fig. 4). Suctioning of the stomach wall is avoided to bring more tissue inside the distal endcap. Instead rotating the helix 3–4 times to capture adequate tissue is recommended. Excessive rotation of the helix could either perforate the gastric wall or capture deeper structures, causing bleeding or other adverse events. Reinforcement sutures are not routinely performed. Since the initial description, several suture patterns, including the "M" pattern, "Z" pattern, "U" pattern, "O" pattern, and triangular and interrupted pattern, have been described. The "U" pattern was the preferred for all cases as it narrows and foreshortens the stomach length by over 40%. A comparative study from the European registry data has

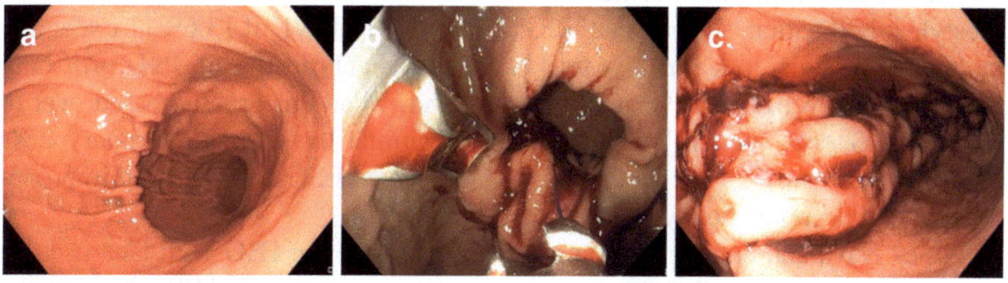

Fig. 3 Endoscopic image of the stomach after ESG. (**a**) Normal stomach before the procedure. (**b**) Continuous "U" pattern suturing was performed using the dual channel overstitch suturing system. (**c**) Sleeve configuration of the stomach after ESG

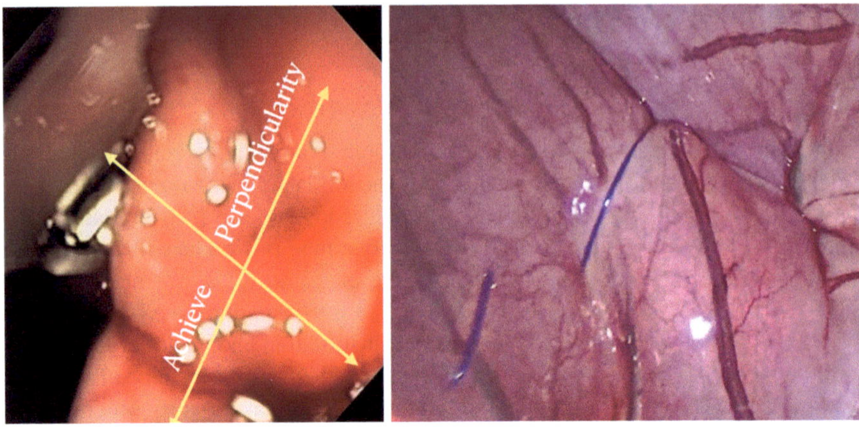

Fig. 4 Performing full-thickness suturing. (**a**) The tissue grasped using the helix is placed perpendicular to the axis of the needle driver assembly to enable the needle to pierce through the serosa when closed. (**b**) Suture can be seen running through the serosal layer after a full-thickness bite

shown better weight loss outcomes with the "U" pattern [8]. Intubating the duodenum or over-insufflating the stomach is not recommended after the procedure to minimize post-procedure symptoms.

Weight-Loss Outcomes after ESG

The American Society for Gastrointestinal Endoscopy (ASGE) and the American Society for Metabolic and Bariatric Surgery (ASMBS) recommended an acceptable efficacy threshold of ≥25% excess weight loss (EWL) or ≥ 10% total body weight loss (TBWL) at 12 months and a safety threshold of ≤ 5% complication rate for endoscopic bariatric therapies [9]. Similarly, the DPP study and Look AHEAD randomized control trial showed that achieving ≥8–10% weight loss at 12 months significantly reduced the incidence of diabetes mellitus, all causes, and cardiovascular mortality [10, 11]. Multiple studies evaluating the results of ESG at 1 year have shown that it has surpassed the guideline recommendations and met the safety standards.

The MERIT trial, a multicenter randomized control study that compared ESG to lifestyle modification, showed that ESG achieved a %TBWL of 13.6% at 1 year and maintained weight loss for 2 years [12]. The patients in the lifestyle arm only achieved a %TWBL of 0.8% at 1 year. However, when this group crossed over to receive ESG, their weight loss trajectory was similar to that of the primary ESG group. Besides, 80% of the participants who received ESG demonstrated improvement in one or more obesity-related comorbidities.

Lopez Nava and colleagues compared the outcomes of ESG with laparoscopic greater curve plication (LGCP) and sleeve gastrectomy (LSG) [13], showing the mean %TBWL at 2 years for ESG, LSG, and LGCP were 18.5%, 28.3%, and 26.9%, respectively. Likewise, Alqahtani et al. and Sharaiha et al. showed that at 3 years and 5 years, ESG achieved a total body weight loss of 14% and 15.9%, respectively, stressing that weight loss could be maintained with good adherence to multidisciplinary follow-up [14, 15].

ESG induces weight loss by interfering with gastric accommodation and impacting the motility function. The multiple full-thickness bites have been shown to decrease gastric emptying for solids by 90 min, with the effect maintained for 1 year [16]. ESG also generated weight loss-dependent changes in gut hormones. Our experiments showed that the ghrelin levels were unaltered, unlike diet-induced weight loss, which contributed to the suppression of hunger after ESG. Also, there was an improvement in insulin resistance, a change in insulin secretory pattern, and a marked reduction in leptin levels following weight loss [17]. Aligned with these observations, Asokkumar and colleagues demonstrated improvement in hypertension, diabetes mellitus, and fatty liver disease 6 months after ESG [18].

Complications with ESG

ESG is a major skill as it is a relatively recent procedure that involves high complexity. A study evaluating the learning curve in ESG showed efficiency for ESG was attained after 38 ESG, with mastery after 55 procedures [19]. Although safe, complications can still occur because of technical and operative factors. Overall, the serious adverse event rate reported with ESG is 2%. A meta-analysis comparing ESG and LSG showed the pooled rate of all adverse events with ESG was 2.9% (95% CI 1.8–4.4), and with LSG was 11.8% (95% CI 8.4–16.4) [20].

The frequently encountered symptoms with ESG include post-procedure nausea and vomiting, which could be managed with symptomatic treatment. Other complications, such as bleeding, perforation, peri-gastric leak, pulmonary embolism, and entrapment of adjacent structures like the gall bladder within the suture, are uncommon. Tips and tricks for successful ESG and the steps to avoid complications had been previously described [21].

Primary Obesity Surgery Endoluminal (POSE)

Incisionless Operating Platform (IOP)

The IOP device used for performing the POSE procedure has four components: (a) transport, (b) g-Lix, (c) g-Prox EZ, and (d) g-Cath EZ (Fig. 5). The transport facilitates the insertion of the accessories and endoscope into the stomach. The outer diameter of the transport is 18 mm, and it has 4 working channels for accessories and CO2 insufflation. It has a side port for inserting the ultra-thin upper endoscope. Unlike other endoscopic procedures, the movement of the distal tip is controlled by the two wheels at the transport handle. The g-Lix is a helical tissue anchor catheter that captures the tissue for plication. The multifunctional g-Prox has three

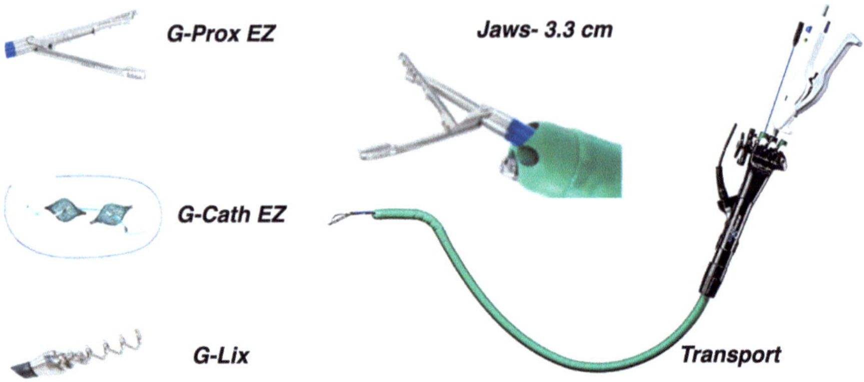

Fig. 5 Components of the incisionless operating platform for POSE 2.0. (**a**) g-Prox with 3.3 cm serrated jaws to capture and advance the helical needle. (**b**) g-Cath EZ Snowshoe anchors that hold the tissue together. (**c**) g-Lix with the helical design to capture the tissue. (D) Transport that mounts the ultra-thin endoscope and accessories for performing the procedure

functions- mobilize the tissue captured by g-Lix to create the plications. Advance the helical needle through the captured tissue to release the snowshoe anchors and trim the excess suture using its cutting mechanism. The g-Prox is loaded with the g-Cath, which contains the snowshoe anchors before application. Each serrated jaw of the rotatable g-Prox is 3.3 mm and can securely capture a large amount of tissue.

POSE 2.0- Technical Description

Unlike ESG, the POSE 2.0 procedure is performed with the patient in supine position and under general anesthesia. Antibiotics are administered before the procedure. The transport device is advanced after examining the stomach for contraindications using a gastroscope. Laparoscopic CO2 insufflation is used to maintain constant pressure and gastric distention (10–12 mm Hg). Once the transport enters the stomach in a straight position, the g-prox and g-lix is advanced through the dedicated accessory channel. Starting at the distal body, capture of the target tissue using the g-lix, and is drawn inside the serrated jaws of the g-prox. The g-prox is loaded with a g-cath snowshoe anchor delivery catheter. The jaw is oriented in the anteroposterior direction for the first plication. Right after the jaws is closed to fix the gastric fold and advance the helical needle in the g-prox through the tissues to release the proximal snowshoe anchors. Each folded plication is approximately 6.6 cm in length and submucosal release of the anchor is avoided. Once released, the needle is withdrawn, the jaws are open releasing the distal anchor and cinching the two anchors together. The excess suture is trimmed using the cutting system in the g-prox. Posteriorly, the g-prox is loaded with a new g-cath and the steps are repeated to complete the desired suture pattern. The objective behind creating these folded plications is to narrow the anteroposterior diameter of the

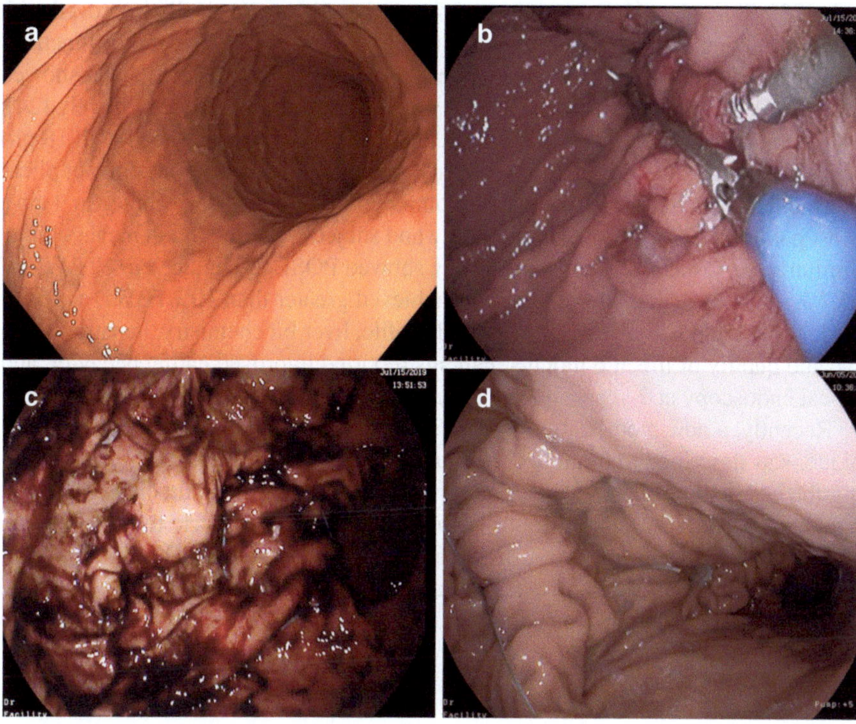

Fig. 6 Endoscopic appearance of the stomach after POSE 2.0. (**a**) Normal stomach before the procedure. (**b**) Creation of plication in the distal body to narrow and shorten the stomach. Each plication is 6.6 cm in length. (**c**) Shortened and narrowed stomach after the procedure. An average of 16–20 plications are placed to reduce the stomach. (**d**) Repeat endoscopy at 1 year, showing intact plications and restricted gastric volume

stomach and to shorten the vertical length [22]. The first two rows are placed with 4–5 plications in the distal body at the incisura, the third row in the proximal body-fundus junction, and the last two rows in the mid-body. Between 16 to 18 snowshoe anchors are used to achieve the configuration, sparing the fundus to serve as a pouch. Upon completion, the stomach is examined with a gastroscope to secure hemostasis (Fig. 6).

Weight-Loss Outcomes after POSE 2.0

The POSE procedure posits that each snowshoe anchor plication is durable and has less suture tension, maintaining the restrictive effect for a longer duration. It has evolved considerably since its initial description. The earlier technique focused on collapsing the fundus to impair the accommodation function using less number of sutures (11 plications). However, the ESSENTIAL randomized control trial failed to meet the predefined weight loss endpoints and achieved a %TBWL of 4.95%

only [23]. Since then, the technique and pattern have been drastically improved with a focus on the gastric body to restrict distention and impact gastric motor function.

Lopez Nava et al. reported the outcome of POSE 2.0 in 46 patients and showed the %TBWL and BMI decline at 1 year was 17.8% and 7 kg/m^{2,} respectively [24]. The median procedure time was 42 min, and the stomach was reduced with 18 plications. Additionally, repeat endoscopy at 1 year in 15 patients showed intact plications and a reduction in gastric length compared to baseline (35.7 cm vs.26.9 cm). Most patients (87%) reported early satiety and subjective reduction in meal volume. Similarly, a prospective multicenter study showed POSE 2.0 induced a %TBWL of 15.7%, with more than 86% of patients achieved greater than 10%TBWL at 1 year [25]. The weight loss also improved lipid profile, liver biochemistry, hepatic steatosis, and quality of life at 6 months. Patients reported improved eating behavior, and repeat endoscopy at 2 years showed fully intact plications in a subset of patients.

Recently, a new modification to POSE 2.0, called the POSE 2.0 enfolding technique, was described to minimize the number of suture plications, thereby improving the cost and efficiency while retaining similar weight loss outcomes [26]. The method involves using two g-lix to capture a large fold of gastric tissue along the greater curve and plicate them using a single snowshoe anchor. The added advantage is that all the plications are staggered linearly along the greater curvature of the stomach, allowing future conversion to sleeve gastrectomy when required. More studies are needed to evaluate the effectiveness of this modified procedure.

Complications with POSE 2.0

Overall, the reported adverse event rate with POSE 2.0 was 2%. All these reports are from high-volume centers with procedures performed by experts. The common symptoms post-procedure are nausea and abdominal pain, which could be managed conservatively. The serious adverse events reported with POSE 2.0 include gastric perforation from the jaws of the g-prox device during advancement [24]. Early recognition of these complications is crucial as endoscopy could treat them in the same setting.

Automatic Endoscopic Gastroplasty

EndoZip Suturing System

Endozip is a robotic automated suturing platform that creates multiple gastric segmentations by opposing the gastric walls under endoscopic guidance with minimal operator interference. The device has several parts: (1) Bougie—designed to capture the tissue using a vacuum and facilitate suturing. The steerable segments of the bougie allow device bending. (2) Insertion Tube–contains a dedicated port for endoscope insertion. It connects the handle to the bougie and contains the power source

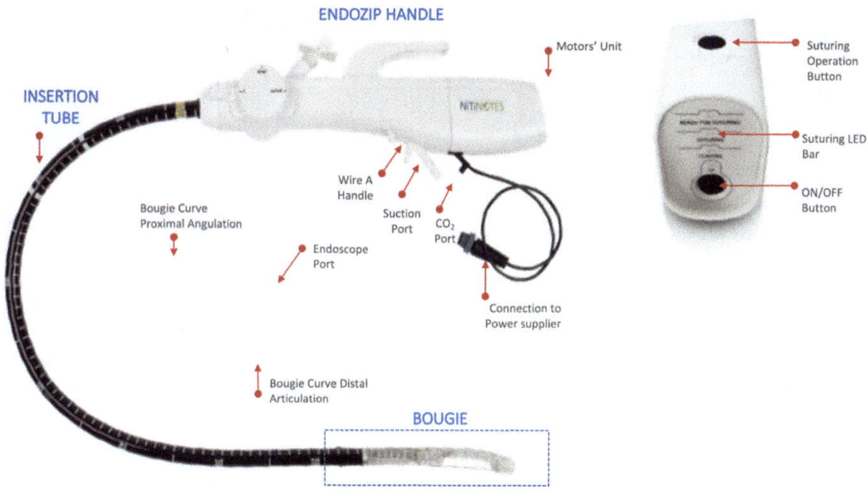

Fig. 7 Design and parts of the automated endoscopic suturing system

and sensors. It also allows CO2 insufflation and deflation. (3) Handle—contains left and right knobs for maneuvering the device to the preferred location in the stomach (4) Endoscope holder fixes the endoscope to the device handle and allows insertion as one unit. (5) The in-built motor unit controls stitching, tightening, clipping, trimming of suture wire. The device is embedded with a custom-designed, auto-driven, helical needle and utilizes a polypropylene suture for plication (Fig. 7).

Endozip-Technical Description

The procedure is performed with the patient in the left lateral position and under general anesthesia. CO_2 insufflation is used and an upper endoscopy is performed to look for contraindications. Once excluded, the device is advanced through an overtube to the desired location. Vacuum is applied to bring the opposing gastric walls inside the bougie. An external pump generates the vacuum, and suturing is performed only when the desired vacuum level is reached (-80Kpa). Once confirmed, suturing is activated by pressing the button on the handle, and the helical needle is driven through the tissue to create the plication. Once completed, upon a second button press, the device tightens and cinches the approximated tissue with an integrated clip. The procedure is repeated till the desired restriction is achieved (Fig. 8).

Weight-Loss Outcomes after Endozip

The first-in-human study using the first-generation Endozip system in 13 patients showed the device was safe and could induce a %TBWL of 16.2% at 6 months with no significant adverse events [27]. A recent prospective multicenter study involving

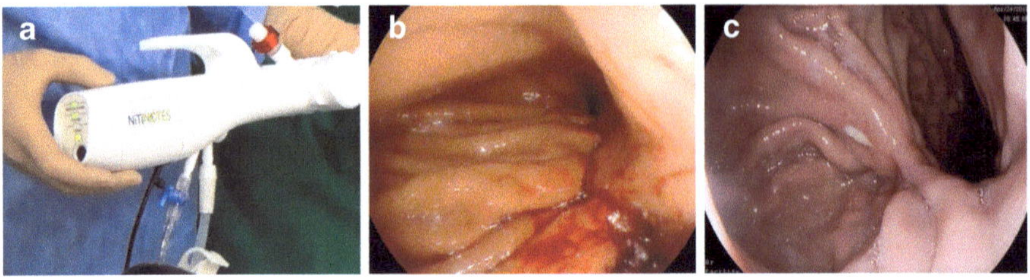

Fig. 8 Endoscopic appearance of the stomach after Endozip procedure. (**a**) The device is advanced into the stomach through an overtube and placed at the desired position. Once confirmed, suturing is activated by pressing the operating button on the handle. (**b**) Endoscopic appearance of the stomach after creating gastric segmentation using the auto-driven helical needle. (**c**) Appearance of the stomach at 6 months after the procedure showing mucosal bridging and gastric restriction

45 patients showed that the automated suturing system achieved a TBWL of 13.2% at 1 year with improvements in HbA1C, liver biochemistry, and quality of life. All the endoscopists involved in the study reported the device was easy to use and suturing could be completed in an average of 30 min [28].

Complications with Endozip

The use of Endozip in obesity is in its early phase. Overall, the reported complication rate from available studies is 4.4%, most of which were managed conservatively [28]. Further studies are needed to understand the device's safety, utility, and usability.

Conclusions

Endoscopic bariatric therapies have emerged as a mainstream treatment option for obesity. The available evidence has confirmed that they are ready for prime time and can induce significant weight loss and improve comorbid illnesses. The continued innovation in the field of bariatric endoscopy is exciting. The future lies in training and expanding the reach of endoscopic bariatric therapies to increase accessibility to combat the ever-expanding obesity pandemic.

Disclosure Statement Dr. Ravishankar Asokkumar is a consultant for Boston Scientific, USA; Dr. Gontrand Lopez-Nava is a consultant with Boston Scientific, USA, and USGI Medical, USA; Dr. Natan Zundel is a consultant for Ethicon, Medtronic, Olympus, GI Windows, Boston Scientific, Boheringer, and LivsMed.

References

1. https://www.who.int/news-room/fact-sheets/detail/obesity-and-overweight.
2. https://asmbs.org/resources/estimate-of-bariatric-surgery-numbers/.
3. Chakhtoura M, Haber R, Ghezzawi M, et al. Pharmacotherapy of obesity: an update on the available medications and drugs under investigation. EClinicalMedicine. 2023;58:101882.
4. Abu Dayyeh BK, Edmundowicz S, Thompson CC. Clinical practice update: expert review on endoscopic bariatric therapies. Gastroenterology. 2017;152:716–29.
5. Jirapinyo P, Hadefi A, Thompson CC, et al. American Society for Gastrointestinal Endoscopy-European Society of Gastrointestinal Endoscopy guideline on primary endoscopic bariatric and metabolic therapies for adults with obesity. Endoscopy. 2024;56:437–56.
6. https://www.nice.org.uk/guidance/ipg783.
7. Lopez-Nava G, Asokkumar R. Step-by-step approach to endoscopic gastroplasty by a novel single-channel endoscopic suturing system. VideoGIE. 2019;4:444–6.
8. Lopez Nava G, Bautista Castano I, Perretta S, et al. European Endoscopic Bariatric Suturing Registry. Gastrointest Endosc. 2019;89:AB278.
9. ASGE/ASMBS Task Force on Endoscopic Bariatric Therapy. A pathway to endoscopic bariatric therapies. Surg Obes Relat Dis. 2011;7:672–82.
10. Bray GA, Culbert IW, Champagne CM, et al. Reduction in the incidence of type 2 diabetes with lifestyle intervention or metformin. N Engl J Med. 2002;346:393–403.
11. Gregg EW, Jakicic JM, Blackburn G, et al. Association of the magnitude of weight loss and changes in physical fitness with long-term cardiovascular disease outcomes in overweight or obese people with type 2 diabetes: a post-hoc analysis of the look AHEAD randomized clinical trial. Lancet Diabetes Endocrinol. 2016;4:913–21.
12. Abu Dayyeh BK, Bazerbachi F, Vargas EJ, et al. Endoscopic sleeve gastroplasty for treatment of class 1 and 2 obesity (MERIT): a prospective, multicentre, randomized trial. Lancet. 2022;400:441–51.
13. Lopez-Nava G, Asokkumar R, Bautista-Castaño I, et al. Endoscopic sleeve gastroplasty, laparoscopic sleeve gastrectomy, and laparoscopic greater curve plication: do they differ at 2 years? Endoscopy. 2021;53:235–43.
14. Alqahtani AR, Elahmedi M, Aldarwish A, et al. Endoscopic gastroplasty versus laparoscopic sleeve gastrectomy: a noninferiority propensity score-matched comparative study. Gastrointest Endosc. 2022;96:44–50.
15. Sharaiha RZ, Hajifathalian K, Kumar R, et al. Five-year outcomes of endoscopic sleeve Gastroplasty for the treatment of obesity. Clin Gastroenterol Hepatol. 2021;19:1051–1057.e2.
16. Vargas EJ, Rizk M, Gomez-Villa J, et al. Effect of endoscopic sleeve gastroplasty on gastric emptying, motility and hormones: a comparative prospective study. Gut. 2023;72:1073–80.
17. Lopez-Nava G, Negi A, Bautista-Castaño I, et al. Gut and metabolic hormones changes after endoscopic sleeve gastroplasty (ESG) vs. laparoscopic sleeve gastrectomy (LSG). Obes Surg. 2020;30:2642–51.
18. Asokkumar R, Lim CH, Tan AS, et al. Safety and early efficacy of endoscopic sleeve gastroplasty (ESG) for obesity in a multi-ethnic Asian population in Singapore. JGH Open. 2021;5:1351–6.
19. Saumoy M, Schneider Y, Zhou XK, et al. A single-operator learning curve analysis for the endoscopic sleeve gastroplasty. Gastrointest Endosc. 2018;87:442–7.
20. Mohan BP, Asokkumar R, Khan SR, et al. Outcomes of endoscopic sleeve gastroplasty: how does it compare to laparoscopic sleeve gastrectomy? A systematic review and meta-analysis. Endosc Int Open. 2020;8:E558–65.
21. Asokkumar R, Babu MP, Bautista I, et al. The use of the OverStitch for bariatric weight loss in Europe. Gastrointest Endosc Clin N Am. 2020;30:129–45.
22. Lopez-Nava G, Asokkumar R, Turró Arau R, et al. Modified primary obesity surgery endoluminal (POSE-2) procedure for the treatment of obesity. VideoGIE. 2020;5:91–3.

23. Sullivan S, Swain JM, Woodman G, et al. Randomized sham-controlled trial evaluating efficacy and safety of endoscopic gastric plication for primary obesity: the ESSENTIAL trial. Obesity (Silver Spring). 2017;25:294–301.
24. Lopez Nava G, Asokkumar R, Laster J, et al. Primary obesity surgery endoluminal (POSE-2) procedure for treatment of obesity in clinical practice. Endoscopy. 2021;53:1169–73.
25. Lopez Nava G, Arau RT, Asokkumar R, et al. Prospective Multicenter study of the primary obesity surgery Endoluminal (POSE 2.0) procedure for treatment of obesity. Clin Gastroenterol Hepatol. 2023;21:81–89.e4.
26. Al Khatry M, Abu Dayyeh BK. The primary obesity surgery Endoluminal 2.0 enfolding technique (POSE 2.0et): modification to enhance efficiency and increase restriction. Obes Surg. 2023;33:1953–4.
27. Lopez-Nava G, Asokkumar R, Rull A, et al. Safety and feasibility of a novel endoscopic suturing device (EndoZip TM) for treatment of obesity: first-in-human study. Obes Surg. 2020;30:1696–703.
28. Boskoski I, Lopez-Nava G, Ravishankar A, et al. Automatic endoscopic gastroplasty for the treatment of obesity: results from a prospective multicenter study. Gastrointest Endosc. 2024;S0016-5107(24):03508–9.

Intragastric Balloons

Rogelio Tioni, Alejandro Marcolini, Carlos Esquivel, and Diego Awruch

Abstract Intragastric balloons (IGBs) are non-surgical devices used for weight loss in individuals with obesity, particularly when other methods have not been successful. These balloons are placed in the stomach through a minimally invasive endoscopic procedure or swallowing it, and filled with saline or gas, occupying space and promoting a feeling of fullness to reduce food intake. Typically, IGBs are kept in the stomach for about 4-12 months and are then removed or they passed away trought the digestive tract. When combined with diet and lifestyle changes, IGBs can lead to significant weight loss and improvements in obesity-related conditions. Side effects, such as nausea and discomfort, are common but usually temporary. Ongoing research aims to enhancenhance IGB effectiveness and safety, positioning them as a valuable, intermediate option for weight management before considering surgical interventions.

Keywords Intragastric balloons (IGBs) · Weight loss · Obesity management · Minimally invasive

Introduction

The ongoing increase in global obesity rates, combined with the scarcity of effective medical treatments for this condition, has driven the development of interventional weight loss therapies. Some individuals, despite being medically eligible for

---

R. Tioni · A. Marcolini · D. Awruch (✉)
Centro de Cirugia Bariatrica y Metabolica del Sanatorio Britanico de Rosario, Rosario, Argentina

C. Esquivel
Servicio de Cirugia Bariatrica y Metabolica Sanatorio Allende, Cordoba, Argentina

F. Schlottmann, M. A. Masrur (eds.), *Endoscopic, Laparoscopic and Robotic Techniques for Foregut Disorders*, https://doi.org/10.1007/978-3-032-00811-4_11

bariatric surgery, might opt not to undergo surgery or may not meet the criteria for surgical candidacy based on current standards or surgeon evaluation.

Examples of patients who do not qualify for surgery include those with obesity-related health issues but whose body mass index (BMI) is below the current thresholds for bariatric surgery, and patients considered high-risk for surgery due to severe obesity or poor overall health. Additionally, individuals in certain age groups or those aiming to improve their health as a preparatory step for other treatments (such as organ transplants or joint replacements) may seek non-surgical weight-loss methods. The available options for these patients are limited.

Currently, pharmacotherapy and medically supervised diet programs offer inconsistent and modest weight loss results and are generally inadequate for long-term weight maintenance and reducing comorbidities. Endoscopic bariatric procedures have emerged as appealing tools for weight loss; however, fewer than 5% of obese patients seeking weight-loss treatment are aware of endoscopic options. Intragastric balloons, introduced nearly 40 years ago, have gained renewed interest with several new devices entering the US market recently.

Intragastric balloon (IGB) therapy has been proposed as a strategy to bridge this treatment gap. Positioned between clinical and surgical interventions, it is currently the most widely used endoluminal obesity therapy.

Indications and Patients Selection

IGB offers a wide range of indications, spanning from overweight patients (body mass index [BMI] 25 to 29.9 kg/m2) to those with obesity who do not qualify for bariatric surgery, and even for super-obese individuals (BMI ≥50 kg/m2) as a preparatory measure before bariatric surgery [1]. Due to its favorable safety profile, IGBs can also be considered for morbidly obese patients who are eligible for bariatric surgery but face high risks of complications or prefer to avoid surgery altogether. Other indications include preparation for non-bariatric surgeries where weight loss is necessary to optimize outcomes, as well as for managing comorbidities.

The minimum BMI requirement for balloon implantation is 27 kg/m2, with no influence on the selection of balloon type. There is no consensus regarding specific age limits for IGB placement, with each patient evaluated on an individual basis. According to the Intragastric Balloon Consensus Statement [2], placement of an IGB in patients under 16 years of age should generally be avoided, except in carefully selected cases post-puberty with multidisciplinary evaluation and parental consent.

Contraindications

Absolute

Gastric, duodenal, and esophageal ulcers are considered absolute contraindications for balloon implantation, regardless of active bleeding, due to the heightened risk of perforation. Previous gastric surgery is also established as an absolute contraindication. Other absolute contraindications include gastric and esophageal varices, hiatal hernia >5 cm, esophageal or gastric pathologies, such as diverticula, gastroparesis, strictures, or achalasia, ongoing anticoagulant therapy, and uncontrolled or untreated psychiatric disorders.

Relative

Relative contraindications encompass gastric angioectasias without active bleeding, eosinophilic esophagitis, familial gastric polyposis, and the use of platelet inhibitors. Grade C or D esophagitis may require treatment prior to considering balloon implantation. History of abdominal surgeries involving resection and anastomosis of the digestive tract, as well as a history of generalized peritonitis.

Not Considered Contraindications

Grade A/B esophagitis, gastritis, hyperplasia, HIV-positive immunocompetent patients, benign polyps, or Helicobacter pylori positivity are not considered contraindications.

Preprocedural Evaluation

It is universally agreed that laboratory tests should be conducted prior to the procedure.

Imaging exams are not deemed mandatory before the procedure unless there is a clinical indication or a request from the anesthesiologist. During endoscopic intragastric balloon placement, the stomach can be assessed as part of the procedure.

Post-implantation, patients are advised to follow a liquid diet initially, transitioning to a solid diet after 1 week. While dietary modifications can enhance and sustain weight loss in patients undergoing IGB therapy, it remains unclear whether other lifestyle changes (e.g., exercise) have the same impact. This is an area warranting further investigation.

After balloon removal, there is no consensus on the minimum clinical follow-up period, but a follow-up of at least 6 months is recommended.

Procedure Description

Intragastric balloons (IGBs) function as space-occupying devices that reduce stomach capacity, delay gastric emptying, and induce satiety. Various models of IGBs exist, including those filled with liquid or air, adjustable or non-adjustable, endoscopic or swallowable, with no significant differences in weight loss outcomes among them.

Preparation A 4-hour fasting period is advised before the procedure. No specific pre-procedure diet is required but is strongly recommended to have a light dinner the night before and clear liquids up to 4 hours before implantation.

Balloon Implant It is recommended to perform de procedure in an outpatient clinic equipped with advanced life support and patient transfer services if needed. In the case to choose for an endoscopic delivered balloon, the use of an adult gastroscope is preferred, with no specific preference for double-channel endoscopes. The patient is positioned in the left lateral position for direct oro-esophageal introduction.

Anesthesia General anesthesia with orotracheal intubation is mandatory. However, there is no consensus on this matter. Most endoscopists prefer deep general sedation without orotracheal intubation or the presence of an anesthesiologist. Some prefer conscious sedation or deep general sedation without orotracheal intubation, administered by an anesthesiologist for the endoscopic ballons.

Balloon Volume The recommended balloon fill volume should range between 500 mL and 599 mL for both liquid-filled adjustable and non-adjustable balloons, with the consideration of potential upward readjustments. During the readjustment session, the volume should be adjusted based on the patient's clinical progress, with a maximum additional volume recommended between 200 to 300 mL. For downward adjustments due to intolerance (such as nausea and vomiting), the minimum fill volume to maintain in the adjustable balloon should be between 100 to 200 mL, aiming to alleviate symptoms and allow for subsequent upward adjustments.

Endoscopic Balloon Removal To prepare for balloon removal, a minimum of 3 days on a liquid diet is advised, followed by an 8-hour fasting period. Consumption of sugar-free carbonated drinks, such as coke, is recommended to help cleanse the stomach of any residual food prior to removal. The preferred tool for balloon removal is a hybrid jaw grasper (combining alligator and rat tooth features). In specific cases, an esophageal overtube may aid in easier removal, and a small amount of vegetable cooking oil can be applied selectively to lubricate the esophagus. Tracheal intubation is strongly recommended in all cases to protect the airway, in experienced surgical suites, the deep sedation can be selected. In case of emergency extraction, orotracheal intubation is mandatory.

Swallowable Gastric Balloon: Allurion Balloon

The Allurion balloon(TM) (Allurion Technologies, Natick, MA, USA) is an intragastric device that requires no anesthesia or upper endoscopy for placement and removal. Enclosed within a capsule, it can be easily ingested after a 4-hour fasting period. This balloon is additionally associated with a bioimpedance scale and a

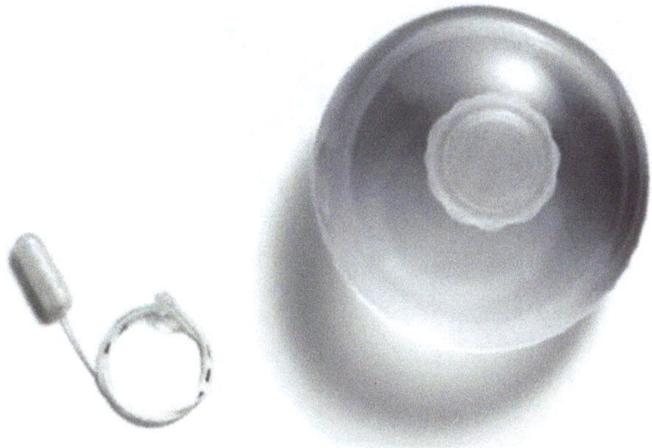

Fig. 1 Swallowable gastric ballon (Allurion)

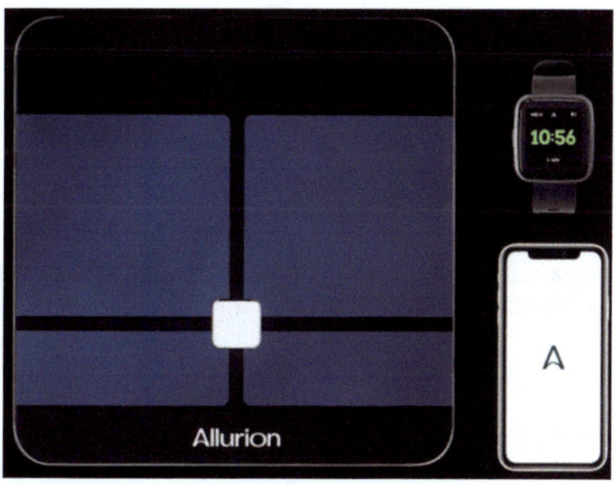

Fig. 2 Bioimpedance scale, smartwatch and movil App

smartwatch, both connected to an application that allows real-time analysis of weight loss outcomes and physical activity performed by the patient (Figs. 1 and 2).

The procedure takes place in the radiology room, the patient ingests the capsule with water, followed by a radiograph to confirm its correct placement. The balloon includes a small radiopaque marker used to verify its correct intragastric positioning via abdominal x-ray before inflation. Subsequently, it is filled with 550 mL of distilled water containing potassium sorbate preservative, delivered through a small catheter. Another radiograph is then taken to verify proper filling and placement (Figs. 3 and 4). Finally, the balloon catheter is disconnected by traction. At approximately 16 weeks ±2 weeks, a valve in the balloon opens, allowing it to self-deflate and be naturally eliminated through the digestive tract.

Dietary Guidelines Patients are instructed to follow a liquid diet for the initial 48 hours. Subsequently, they gradually transitioned to a semi-solid diet including items like thin soups, yogurt, puréed vegetables, and mashed potatoes during the first week. All patients are encouraged to engage in regular physical activity starting from the second day after insertion.

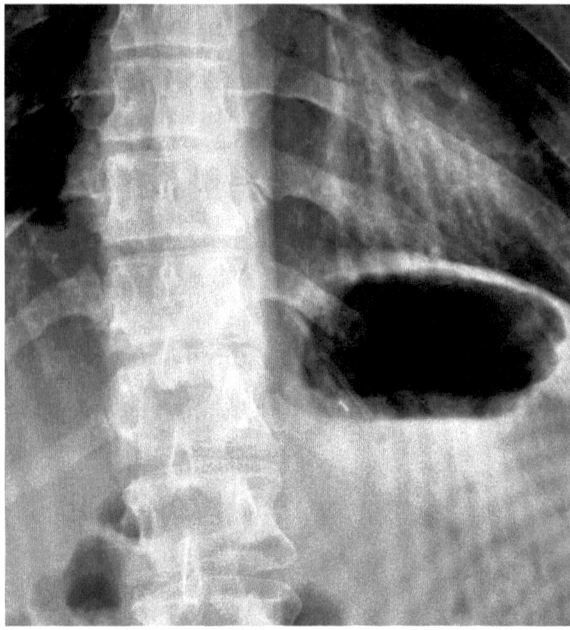

Fig. 3 Swallowable gastric balloon before filling

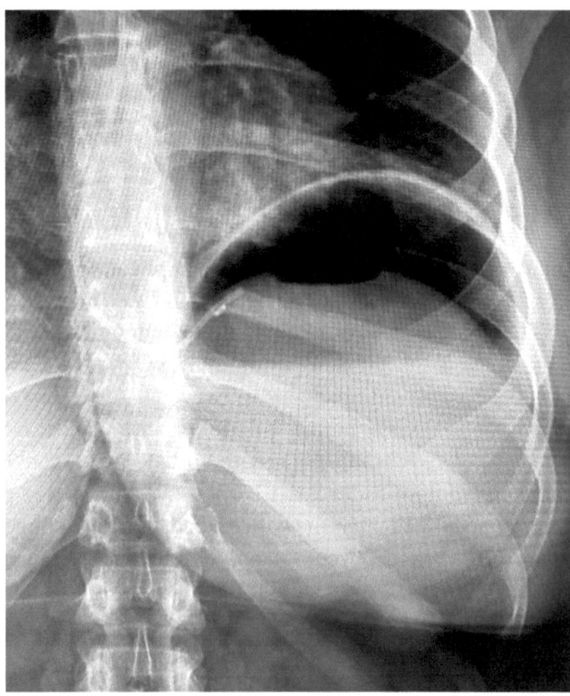

Fig. 4 Swallowable gastric balloon after filling

Legal Considerations Consensus was reached regarding the necessity of obtaining a specific informed consent document where the follow-up protocol is detailed. Failure to follow up among patients who have undergone traditional balloon procedures, where patients do not return for balloon removal, may potentially result from spontaneous emptying and migration into the intestines, leading to intestinal obstruction. Therefore, if a patient fails to attend their scheduled balloon removal appointment, proactive measures such as contacting them via telephone, email, or sending a registered letter should be implemented.

Postimplant Follow-Up

During the adaptation period, medications recommended to alleviate symptoms include ondansetron, hyoscine, corticosteroids, proton pump inhibitors (PPIs), analgesics, and dimenhydrinate, typically prescribed for 3 to 5 days following implantation.

Specifically for the swallowable gastric balloon, to reduce nausea and vomiting, a combination of netupitant and palonosetron can be administered at least 1 hour before the procedure, this is suggested for all kind of IGB.

The use of proton pump inhibitors (PPIs) should be continued throughout the treatment. Metoclopramide is used only in medical indication when the main symptom is nausea during the adaptation period due to its potential to increase gastrointestinal motility and exacerbate symptoms. Similarly, anti-inflammatory drugs should be avoided to mitigate the risk of gastric ulcers.

Patients should refrain from air travel and strenuous physical activities immediately after IGB implantation, but these activities may be resumed after the adaptation period. Additionally, consumption of carbonated drinks is discouraged during treatment. Is its prohibited scuba dive and strongly recommended to avoid sports with high active contact to the abdomen as well as extreme yoga flexing positions.

Efficacy and Clinical Results

Based on current evidence, the average percentage of total body weight loss (%TBWL) achieved was 17.66 ± 2.5% (range: 11.87–25.00%). The mean total weight loss (TBWL) was 17.13 ± 1.5 kg (range: 11.60–22.60 kg). The mean reduction in BMI was 5.73 ± 1.7 kg/m2 (range: 4.0–8.1 kg/m2). The failure rate, defined as the percentage of patients achieving %TBWL <10%, was 11.20 ± 2.0% (range: 0–38%).

The Allurion Balloon has shown an excellent safety profile. By 4 months, the balloon demonstrated significant efficacy with mean total weight loss (WL) of 13.5 ± 5.8 kg and mean reduction in BMI (BMIL) of 4.9 ± 2.0 points. Percentage of total body weight loss (%TBWL) was 14.2 ± 5.0%.

Sequential Implants There is no limit to the number of sequential balloon implants as long as the patient continues to meet the criteria for the procedure. For patients opting for a second balloon for weight loss, it is recommended simultaneous implantation with removal of the existing balloon, while others suggest a 2/3-month interval between procedures. If a patient desires a second balloon after an interval from the first, it is recommended switching to an adjustable balloon if the initial one was liquid-filled.

Metabolic and Medical Improvements Short-term use of IGBs has shown improvements in several metabolic parameters and medical comorbidities compared to non-invasive weight loss measures. Data from 5 randomized controlled trials (RCTs) and 18 observational studies indicate that IGB therapy significantly reduces hemoglobin A1c and fasting blood glucose levels more effectively than non-invasive methods alone. Significant improvements were particularly noted in patients with initial fasting blood glucose levels >100 mg/dL, hemoglobin A1c >6.5%, and BMI >40 kg/m2. Additionally, IGB use contributed to improvements in abnormalities observed in liver function tests among patients undergoing weight loss treatment [1]. Diabetes, hypertension, and dyslipidemia all showed statistically significant rates of remission in patients using IGB for weight loss compared to those pursuing non-invasive methods.

Post-Removal Care Following IGB removal, it is recommended subsequent weight-loss or maintenance therapies such as dietary interventions, pharmacotherapy, sequential IGB placement, or bariatric surgery. Treatment decisions should be based on patient discussions about their clinical status, preferences, and the safety profiles of various strategies, emphasizing shared decision-making.

Combination Therapies The use of combined therapies involving Intragastric Balloons (IGB) and anti-obesity medications has shown promising results in enhancing weight loss outcomes under medical supervision [3, 4].

A recent randomized controlled trial investigated the combination of semaglutide, administered at 2.4 mg/day, with an intragastric balloon. The study demonstrated that patients receiving the combined treatment exhibited a significant improvement in weight loss compared to those receiving the IGB alone. Specifically, the combined treatment group achieved a mean total weight loss (TWL) of 16.1% compared to 11.3% in the IGB-only group at 6 months. Additionally, the combined approach showed improvements in metabolic parameters, including reductions in HbA1c and blood pressure.

Further, a study by Pi-Sunyer et al. evaluated the combination of IGB with 3.0 mg/day subcutaneous liraglutide in a randomized, controlled trial involving 3,731 nondiabetic patients with a BMI $\geq$ 30 or $\geq$ 27 kg/m^2 with dyslipidemia or hypertension. The study reported significant weight loss and reductions in blood pressure and prediabetes prevalence after 56 weeks, emphasizing the effectiveness of this combined approach in promoting substantial and clinically meaningful weight loss. Another randomized controlled trial investigated the addition of liraglutide 3 mg/day to IGB versus IGB alone over 6 months, demonstrating superior outcomes in the pharmacotherapy group (total weight loss 10%: mean difference 14.72%; 95% confidence interval, 8.81 to 21.26; weight loss in kilograms: mean difference 3.8 kg loss; 95% CI, 2.43–5.17 kg loss; decrease in BMI: mean difference 1.32 kg/m2 decrease; 95% CI, 0.92 kg/m2 increase to 1.72 kg/m2 decrease).

These findings suggest that combining IGB with modern pharmacotherapies like GLP-1 analogues significantly enhances weight loss outcomes.

IGB Complications

Adverse Events early versions of IGB were associated with significant adverse events, leading to their removal from the US market in the 1980s and 1990s. Therefore, understanding the adverse events linked with newer IGB models introduced in the past two decades is crucial. The most common major adverse event necessitating balloon removal was gastric ulcer (0.4%), predominantly seen with the Spatz 2 balloon (27%). Other major complications occurred at rates below 0.10%: perforation (0.10%, 50% during removal, 40% during treatment, and 10% during implantation), bronchial aspiration (0.08%), gastric bleeding (0.04%), symptomatic hyperinflation (0.03%), and migration leading to intestinal obstruction (0.02%). Rare major complications such as acute pancreatitis or renal failure were reported anecdotally (0.02%). The most common minor adverse effects included esophagitis (3.7%), spontaneous balloon deflation (1.19%), migration with spontaneous expulsion (0.56%), fungal infection (0.50%), ulceration and non-bleeding ulcer (0.42% and 0.10%), and asymptomatic hyperinflation (0.04%). Early removal due to intolerance occurred in 3.6% of cases. It's worth noting that prophylactic use of antifungal drugs to prevent hyperinflation is not recommended, as there is insufficient scientific evidence linking this adverse event to fungal infection. Serious adverse events, such as small bowel obstructions, were rare (0.16%), predominantly occurring with earlier generations of the Allurion balloon (Fig. 5).

Premature Balloon Removal it refers to explantation within 1 month of implantation, typically due to adverse events or patient request. Consensus guidelines recommend IGB removal in cases of moderate or severe pancreatitis, gastrointestinal bleeding, gastric ulcer with a non-adjustable balloon, recurrent antral impaction, symptomatic hyperinflation, and recurrent electrolyte disturbances. In instances of antral impaction (Fig. 6), repositioning the balloon may be attempted initially, but recurrent occurrences warrant balloon removal. During pregnancy, removal of the balloon is generally advised, typically in the second trimester, with guidance from an obstetrician on the optimal timing. In the event of a thromboembolic event, prompt balloon removal is recommended.

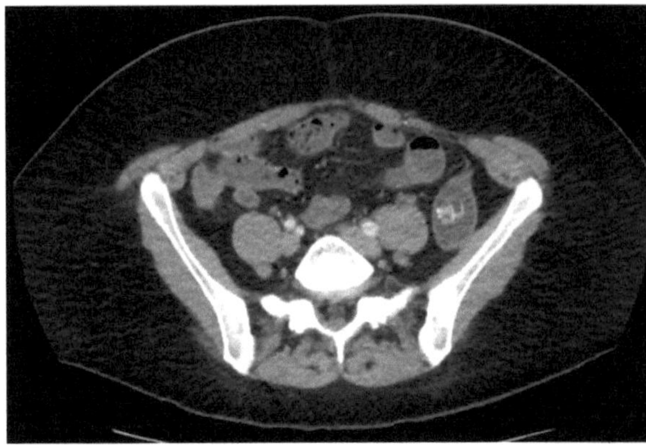

Fig. 5 Intestinal sub-occlusion secondary to digestive elimination of the ingestible intragastric balloon

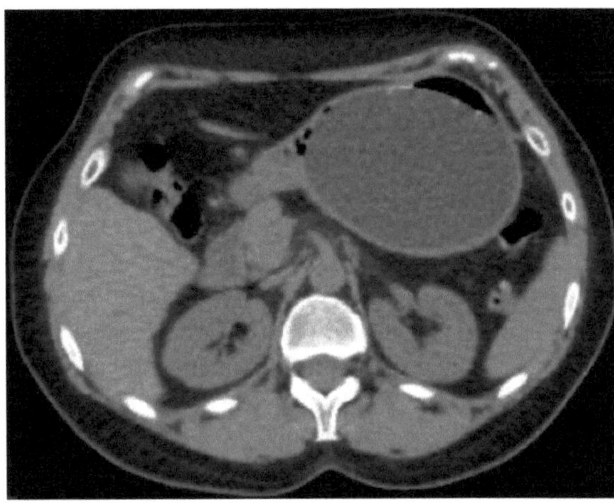

Fig. 6 Antral impactation

Severe erosive esophagitis necessitates caution, and balloon removal should be delayed until appropriate treatment has been initiated to minimize the risk of esophageal tear or perforation during removal. Similarly, in cases of Mallory-Weiss Syndrome, retaining the balloon is advisable due to the heightened risk of bleeding during its removal.

Conclusions

Intragastric balloons (IGBs) have been available in the US market since 1982, yet there remains a scarcity of specific guidelines or consensus documents addressing their efficacy, safety, and role in weight-loss therapy. Key evidence gaps include the long-term efficacy of IGB therapy beyond one year, encompassing not only sustained weight loss but also improvements in metabolic parameters and medical comorbidities. However, clinical studies have shown significant short- and mid-term weight loss with the gastric balloon, leading to improvements in obesity-related comorbidities such as type 2 diabetes, hypertension, and sleep apnea. This not only enhances patients' quality of life but also reduces long-term healthcare costs. Variables such as the filling medium (liquid vs gas) and the potential benefits of concurrent dietary interventions, pharmacotherapy, or sequential balloon placements for sustained outcomes warrant further investigation. The optimization of intraoperative anesthetic protocols and antiemetic regimens, both pre- and post-operatively, represents an important research area to enhance IGB tolerability. Additionally, the management of micronutrient deficiencies in individuals undergoing IGB placement requires additional study to ensure comprehensive patient care. Its endoscopic/ingestible placement reduces surgical risks, shortens recovery times, and decreases postoperative complications, allowing patients to quickly resume their daily activities. The reversibility of the gastric balloon is another significant advantage. As a temporary device, it can be removed after a set period, allowing for assessment of results and future treatment planning. This flexibility is particularly beneficial for patients seeking non-permanent solutions or those evaluating their ability to maintain weight loss through lifestyle changes. In summary, the gastric balloon therapy offers a significant advancement in obesity treatment, providing a less invasive, effective, and flexible solution. Its multidisciplinary approach can lead to substantial health and well-being improvements, solidifying its role as a valuable tool in combating obesity. Furthermore, the combination of IGBs with the new anti-obesity drugs will probably engage more patients to take this serious chronic illness as it is and in advice with multidisciplinary teams and weareable techs increase the results in weight loss and long term control of obesity.

References

1. Zerrweck C, Maunoury V, Caiazzo R, et al. Preoperative weight loss with intragastric balloon decreases the risk of significant adverse outcomes of laparoscopic gastric bypass in super-super obese patients. Obes Surg. 2012;22(5):777–82.
2. Espinet Coll E, Del Pozo García AJ, TurróArau R, Nebreda Durán J, Cortés Rizo X, Jiménez S, et al. Spanish Intragastric balloon consensus statement (SIBC):practical guidelines based on experience of over 20 000 cases. Rev Esp Enferm Dig. 2023;115:22–34.
3. Reulen R, Zeegers M, Jenkinson C. Effect of swallow balloon therapy with the combination of Semaglutide Oral formulation: a randomised double-blind single-Centre study. Obes Surg. 2024;34:198–205.
4. Pi-Sunyer X, Astrup A, Fujioka K, et al. A randomized, controlled trial of 3.0 mg of liraglutide in weight management. N Engl J Med. 2023;373(1):11–22.

Sutureless Duodenal-Ileal Anastomosis with Self-Assembling Magnets

Sofia Bertona, Francisco Schlottmann, and Rudolf Buxhoeveden

Abstract Over the past 20 years, laparoscopic and endoscopic procedures have advanced significantly, leading to better outcomes for patients. One notable innovation has been the introduction of magnetic devices for the creation of gastrointestinal anastomoses. Magnets are now used for bariatric surgery providing promising results.

Keywords Magnets · Bariatric surgery · Obesity · Anastomosis

Introduction

Obesity prevalence has risen dramatically over the last decades. From 2000 to 2019, obesity-related Disability-Adjusted Life Years (DALYs) rose at an annual rate of 0.48%. Projections suggest that these DALYs will increase by 39.8% between 2020 and 2030 [1]. Obese patients who undergo bariatric surgery are more likely to experience remission of obesity-related complications, as compared to those who received medical treatment [2].

Minimally invasive gastrointestinal surgery has undergone vast progress during the last two decades. One of the key developments in this field is the use of magnetic devices to create an intestinal anastomosis. Self-assembling magnetic octagons using minimally invasive techniques (endoscopy and laparoscopy) have been used to create a diversion through a process called compression anastomosis. The tissues

S. Bertona · R. Buxhoeveden
Department of Surgery, Hospital Alemán of Buenos Aires, Buenos Aires, Argentina
e-mail: sbertona@hospitalaleman.com; rbuxhoeveden@hospitalaleman.com

F. Schlottmann (✉)
Department of Surgery, Hospital Alemán of Buenos Aires, Buenos Aires, Argentina

Department of Surgery, University of Illinois at Chicago, Chicago, IL, USA

F. Schlottmann, M. A. Masrur (eds.), *Endoscopic, Laparoscopic and Robotic Techniques for Foregut Disorders*, https://doi.org/10.1007/978-3-032-00811-4_12

between the two segments of the intestine heal and the tissue within the magnet ultimately experience necrosis. Once the anastomosis is formed, the mated magnet complex is released into the bowel to be excreted with the feces. This technique has demonstrated to be feasible and safe for obese patients. This novel approach allows for the creation of a durable and large-caliber anastomosis, which is crucial for ensuring long-term effectiveness in metabolic surgery [3–7].

Procedure Description

Position of the Patient and Surgical Team

After induction of general endotracheal anesthesia, the patient should be in low lithotomy position with the lower extremities extended on stirrups and with the knees flexed around 20°–30°. We strongly suggest the use of pneumatic compression devices for legs to reduce the risk of deep vein thrombosis. During the entire operation, the surgeon stands between the patient's legs. Both arms are left abducted and secured on a board with adequate padding. The surgeon stands on the patient's right side, and the 1st and 2nd assistant on the patient's left side and between the legs, respectively.

Pneumoperitoneum and Trocar Placement

The Veress needle is placed at Palmer's point (3 cm below the left costal margin in the mid-clavicular line) and pneumoperitoneum is established at 12 mmHg. A total of five laparoscopic ports (two 10 mm and three 5 mm) are commonly used for the operation.

Laparoscopic Approach

The ileocecal valve (ICV) is identified, and an ileum loop 300 cm away from the ICV is grasped. A 5-mm enterotomy is created as shown in Fig. 1, and the magnet is delivered with a laparoscopic deployment tool at the site of the enterotomy (Figs. 2, 3 and 4).

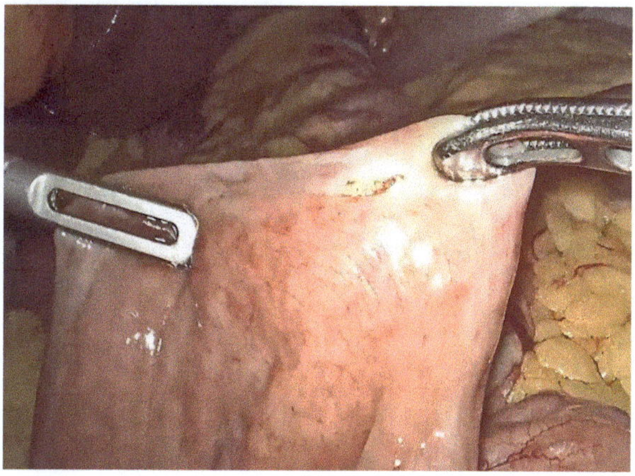

Fig. 1 Laparoscopic enterotomy

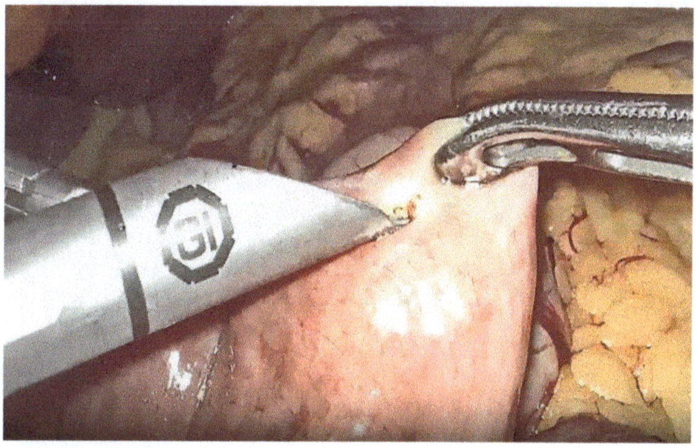

Fig. 2 Laparoscopic tool for magnet delivery

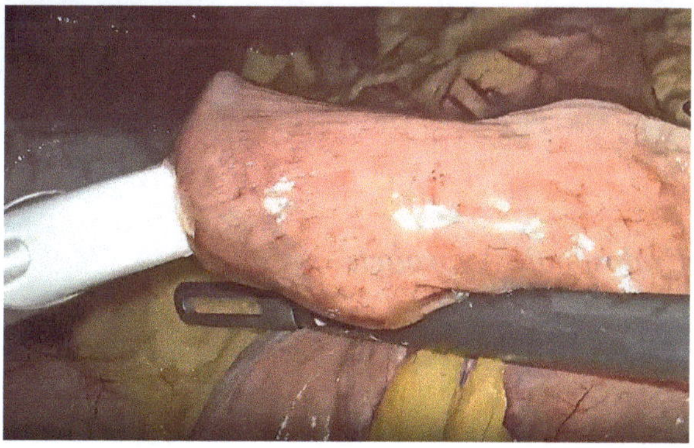

Fig. 3 The magnet is positioned at the site of the enterotomy

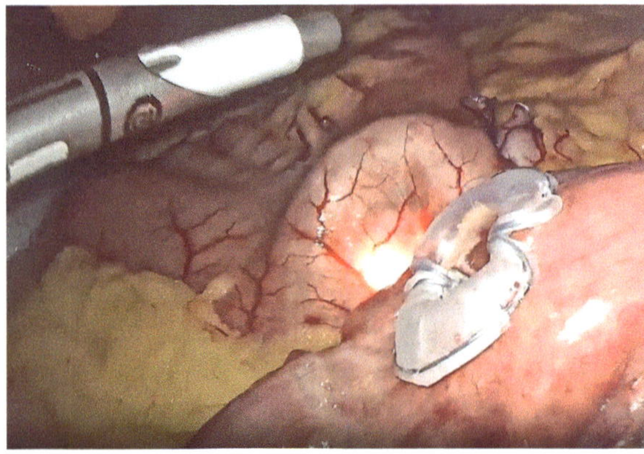

Fig. 4 The magnet is already delivered in the small bowel

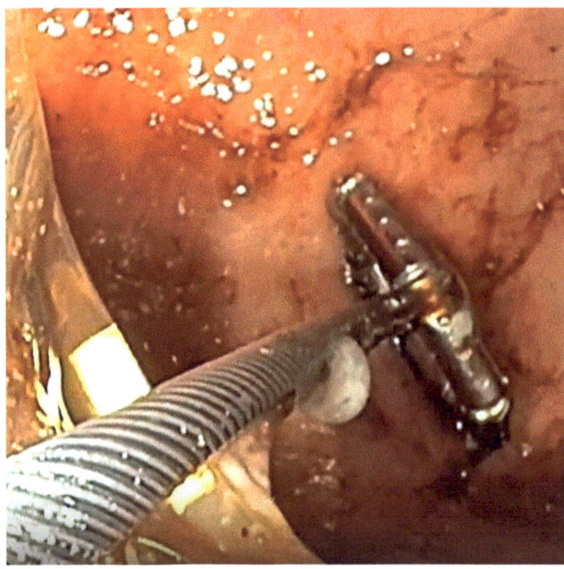

Fig. 5 Endoscopy delivery of the magnet in the duodenum

Endoscopic Approach

An upper endoscopy is then performed, delivering the magnet in the duodenum (2 cm distal to the pylorus) with an endoscopic deployment tool (Fig. 5). The ileum loop with the inserted magnet is then approximated towards the duodenum, and both magnets are coupled under laparoscopic guidance (Fig. 6).

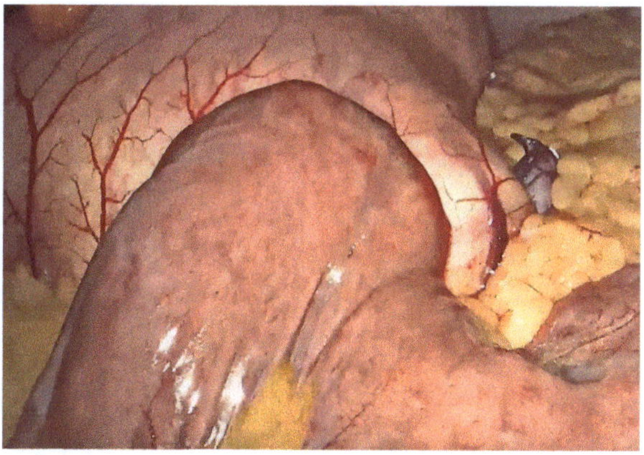

Fig. 6 Laparoscopic engagement of both magnets

Final Inspection

After adequate hemostasis is achieved, instruments and trocars are removed from the abdomen under direct vision. The fascia of the 10–12 mm ports should be closed.

Postoperative Care

Patients are extubated immediately after completion of the procedure. Patients are fed the morning after the operation with clear liquids and usually discharged after 24 h, with instructions to continue with liquid/soft diet for the first 2 weeks, with no specific dietary restrictions thereafter.

Follow Up

An abdominal X-ray is performed at 2 and 4 weeks after the procedure to determine the localization and/or expulsion of the magnets (in case the patient did not notice the magnets in the toilet) (Fig. 7). Follow-up endoscopies are performed at 2 and 12 months after device placement to confirm patency of the anastomosis (Fig. 8).

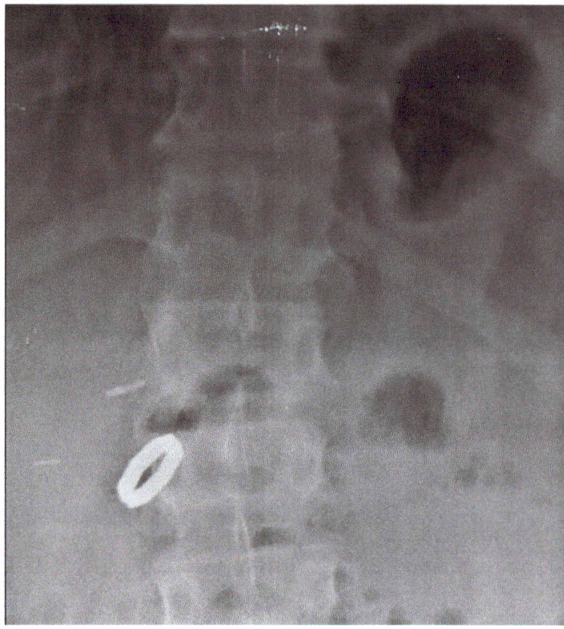

Fig. 7 Abdominal X-ray at 2 weeks

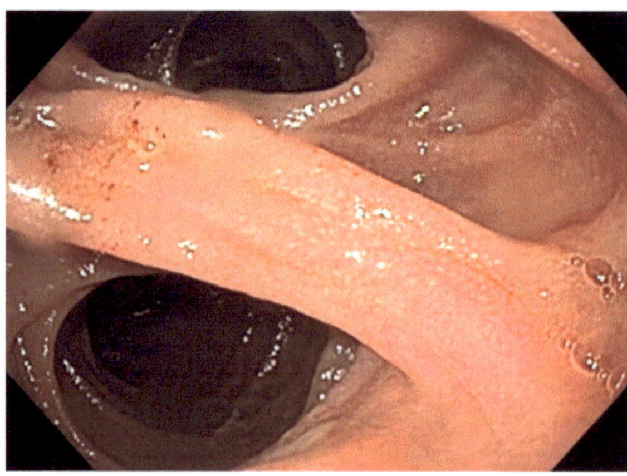

Fig. 8 Upper endoscopy at 12 months confirming patency of the anastomosis and healthy appearing mucosa

Conflicts of Interest The authors have no conflicts of interest.

References

1. Chong B, Jayabaskaran J, Kong G, et al. Trends and predictions of malnutrition and obesity in 204 countries and territories: an analysis of the global burden of disease study 2019. EClinicalMedicine. 2023;57:101850.
2. Jakobsen GS, Småstuen MC, Sandbu R, et al. Association of Bariatric Surgery vs medical obesity treatment with long-term medical complications and obesity-related comorbidities. JAMA. 2018;319(3):291–301.
3. Schlottmann F, Ryou M, Lautz D, et al. Sutureless Duodeno-Ileal anastomosis with self-assembling magnets: safety and feasibility of a novel metabolic procedure. Obes Surg. 2021;31(9):4195–202.
4. Marrache MK, Itani MI, Farha J, et al. Endoscopic gastrointestinal anastomosis: a review of established techniques. Gastrointest Endosc. 2021;93(1):34–46.
5. Ryou M, Agoston AT, Thompson CC. Endoscopic intestinal bypass creation by using self-assembling magnets in a porcine model. Gastrointest Endosc. 2016;83(4):821–5.
6. Machytka E, Bužga M, Zonca P, et al. Partial jejunal diversion using an incisionless magnetic anastomosis system: 1-year interim results in patients with obesity and diabetes. Gastrointest Endosc. 2017;86(5):904–12.
7. Arau RT, Ortega A, Diez-Caballero A, et al. Duodeno-ileal diversion with self-forming magnets in a sutureless neodymium anastomosis procedure (SNAP) for weight recidivism after sleeve gastrectomy: feasibility and 9-month results. Surg Endosc. 2024;38(9):5199–206.

Revisional Bariatric Procedures

Nicholas J. Skertich, Scott Schimpke, and Philip Omotosho

Abstract Metabolic and bariatric surgery is the most effective treatment for severe obesity. However, recurrent weight gain occurs at varying rates depending on the initial procedure and other factors. Revisional bariatric surgery can be done safely and effectively offering patients additional options for treatment of obesity and obesity related diseases. In this chapter, we describe minimally invasive reoperative approaches to address recurrent weight gain after laparoscopic adjustable gastric banding (LAGB), sleeve gastrectomy (SG), and Roux-en-Y gastric bypass (RYGB); specifically, the conversion procedures of LAGB to SG, LAGB to RYGB, SG to RYGB, and SG to biliopancreatic diversion with duodenal switch (BPD-DS), as well as the revision of RYGB via type I distalization.

Keywords Revisional bariatric surgery · Reoperation · Conversion · Adjustable gastric band removal · Adjustable gastric band to sleeve gastrectomy · Adjustable gastric band to Roux-en-Y gastric bypass · Sleeve gastrectomy to Roux-en-Y gastric bypass · Sleeve gastrectomy to biliopancreatic diversion with duodenal switch · Roux-en-Y gastric bypass distalization

Introduction

Inadequate weight loss or recurrent weight gain occurs in up to 35% of patients who have undergone bariatric surgery [1]. Although various definitions exist, inadequate weight loss can be defined as having a percent excess weight loss (%EWL) less than 50% for SG and RYGB and less than 25% for LAGB. Recurrent weight gain can be defined as having a %EWL less than 50% after achieving %EWL greater than 50%

N. J. Skertich · S. Schimpke · P. Omotosho (✉)
Departent of Surgery, Division of Minimally Invasive and Bariatric Surgery,
Rush University Medical Center, Chicago, IL, USA
e-mail: Philip_Omotosho@rush.edu

F. Schlottmann, M. A. Masrur (eds.), *Endoscopic, Laparoscopic and Robotic Techniques for Foregut Disorders*, https://doi.org/10.1007/978-3-032-00811-4_13

and/or a body mass index (BMI) greater than 35 kg/m^2 after achieving a BMI less than 35 kg/m^2 or a 10% weight gain from weight loss nadir [2]. Between 6% and 27% of bariatric surgery patients undergo revisions, which can be subdivided into conversions and corrective operations [3, 4]. In this chapter we will discuss the conversions of a LAGB to SG, LAGB to RYGB, SG to RYGB, SG to BPD-DS and the revision of RYGB via type I distalization.

Once popular, LAGB only made up 1% of bariatric procedures performed in 2022 [5]. If recurrent weight gain occurs, revisions can be completed in one or two stages. In the latter, the LAGB is removed in the operating room and the conversion takes place typically 3 months later after an upper GI is obtained to assess for reflux and pseudoachalasia. While a one stage procedure is less demanding on the patient, limits weight regain by avoiding a period of non-restriction, and only requires adhesiolysis once, a two stage approach in theory allows for band-related gastric inflammation to decrease, thinning of the residual band capsule, improvement in vascularization of the previously fibrotic stomach, and possible resolution of prior band-induced esophageal dilation [6]. A two-stage approach is pursued when converting to SG for the aforementioned reasons and due to a reported higher leak rate in a one stage LAGB to SG approach [6]. When converting to RYGB, a single-stage approach is generally adopted. LAGB to SG or RYGB can achieve effective weight loss results (up to 13%EWL and 46%EWL at 5 years respectively) and comorbidity resolution [7].

SG is now the most common bariatric procedure performed, accounting for 57.5% of cases in 2022 [5]. SG was initially performed as the first stage in a two-stage duodenal switch procedure; however, it was found to have substantial weight loss and comorbidity control by itself. Unfortunately, weight recidivism occurs in up to 27.8% of patients, with 13.1% of patients having a revision due to recurrent weight gain [8]. Conversion to RYGB and BPD-DS can lead to 50% and 60%EWL respectively [9, 10]. Both conversion procedures demonstrate improvement in comorbidities, but %EWL may not be as robust compared to primary RYGB or BPD-DS. In our practice, conversion to RYGB is preferred if the patient has clinically significant gastroesophageal reflux disease (GERD) as it can successfully treat the reflux and does not have a high-pressure system with competent pylorus like the BPD-DS [10]. It also is associated with fewer perioperative and long-term complications. We reserve conversion to BPD-DS for patients with high BMIs, without GERD who clearly understand the long-term risks of nutritional deficiencies.

RYGB has been considered the gold-standard bariatric procedure with excellent %EWL and improvement or resolution of comorbidities such as diabetes, hypertension, and dyslipidemia [11]. However, inadequate weight loss or recurrent weight gain can occur in up to one third of patients who undergo RYGB [1]. In this case, revision via distalization can be considered to bypass additional bowel and increase malabsorption. Type I distalization is performed by dividing the Roux or alimentary limb (AL) and moving it distally, thereby shortening the common channel (CC) and total alimentary limb length (TALL) and elongating the biliopancreatic limb (BPL).

Type II distalization is performed by dividing the BPL and moving it distally, elongating the AL and shortening the CC keeping the TALL constant [1]. However, these procedures are fraught with mixed results and potential for severe protein-calorie malnutrition and vitamin deficiencies if the CC is too short. In small studies, Type I distalization has led to acceptable %EWL ranging from 40% up to 60% of patients and can lead to comorbidity resolution [1, 12]. A type I distalization is preferred with a 200 cm CC, 150 cm AL and 350 cm TALL, which is described below.

In all patients undergoing a revision, a thorough pre-operative work-up is completed. This starts with a review of the patient's nutritional, behavioral, and medical histories, followed by repeat nutritional counseling and psychological evaluation and counseling. Prior operative reports are reviewed when available, and an UGI and EGD are obtained on all patients.

Procedural Descriptions

At our institution, both laparoscopic and robotic-assisted revisional surgery are performed. Below description of laparoscopic approaches for LAGB removal, LAGB to SG, LAGB to RYGB and SG to RYGB are detailed. Robotic approaches for SG to BPD-DS and type I distalization of a RYGB are described.

Patient Positioning

For all procedures described, the patient is positioned supine on the operating table with arms extended. A footboard is positioned so that the feet lie flat with appropriate padding. Sequential compression devises are placed and two grams of cefoxitin as well as 40 mg enoxaparin are given intravenously before the induction of anesthesia. General endotracheal anesthesia is used. An orogastric tube is inserted to decompress the stomach (with exception of distalization procedures).

Pneumoperitoneum

The abdomen is prepared in typical sterile fashion, and access to the peritoneal cavity is obtained via a Veress needle in the left upper quadrant just inferior to the costal margin in the midclavicular line. Following a satisfactory saline-drop test, the abdomen is insufflated with carbon dioxide gas to a pressure of 15 mmHg to establish pneumoperitoneum. Port placement varies somewhat by procedure and by approach, i.e. conventional laparoscopic versus robotic-assisted.

Operative Technique: Adjustable Gastric Band Conversions

Adjustable Gastric Band Removal

Port Placement

The Veress needle is changed to a 5-mm port via optical entry. A 5-mm 45-degree laparoscope is used. Additional trocars are placed under direct vision: a 5-mm trocar for the camera superior and to the left of the umbilicus, a 12-mm trocar in the right hemiabdomen in the midclavicular line, and a 5-mm trocar along the right subcostal margin (Fig. 1a). The patient is then placed in the reverse Trendelenburg position.

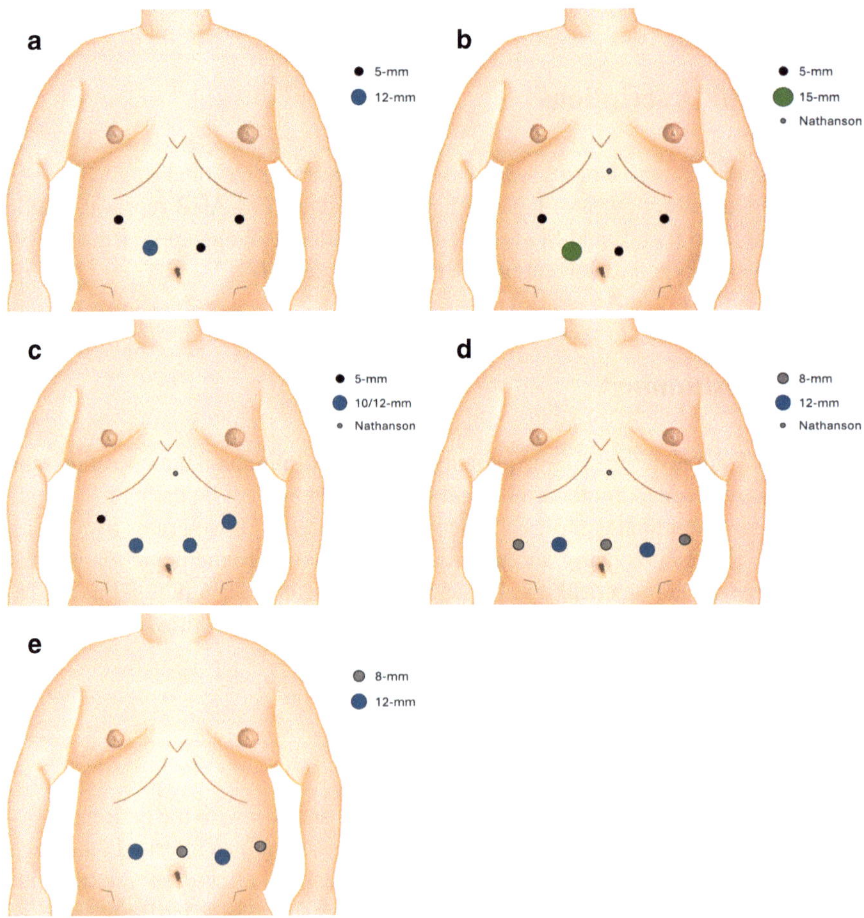

Fig. 1 Port placement for (**a**) adjustable gastric band removal, (**b**) adjustable gastric band to sleeve gastrectomy, (**c**) adjustable gastric band to Roux-en-Y gastric bypass and sleeve gastrectomy to Roux-en-Y gastric bypass, (**d**) sleeve gastrectomy to biliopancreatic diversion with duodenal switch (robotic assisted), (**e**) Roux-en-y gastric bypass distalization (robotic assisted)

Band Removal

The left lobe of the liver is retracted in an atraumatic fashion to expose the band and esophagogastric junction (Fig. 2). The inflammatory capsule/scar covering the band is divided with an L-hook using electrocautery to expose the band buckle (Fig. 3). Once the buckle is exposed and enough of the capsule divided, the band is cut with laparoscopic scissors (Fig. 4). The band tubing is cut midway along its length, and the band is removed and withdrawn from the peritoneal cavity via the 12-mm port site. It is prudent at this point to evaluate for evidence of slippage or erosion by inspecting the stomach closely. Brownish discoloration of the inner aspect of the band upon inspection should raise

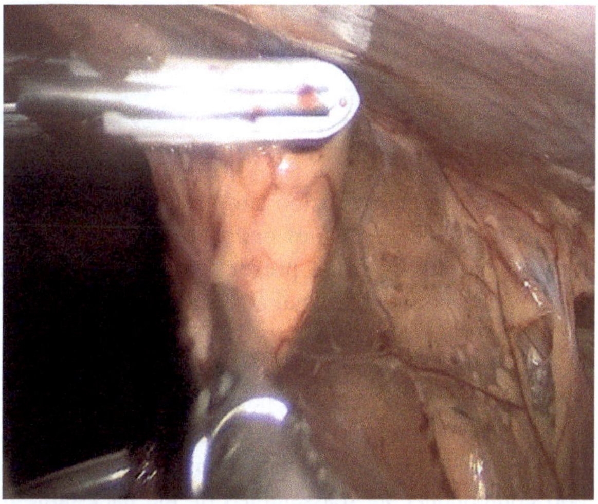

Fig. 2 Take down of adhesions and exposure of the adjustable gastric band and esophagogastric junction

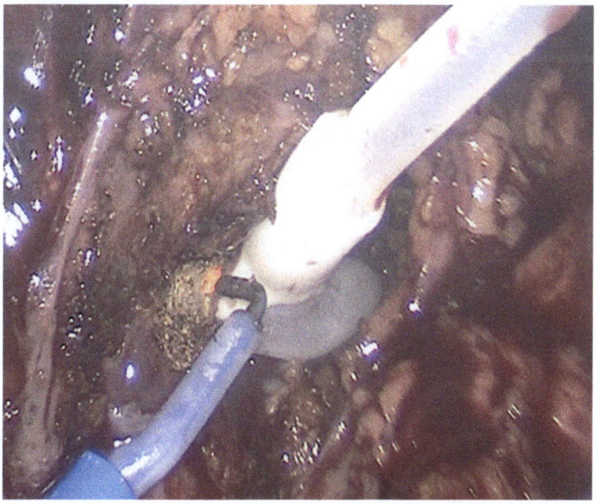

Fig. 3 Adhesiolysis of inflammatory capsule with L-hook via electrocautery

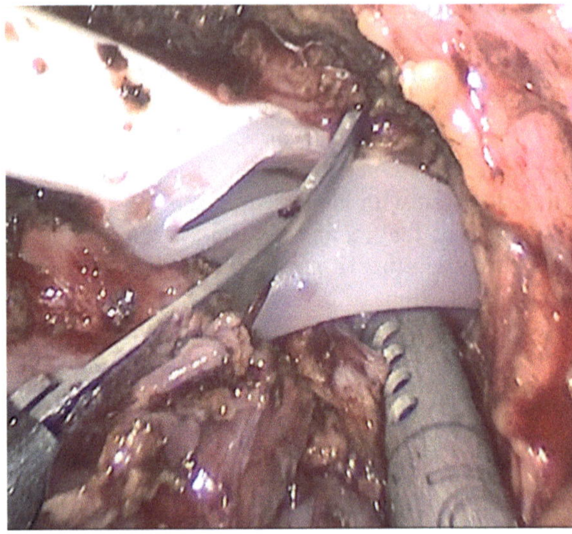

Fig. 4 Exposure of the adjustable gastric band buckle and transection of the band

suspicion for occult erosion and prompt upper endoscopy for a more complete assessment. Liberal use of endoscopy is applied should any concern arise. If gastro-gastric plication is present, it is taken down via sharp dissection to allow the stomach to lie in normal anatomical position.

Attention is then turned to the subcutaneous port. The previous skin incision overlying the subcutaneous port is reopened and dissection is carried through the subcutaneous tissue onto the port surface. The capsule over the port is taken down with electrocautery, and the port is grasped. The capsule is completely dissected off and the port and it, with the remaining tubing, is removed. The band, its tubing, and port components are reassembled on the back table to ensure that the device has been completely removed. The trocars are then removed, the abdomen desufflated, and skin closed.

Adjustable Gastric Band to Sleeve Gastrectomy

LAGB to SG procedures is typically performed in two stages. First, the band is removed. Next, an UGI study 2 months after removal is completed to assess for reflux and persistent pseudoachalasia. Lastly, the SG is performed 3 months post-removal.

Port Placement

Port placement is similar to that described for LAGB removal but a 15-mm port is used instead of a 12-mm port in the right hemiabdomen. Additionally, a Nathanson retractor is placed in the subxiphoid region to retract the liver (Fig. 1b).

Sleeve Creation

Often post-band removal, adhesions between the liver and stomach and/or omentum require lysis (Fig. 5). These are taken down via sharp dissection and/or with a vessel sealing device. Any remaining gastro-gastric plication is taken down via sharp dissection to ensure that the stomach is restored to its normal anatomic position (Fig. 6). Next, the entire greater curve of the stomach is freed as with a primary SG. We come through the gastrocolic omentum starting 5 cm proximal to the pylorus with a vessel sealing device and carry the dissection up around the greater curve of the stomach to the angle of His, taking the short gastric vessels along the way (Fig. 7). A 38–40 Fr bougie is then used to size the sleeve and the stomach is divided from 5 cm proximal to the pylorus to the angle of His by sequential firings of a reinforced stapling device (Fig. 8).

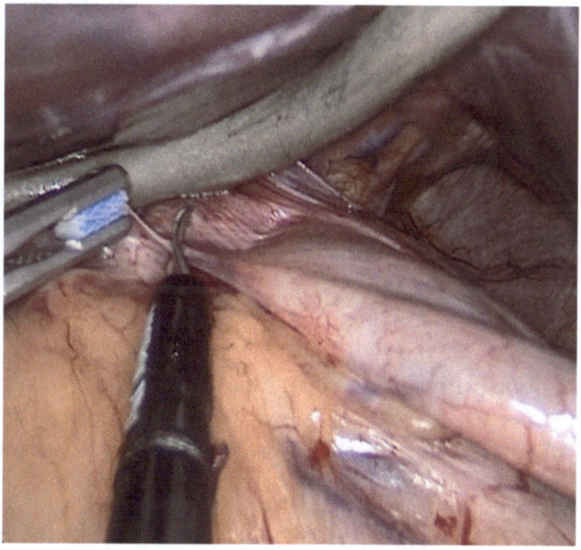

Fig. 5 Adhesiolysis of adhesions between the liver and stomach during conversion from adjustable gastric band to sleeve gastrectomy or adjustable gastric band to Roux-en-Y gastric bypass during a second stage procedure

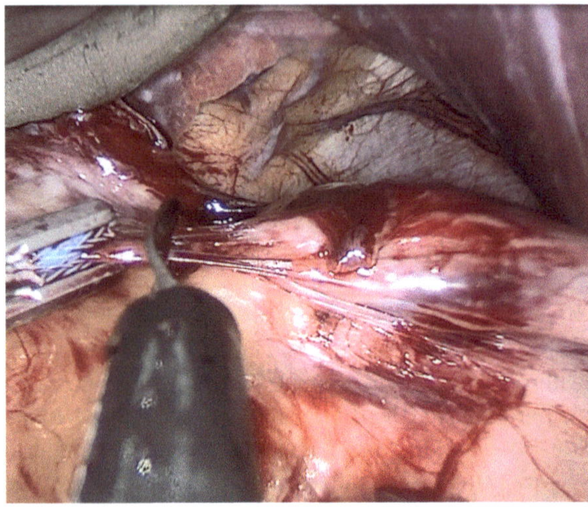

Fig. 6 Take down of fundic plications from prior adjustable gastric band

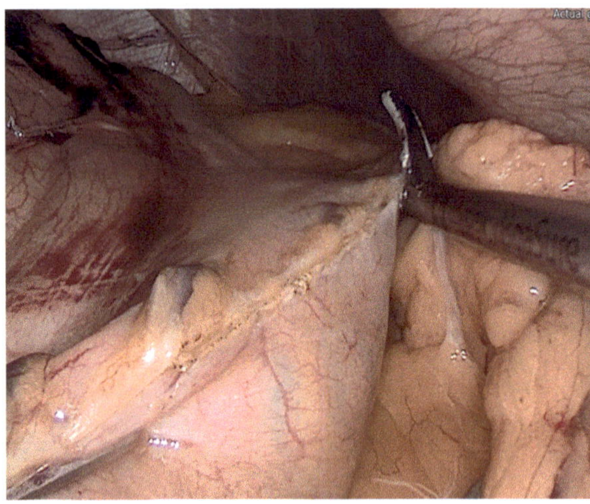

Fig. 7 Dissection of the greater curve of the stomach to the angle of His with division of the short gastric vessels via vessel sealing device

Intraoperative Endoscopy, Final Inspection, Trocar Removal, and Closure

An upper endoscopy is performed with air insufflation leak test checking for bleeding, narrowing, and leak. The specimen is removed through the 15-mm port site. The fascia is closed with suture via a transfascial closure device. The remaining trocars and Nathanson retractor are removed and the skin is closed as the surgeon prefers.

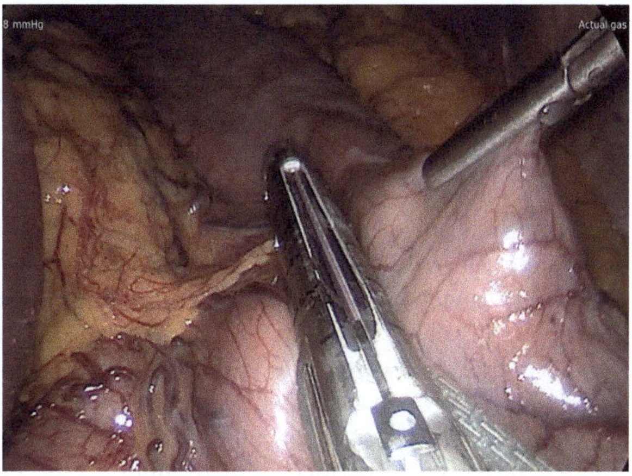

Fig. 8 Sleeve creation with sequential endoscopic GIA purple load staple fires with reinforcement along the greater curve of the stomach to create a sleeve gastrectomy

Adjustable Gastric Band to Roux-en-Y Gastric Bypass

LAGB to RYGB is completed in one stage. However, preoperatively it is discussed with the patient the possibility that intraoperative findings could preclude safely proceeding in a single stage, in which case band removal will constitute the first stage, followed by the RYGB at a later date.

Port Placement

Pneumoperitoneum is achieved as above. The Veress needle is removed, and a 10/12-mm trocar is inserted in the same location. A 10-mm, 45-degree laparoscope is inserted, and we inspect the abdomen to ensure no injury to intra-abdominal viscera from the access technique. Additional trocars are then placed: a 10/12-mm port in the periumbilical position, a 5-mm port just below the right costal margin, and another 10/12-mm port in the right hemiabdomen between the right costal margin and the umbilicus. A Nathanson retractor is positioned in the subxiphoid region to retract the liver (Fig. 1c).

Initial Inspection and Band Removal

The abdomen is inspected for adhesions and to assess whether the procedure can be completed in one stage. The band is then removed, as described above. Adhesiolysis is carried out as necessary.

Division of Small Bowel, Creation of Jejunojejunostomy

This is completed in the same fashion as if done for a primary RYGB. The greater omentum is reflected to the upper abdomen and the transverse colon and mesocolon are lifted to expose the ligament of Treitz. A 50–75 mm length of jejunum is measured from the ligament of Treitz. The jejunum is divided with a 60-mm endoscopic GIA tan load stapler. The ultrasonic scalpel is used to divide the intervening mesentery, being careful to preserve adequate blood supply to both the proximal and distal ends of the divided small bowel. The distal end of the jejunum is measured for a length of 150 cm for use as the Roux limb, and a side-to-side jejunojejunostomy is created at this point with the biliopancreatic limb, using two sequential firings of a 45-mm endoscopic GIA tan load stapler. The common enterotomy is closed using a 60-mm endoscopic GIA tan load stapler. The mesenteric defect is closed using a continuous 0 non-absorbable, braided suture.

Creation of Gastric Pouch

This is completed in the same fashion as if done for a primary RYGB. If adhesions or gastro-gastric plications are present, they are taken down as above with the removal of the band (Figs. 5 and 6). The patient is placed in the reverse Trendelenburg position. Utilizing a perigastric approach, dissection of the lesser curvature fat is undertaken approximately 4–5 cm distal to the esophagogastric junction until the lesser sac is clearly entered and the posterior wall of the stomach is exposed. This may also require dissection from the greater curvature if significant adhesions are present. A 5 cm long tubular gastric pouch is then created using sequential applications of an Laparoscopic purple load stapler with staple line reinforcement, angling toward the angle of His. If significant fibrosis is present, a thicker (black) staple load may be necessary. If at any point there is concern for narrowing from prior fibrosis or scarring, intraoperative endoscopy is used to ensure that the pouch does not have a distal stricture.

Creation of Gastrojejunostomy

We create an antecolic end-to-side gastrojejunostomy using a 45-mm laparoscopic purple load stapler inserted to the 25 mm mark. A 32Fr Ewald dilator (or similar sizing device) is placed across the anastomosis and remains in place for the closure of the common enterotomy. The common enterotomy is oversewn in two layers using running 2-0 absorbable, braided sutures placed on the medial and lateral aspects of the common enterotomy. These sutures are then run in opposite directions and tied in place. After completion of the anastomosis the Ewald dilator is removed and attention is returned to the transverse mesocolon where Petersen's defect is identified. This space between the Roux limb mesentery and the transverse mesocolon is closed using a 0 permanent, braided suture in a purse-string manner.

Intraoperative Endoscopy, Final Inspection, Trocar Removal, and Closure

We then proceed with upper endoscopy after clamping the alimentary limb. We ensure the staple line is hemostatic, the gastrojejunostomy is patent, and an air-leak test is performed. If satisfactory, the trocars and Nathanson retractor are removed under direct visualization. The trocar sites are closed with a 4-0 absorbable, monofilament suture.

Operative Technique: Sleeve Conversions

Sleeve Gastrectomy to Roux-en-Y Gastric Bypass

Port Placement, Initial Inspection, Division of Small Bowel and Creation of Jejunojejunostomy

A similar port configuration is utilized as in conversion from LAGB to Roux-en-Y gastric bypass (Fig. 1c). The abdomen is surveyed to ensure that a RYGB can be safely performed. If there are adhesions to the liver, stomach or prior omentopexy, these are taken down first (Figs. 9 and 10). Once completion of a RYGB is deemed feasible, procedure continues in standard fashion, as described above, the ligament of Treitz is identified, the biliopancreatic limb, is measured the jejunum is transected, measure the Roux limb is measured, the jejunojejunostomy is completed and the mesenteric defect is closed.

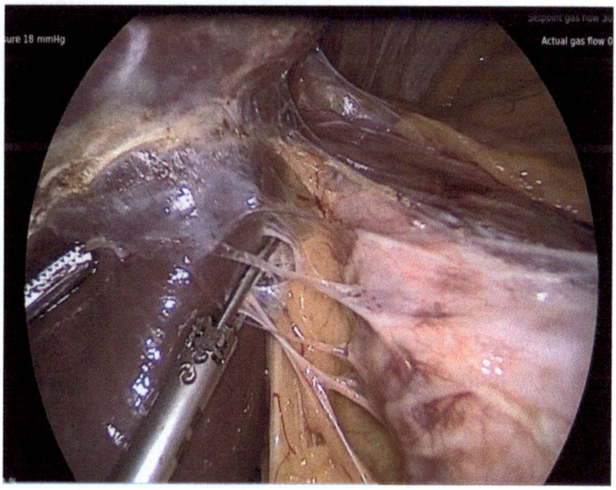

Fig. 9 Adhesiolysis of prior adhesions to the liver for sleeve conversions

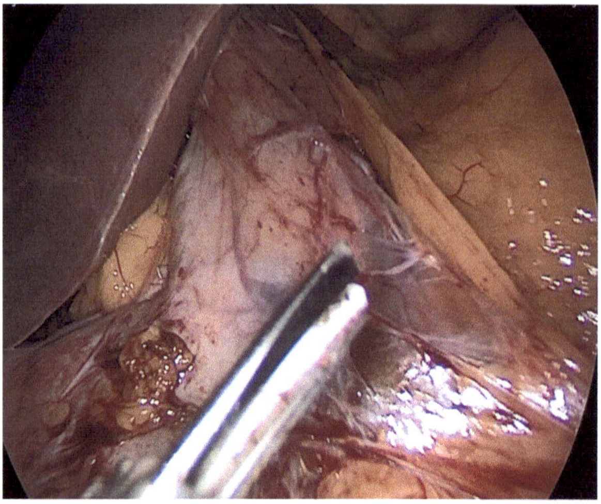

Fig. 10 Adhesiolysis of prior omentopexy, if present, or omentum, if adhered, for sleeve conversions

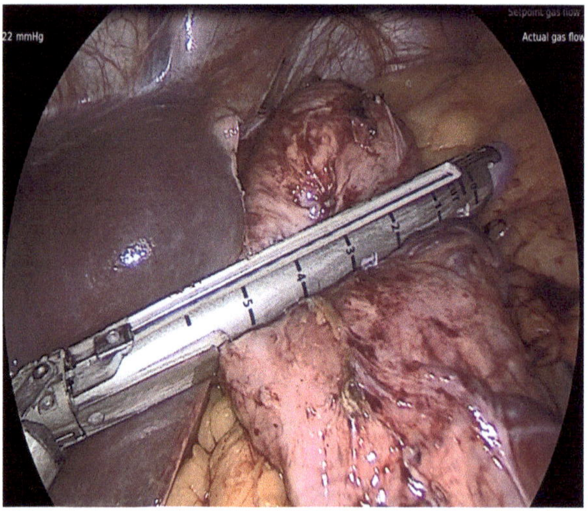

Fig. 11 Transection of prior sleeve using an 60 mm endoscopic GIA purple load non-reinforced stapler to create a 5 cm gastric pouch

Creation of Gastric Pouch and Gastrojejunostomy

Next adhesiolysis between any remaining gastrohepatic or gastroomental adhesions is completed. The lesser curvature fat is dissected at the level of the second terminal vessel branches approximately 5 cm distal to the gastroesophageal junction. The lesser sac is clearly entered, and the posterior wall of the stomach is exposed. A 60-mm laparoscopic purple load non-reinforced stapler is used to come across the sleeved stomach (Fig. 11). Additional staple loads are used if needed to ensure an appropriately sized pouch, particularly if significant dilation of the sleeve is encountered. An antecolic end-to-side gastrojejunostomy is then created. A gastrotomy is

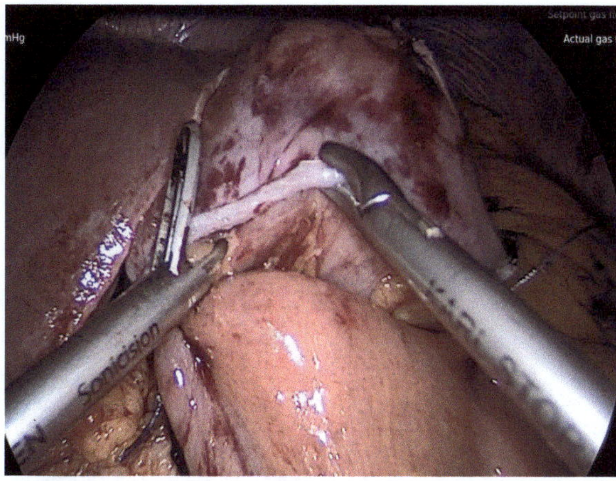

Fig. 12 A gastrotomy is made at the medial aspect of the staple line for gastrojejunostomy creation

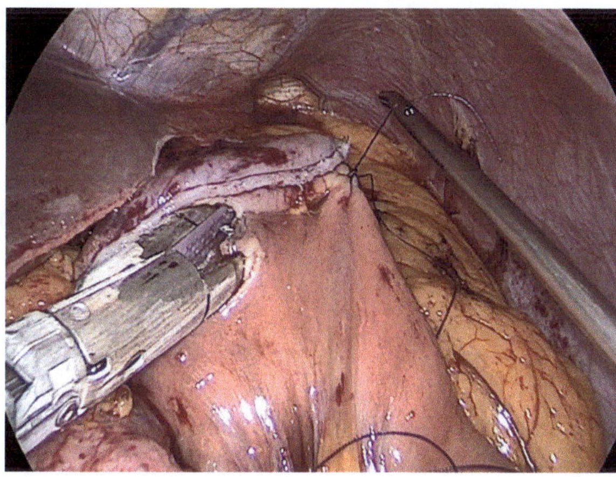

Fig. 13 Gastrojejunostomy creation between newly created gastric pouch and small intestine using a 45-mm endoscopic GIA purple load non-reinforced stapler inserted to the 25 mm mark

made at the medial aspect of the prior staple line (Fig. 12). An antecolic gastrojejunostomy is created with a 150 cm Roux limb as described above (Fig. 13). The common enterotomy is oversewn in two layers over a 32Fr Ewald dilator (or similar sizing device) using running 2-0 absorbable, braided sutures run in opposite direction (Fig. 14). Petersen's defect is closed using an 0 permanent, braided suture in a purse-string manner.

Intraoperative Endoscopy, Final Inspection, Trocar Removal, and Closure

As above, an upper endoscopy is performed to ensure the staple line is hemostatic and the gastrojejunostomy patent. An air-leak test is performed. The trocars and Nathanson retractor are removed under direct visualization and the trocar sites are closed with 4-0 absorbable, monofilament sutures.

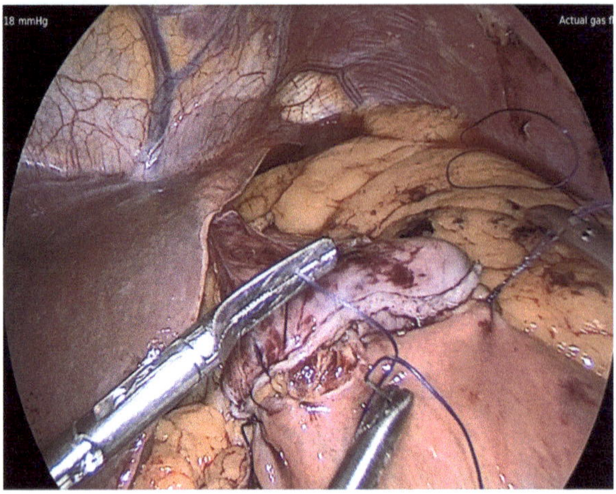

Fig. 14 Closure of the common enterotomy in two layers using running 2-0 absorbable, braided sutures during sleeve conversion to Roux-en-Y gastric bypass

Sleeve Gastrectomy to Biliopancreatic Diversion with Duodenal Switch (Robot-Assisted)

Most conversions to BPD-DS are performed via a robotic-assisted technique. Pre-operatively indocyanine green (ICG) is given to identify the common bile duct (CBD) during duodenal dissection.

Port Placement

Access to the peritoneal cavity is gained via Veress needle in the left upper quadrant as described above. The abdomen is entered with a 12-mm optical trocar, which is later exchanged for a 12-mm robotic port, in the right mid-abdomen. The abdomen is inspected for injuries to the intra-abdominal viscera. Additional trocars are then placed, all under direct visualization: an 8-mm port is placed in the periumbilical position for the camera, an 8-mm port in the left lateral abdomen, a 12-mm port in the left hemi-abdomen between the left lateral port and the umbilicus, and an 8-mm assist port in the right lateral abdomen. A stab incision is made in the subxiphoid region, and a Nathanson retractor is inserted to retract the liver (Fig. 1d). The robot is then docked.

Initial Inspection

The abdomen is surveyed to ensure that a BPD-DS can safely be performed. If there are adhesions to the stomach or prior omentopexy these are taken down first (Fig. 10). Once completion of a BPD-DS is deemed feasible, BPD-DS is performed in standard fashion.

Measuring the Common Channel and Biliopancreatic Limb

The terminal ileum is identified and a marking stitch is placed 200 cm proximal to the ileocecal junction. Then, an additional 150 cm are measured proximally (350 cm from the ileocecal junction) and two marking stitches are placed in order to maintain proximal and distal configuration.

Duodenal Dissection and Creation of the Duodenoileostomy

The patient is placed in the reverse Trendelenburg position. Then the duodenal dissection continues using a greater curvature technique. The greater curve of the stomach is dissected distally with a vessel sealer. Care is taken to avoid injury to the stomach, pylorus, or duodenum. The posterior surface of the pylorus and duodenum are freed. Firefly™ technology is used during this time to identify the CBD to avoid injury. At completion, 2–3 cm of duodenum is cleared of attachments circumferentially distal to the pylorus. The dissection extends to the point of the gastroduodenal artery. Hemostasis is achieved and the duodenum is transected with a 60-mm robotic white load stapler. The previously marked bowel at 350 cm proximal to the ileocecal junction is then brought up and an end-to-side duodenoileostomy is created. This is completed using the omega-loop technique. Cautery scissors are used to create two enterotomies, one on the duodenal bulb and another on the ileum. The posterior outer layer is created using a running 3-0 absorbable V-loc suture (Fig. 15) and the posterior and anterior inner layers are closed with two additional running 3-0 absorbable V-loc sutures which are tied to each other on the anterior wall (Fig. 16). The omega loop is then divided, thus freeing the biliopancreatic limb, just proximal to the duodenoileostomy using a 60-mm robotic white load stapler.

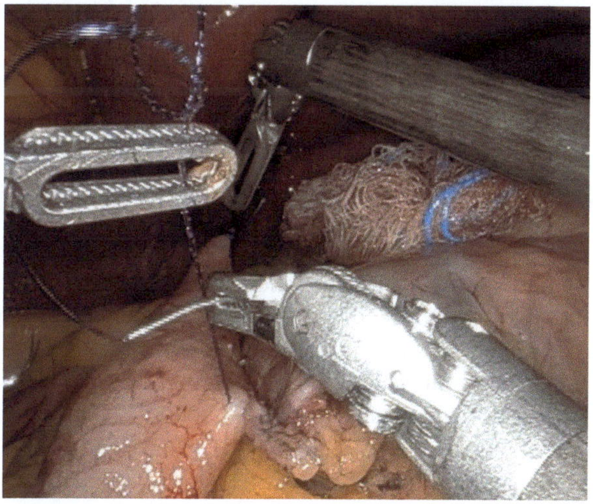

Fig. 15 Outer layer anastomosis creation of the duodenoileostomy using a running 3-0 absorbable V-loc suture

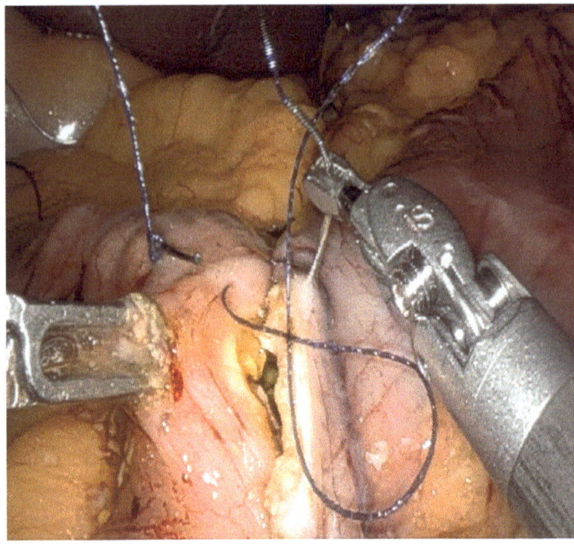

Fig. 16 Inner layer anastomosis creation of the duodenoileostomy using two, running 3-0 absorbable V-loc sutures

Ileoileostomy Creation

The prior marking stitch placed at 200 cm is identified by marching distally from the duodenoileostomy along the Roux limb. A side-to-side stapled anastomosis is then created with the biliopancreatic limb. Enterotomies are made in each limb with cautery scissors and the anastomosis is created with one fire of a 60-mm robotic white load stapler. Care is taken to ensure proper configuration and that the mesentery of each loop of bowel lies flat. The common enterotomy is closed transversely in one layer with a running 3-0 absorbable V-loc suture. The mesenteric defect of the ileoileostomy is then closed with a running 2-0 non-absorbable V-loc suture.

Intraoperative Endoscopy, Final Inspection, Trocar Removal, and Closure

An upper endoscopy is performed. The scope is advanced into the gastric sleeve and through the duodenoileostomy to ensure that the staple line is hemostatic and duodenoileostomy is patent. An air leak test is performed under visualization by insufflating with the endoscope and submerging the staple line under saline irrigation. The robot is undocked, and the liver retractor is removed under direct visualization. The irrigation fluid used for the leak test is removed from the peritoneal cavity. The trocars are removed, and all the carbon dioxide gas is evacuated. Skin at all port sites is closed with an absorbable, monofilament suture.

Operative Technique: Roux-en-Y Gastric Bypass Distalization (Robotic Assisted)

Most RYGB distalizations (most commonly Type I) are performed via the robotic approach. Port placement are similar to the describe for SG to RYGB revision (Fig. 1c).

Port Placement

Access to the peritoneal cavity is gained via Veress needle in the left upper quadrant. The abdomen is entered with a 12-mm optical trocar, which is later exchanged for a 12-mm robotic port, in the right mid-abdomen. The abdomen is inspected for injuries to the intra-abdominal viscera. Additional trocars are then placed, all under direct visualization: an 8-mm port is placed in the periumbilical position for the camera, an 8-mm port in the left lateral abdomen, a 12-mm port in the left hemi-abdomen between the left lateral port and the umbilicus, and a Nathanson retractor is inserted to retract the liver only if needed (Fig. 1c). The robot is then docked.

Initial Inspection and Limb Measurement

Inspection to identify adhesions and adhesiolysis is performed as necessary. Next, the Roux limb is identified and measured (Fig. 17). We construct antecolic Roux limbs in our practice. Roux limbs typically measure between 75 and 150 cm.

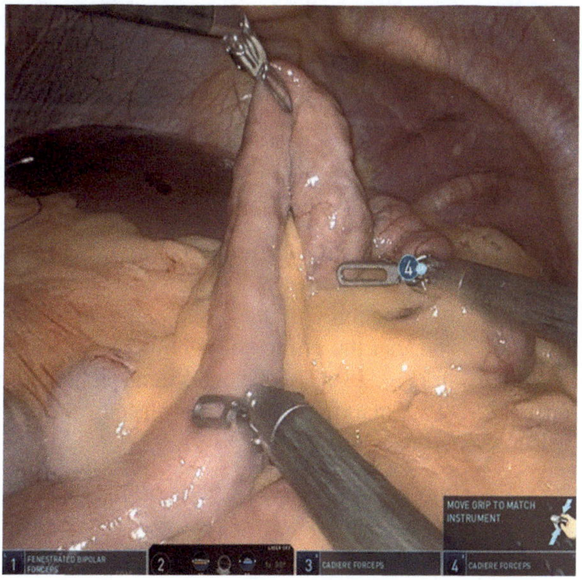

Fig. 17 Identification and measurement of the prior Roux limb

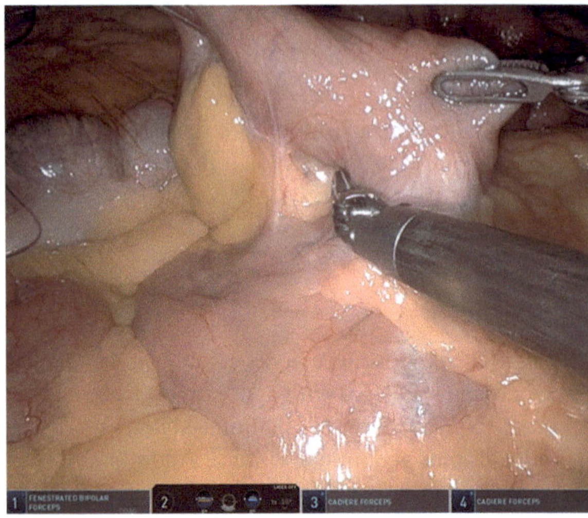

Fig. 18 Identification of prior jejunojejunal mesenteric defect at site of jejunojejunostomy

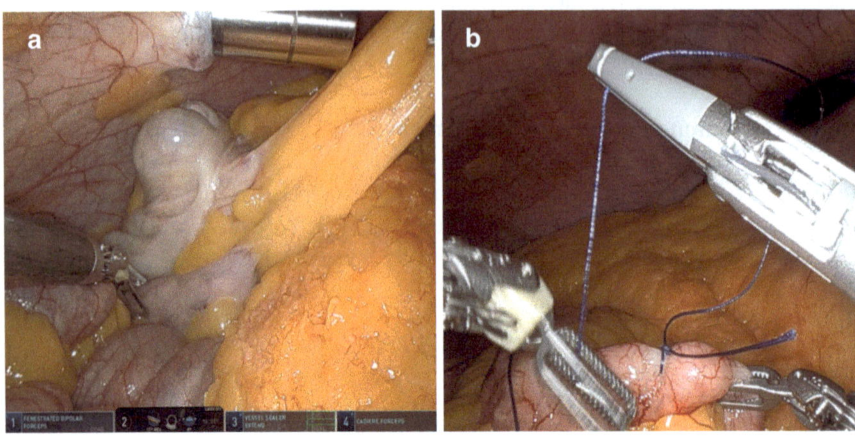

Fig. 19 Identification of the terminal ileum (**a**) and marking future site of common channel anastomosis 200 cm proximally with a short (marking distal) and long (marking proximal) sutures (**b**)

Following, the biliopancreatic limb can be measured, which is often between 50 and 75 cm. Next, we check to ensure no internal hernias are present (between the Roux limb and colon and through the jejunojejunal mesentery at the prior jejunojejunostomy site) and that the entire small bowel is free of adhesions before proceeding with revision (Fig. 18). The terminal ileum is identified, and 200 cm is measured retrograde. Two marking sutures are placed, one short marking distal, one long marking proximal (Fig. 19a, b).

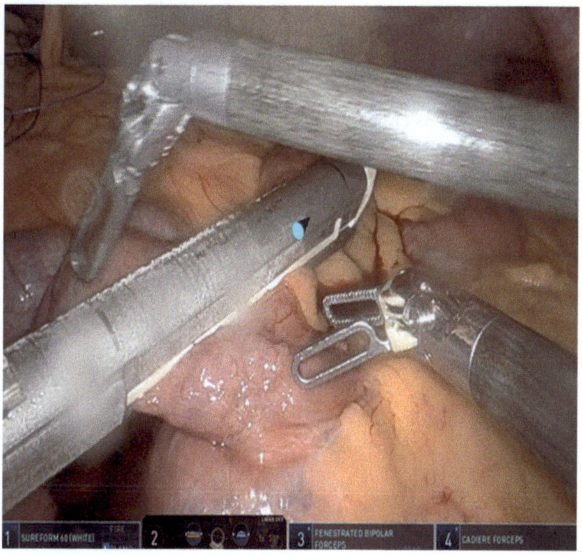

Fig. 20 Transection of Roux-limb proximal to the prior jejunojejunostomy with a 60-mm robotic white load stapler

Roux-Limb Transection and Jejunoileostomy Creation

The Roux limb is identified as it enters the jejunojejunostomy and it is transected just proximal to the anastomosis with a 60-mm robotic white load stapler (Fig. 20). A side-to-side anastomosis is created between the Roux limb and the previously marked common channel (200 cm proximal to the ileocecal valve). Enterotomies are created in both limbs and the anastomosis is made with a 60-mm robotic white load stapler (Fig. 21). The common enterotomy is closed with a continuous running 3-0 absorbable V-loc suture in two layers (Fig. 22). The initial layer is run with full thickness bites, the second layer is run in Lembert fashion. This results in a 150 cm Roux limb, a long biliopancreatic limb (unmeasured) and a 200 cm common channel making a 350 cm total alimentary limb length. The mesenteric defect is closed with a running 3-0 non-absorbable V-loc suture (Fig. 23).

Final Inspection, Trocar Removal, and Closure

An upper endoscopy is not routinely performed for distalizations. The robot is undocked and the liver retractor is removed under direct visualization. The trocars are removed and all the carbon dioxide gas is evacuated. Skin at all port sites is closed with absorbable, monofilament sutures.

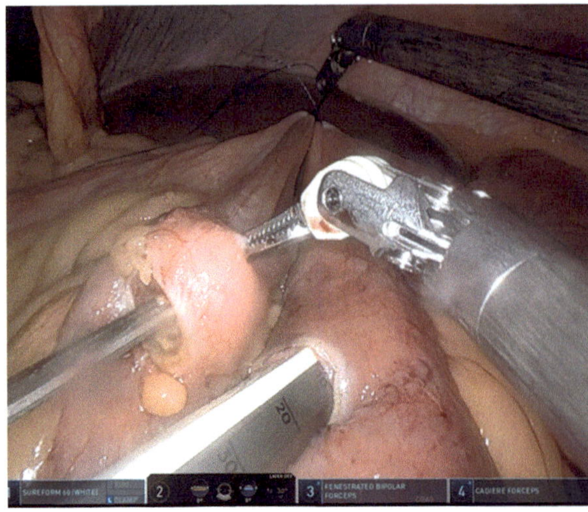

Fig. 21 Enterotomies are made in the prior Roux limb and the new common channel and a jejunoileostomy is created using a 60-mm robotic white load stapler

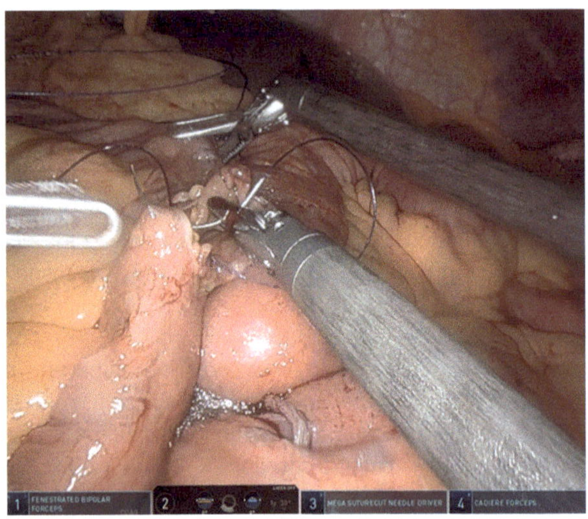

Fig. 22 Closure of the common enterotomy with a running 3-0 absorbable V-loc suture in two layers

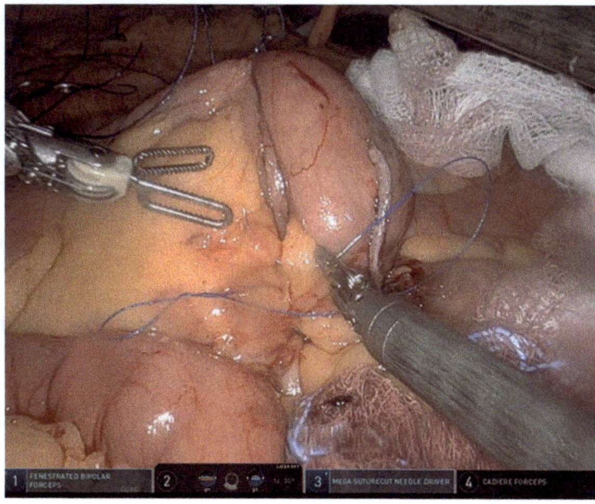

Fig. 23 Closure of the mesenteric defect of the jejunoileostomy using a running 3-0 non-absorbable V-loc suture

Conclusions

Operative revisions may be necessary following initial bariatric surgery due to inadequate weight loss or recurrent weight gain. The safety of revisional procedures is well-demonstrated in the literature [4, 13]. Efficacy depends on the primary procedure and the chosen conversion or revision. Often, revisional surgery does not achieve the same weight loss outcome as the primary intervention but can achieve similar improvement or resolution of comorbidities [3, 7].

Conflict of Interest Nicholas J. Skertich, Scott Schimpke and Philip Omotosho declare that they have no conflicts of interest.

References

1. Aleassa EM, Papasavas P, Augustin T, et al. American Society for Metabolic and Bariatric Surgery literature review on the effect of Roux-en-Y gastric bypass limb lengths on outcomes. Surg Obes Relat Dis. 2023;19(7):755–62.
2. Majid SF, Davis MJ, Ajmal S, et al. Current state of the definition and terminology related to weight recurrence after metabolic surgery: review by the POWER task force of the American Society for Metabolic and Bariatric Surgery. Surg Obes Relat Dis. 2022;18(7):957–63.
3. Franken RJ, Sluiter NR, Franken J, et al. Treatment options for weight regain or insufficient weight loss after sleeve gastrectomy: a systematic review and meta-analysis. Obes Surg. 2022;32(6):2035–46.
4. Sudan R, Nguyen NT, Hutter MM, et al. Morbidity, mortality, and weight loss outcomes after reoperative bariatric surgery in the USA. J Gastrointest Surg. 2015;19(1):171–8. discussion 178-9
5. Clapp B, Ponce J, Corbett J, et al. American Society for Metabolic and Bariatric Surgery 2022 estimate of metabolic and bariatric procedures performed in the United States. Surg Obes Relat Dis. 2024;20(5):425–31.

6. Zadeh J, Le C, Ben-David K. Safety of adjustable gastric band conversion surgery: a systematic review and meta-analysis of the leak rate in 1- and 2-stage procedures. Surg Obes Relat Dis. 2020;16(3):437–44.
7. Carbonaro J, McLaughlin T, Seip R, et al. Five-year outcomes of revisional bariatric surgery: gastric band to sleeve gastrectomy or to Roux-en-Y gastric bypass. Surg Endosc. 2024;38(5):2719–25.
8. Clapp B, Wynn M, Martyn C, et al. Long term (7 or more years) outcomes of the sleeve gastrectomy: a meta-analysis. Surg Obes Relat Dis. 2018;14(6):741–7.
9. Lind R, Ghanem OM, Ghanem M, et al. Duodenal switch conversion in non-responders or weight recurrence patients. Obes Surg. 2022;32(12):3984–91.
10. Shen MR, Hammoud MM, Bonham AJ, et al. Conversion of sleeve gastrectomy to Roux-en-Y gastric bypass: impact on reflux and weight loss. Surg Obes Relat Dis. 2024.
11. Courcoulas AP, Patti ME, Hu B, et al. Long-term outcomes of medical management vs bariatric surgery in type 2 diabetes. JAMA. 2024;331(8):654–64.
12. Shah K, Nergard BJ, Fagerland MW, Gislason H. Failed roux-en-Y gastric bypass-long-term results of Distalization with Total alimentary limb length of 250 or 300 cm. Obes Surg. 2023;33(1):293–302.
13. Giannopoulos S, Li WS, Kalantar Motamedi SM, et al. Outcome comparison between primary and revisional bariatric surgery: a propensity-matched analysis. Surgery. 2024;175(3):592–8.

Selected Readings

14. Sudan R, Nguyen NT, Hutter MM, et al. Morbidity, mortality, and weight loss outcomes after reoperative bariatric surgery in the USA. J Gastrointest Surg. 2015;19:171–9.
15. Carbonara J, McLaughlin T, Seip R, et al. Five-year outcomes of revisional bariatric surgery: gastric band to sleeve gastrectomy or to Roux-en-Y gastric bypass. Surg Endosc. 2024;38(5):2719–95.
16. Franken RJ, Sluiter NR, Franken J, et al. Treatment options for weight regain or insufficient weight loss after sleeve gastrectomy: a systematic review and meta-analysis. Obes Surg. 2022;32(6):2035–46.
17. Aleassa EM, Papasavas P, Augustin T, et al. American society for metabolic and bariatric surgery literature review on the effect of Roux-en-y gastric bypass limb lengths on outcomes. Surg Obes Relat Dis. 2023;19:755–62.

Robotic Sleeve Gastrectomy and Kidney Transplant

Maria Jimena Alaniz, Ivo Tzvetanov, and Enrico Benedetti

Abstract Obesity is a major risk factor for cardiovascular disease, diabetes, and end-stage renal disease, complicating kidney transplantation (KT) eligibility. Therefore, addressing obesity in KT candidates improves graft success and long-term patient health. Moreover, bariatric surgery is a proven intervention for weight loss and can be integrated into KT care before, during, or after transplantation, depending on clinical condition. Sleeve gastrectomy is the preferred procedure for its compatibility with immunosuppressive therapy, excellent weight loss outcomes, and lower morbidity.

Keywords Obesity · Weight loss · Robotic kidney transplantation · Sleeve gastrectomy · Robotics in transplantation

Introduction

Obesity has been consistently rising for the last two decades [1]. Bariatric surgery is an established weight loss intervention as its results are more efficient than medical weight loss [2, 3]. These procedures are recommended for individuals with BMI >40 kg/m^2 or BMI >35 kg/m^2 with at least one obesity-related comorbidity [4].

As obesity implies a major risk for cardiovascular disease, diabetes, and chronic kidney disease, the prevalence for end-stage renal disease (ESRD) in obese patients is also increasing [5]. Due to postoperative complications, a BMI >35 kg/m^2 is considered a relative contraindication when it comes to listing a patient for a kidney transplantation (KT). In the last two decades, minimally invasive surgery (MIS) demonstrated significant decrease of surgical complications in obese population,

M. J. Alaniz · I. Tzvetanov (✉) · E. Benedetti
Division of Transplantation, Department of Surgery, University of Illinois at Chicago, Chicago, IL, USA
e-mail: malaniz@uic.edu; itzveta@uic.edu

F. Schlottmann, M. A. Masrur (eds.), *Endoscopic, Laparoscopic and Robotic Techniques for Foregut Disorders*, https://doi.org/10.1007/978-3-032-00811-4_14

achieving comparable graft and patient survival with non-obese patients [5–7]. This has allowed transplantation in obese population possible.

In KT candidates, bariatric surgery proved to be highly effective and could be applied in three different scenarios depending on the patients' clinical condition. The weight loss intervention can be performed before, during or after actual KT [8]. For patients that do not have the opportunity for living donor (LD) it is beneficial to perform a weight loss intervention before KT. When a LD is available, especially when the recipient is not on dialysis, Pre-emptive kidney transplant is the best opportunity to achieve excellent long-term results. These are the ideal candidate for simultaneous KT and weight loss surgery to address kidney failure and obesity at the same time [9, 10].

Sleeve gastrectomy (SG) is the preferred intervention in a setting of combined KT and Bariatric Surgery, because there is no related malabsorption and hence does not impact immunosuppressive drugs pharmacokinetics. Furthermore, it offers patients the possibility to drink enough water to gain independence from intravenous fluid replacement. During a combined surgical approach, SG should be preferentially performed before transplantation to decrease excessive pneumoperitoneum exposure of the kidney graft.

Procedure Description

Anesthesia and Patient Positioning

The patient is placed in a supine position. General anesthesia is induced through endotracheal intubation. The patient is monitored throughout the procedure with electrocardiogram, oximetry and arterial line. Prophylactic antibiotics and heparin must be given at the time of induction. Special attention is paid to securing the patient to the table and relieving any pressure or hyperextension of the joints. Given the patient will remain in steep Trendelenburg position for an extended period, the best option to achieve stability is to maintain the legs flexed at the knee joint, supported over leg rest. Additionally, shoulder support could be applied, and arms are tucked along the body.

Communication between surgical and anesthesia team regarding fluid management and ventilation settings is particularly important. Patients with higher BMI tend to respond to the pneumoperitoneum and positioning with a significant but temporary, initial desaturation. Proper ventilation management allows for MIS approach.

Pneumoperitoneum and Port Placement

A 5 mm supraumbilical midline incision is made, following the insertion of an Opti-View trocar under direct visualization with a 5 mm 0-degree angle camera. Pneumoperitoneum is created and abdominal cavity is examined with the scope. If no pathology is identified, the procedure continues as planned. The presence of adhesions from previous surgeries or peritoneal dialysis are not considered contra-indications for MIS approach and they must be addressed properly.

Before placement of any additional trocar, transplant and bariatric teams, both agree on port positioning, so no extra additional ports are placed when Robotic-assisted Kidney Transplant (RAKT) takes place. Under direct visualization using Safe Track technique, an 8 mm port is placed in the right anterior axillary line, just below the costal margin and two 8 mm are placed at the level of the umbilicus along the midclavicular line, and 5 cm higher on the left anterior axillary line. Additionally, a 5 mm incision is made in the epigastric area to insert the Nathanson liver retractor which is used to elevate the left lobe of the liver anteriorly. This device is secured to the patient's bed. The patient is positioned in a 30-degree reverse Trendelenburg position (Fig. 1).

Finally, when reaching 15 mmHg of pneumoperitoneum, the robotic system is docked from the right side of the patient.

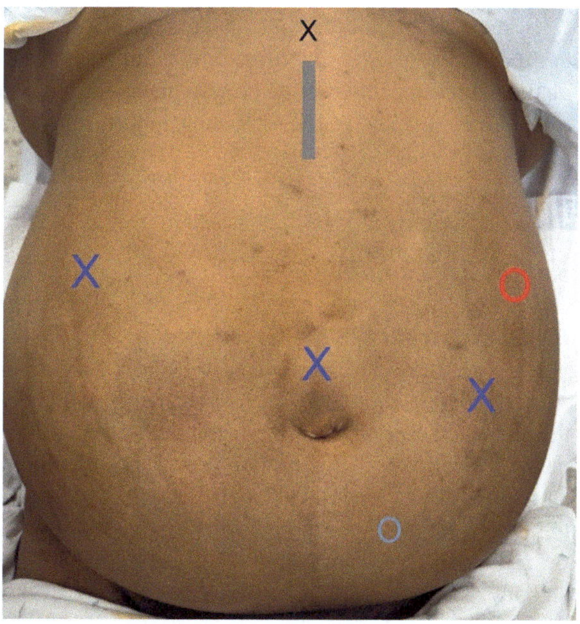

Fig. 1 Port placement. Ports marked as blue cross are used for both surgical procedures; Red circle is used for Sleeve gastrectomy and grey circle represents a left lower quadrant robotic port and midline incision (Gray line) for Hand-assistance device used for kidney transplant

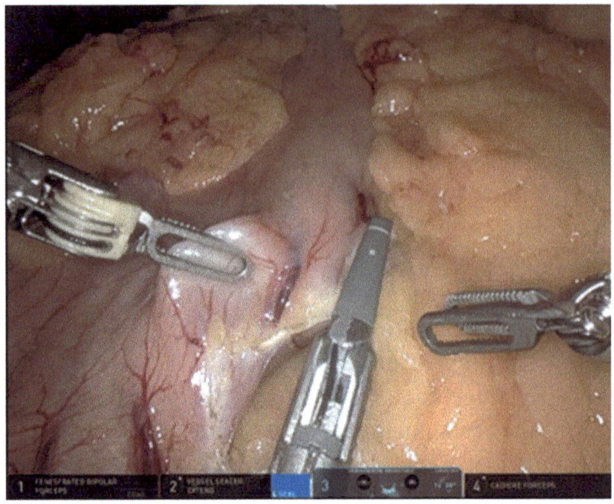

Fig. 2 Dissection of the gastrocolic omentum

Sleeve Gastrectomy

An initial inspection is performed to identify any hiatal hernia.

The gastric pylorus is also identified and about 4–6 cm proximal to it, dissection starts with the division of the gastrocolic omentum close to the greater curvature all the way to the angle of His (Fig. 2). Special care must be taken into consideration while dividing the short gastric arteries.

After stomach greater curvature is mobilized, a 36-French bougie tube is placed in an orogastric fashion and is positioned towards the pylorus (Fig. 3).

Firing a 60 mm robotic blue load robotic stapler, approximately 4–6 cm proximal to the pylorus, the sleeve gastrectomy is initiated. The vertical gastrectomy is completed with sequential robotic blue staplers, until the stomach excess is totally separated (Figs. 4 and 5). The specimen is removed from the abdomen and sent to pathology.

Kidney Transplant

Bench Preparation of the Graft

After donor nephrectomy is completed at the same time in an operative room nearby, the kidney is prepared for implantation. It is important to perform precise and detailed small vessels ligation, to prevent reperfusion bleeding which can represent an important challenge in a robotic surgery setting. Initially, dissection starts with the renal vein, and all vein contributors are dissected and double ligated with silk ties. Afterwards, the renal artery is dissected towards the hilum for sufficient length and any artery branch not supplying the kidney graft or the ureter must be ligated.

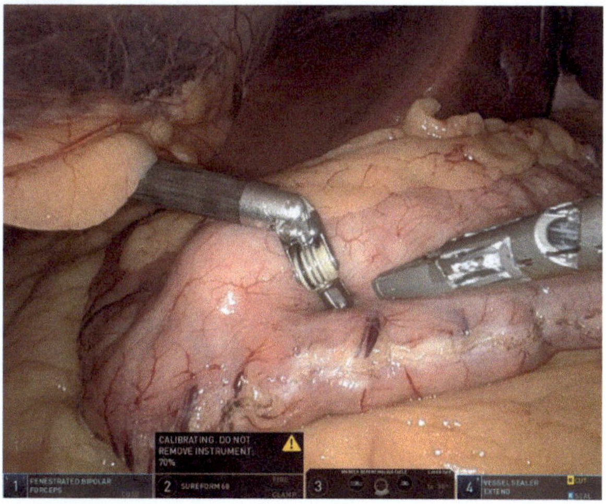

Fig. 3 Orogastric introduction of a 36-French bougie tube, guided toward the pylorus after mobilization of the stomach

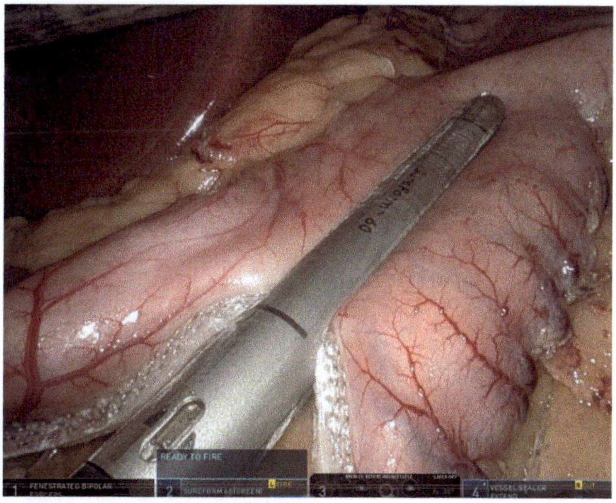

Fig. 4 Sleeve gastrectomy creation

The adipose capsule can be removed using multiple silk ties or a Ligasure device. Ureter spatulation is performed in about 5 mm length and a 6.0 Prolene stitch with a knot placed on it to facilitate handling. After the backbench is completed, the renal artery and vein are marked with a marking pen to facilitate orientation, and the graft is stored in a cold preservation solution.

Robotic Kidney Transplantation

After completing SG, the robotic arms must be repositioned. A 5–7 cm upper midline incision is made, and Hand-assistance device is positioned for graft delivery and occasionally, hand assistance. An additional 8 mm port is placed on the left

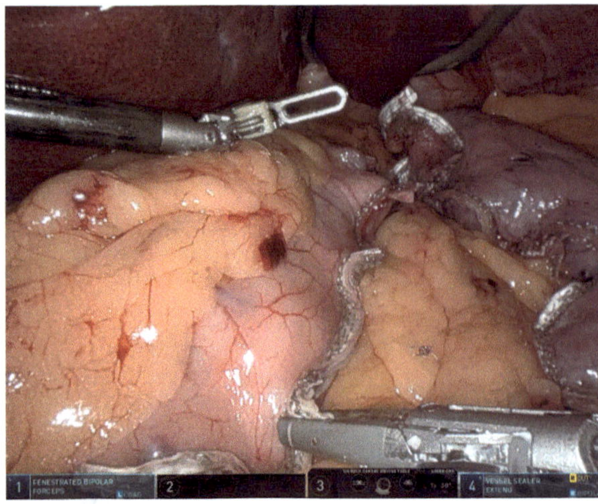

Fig. 5 Sleeve gastrectomy completion

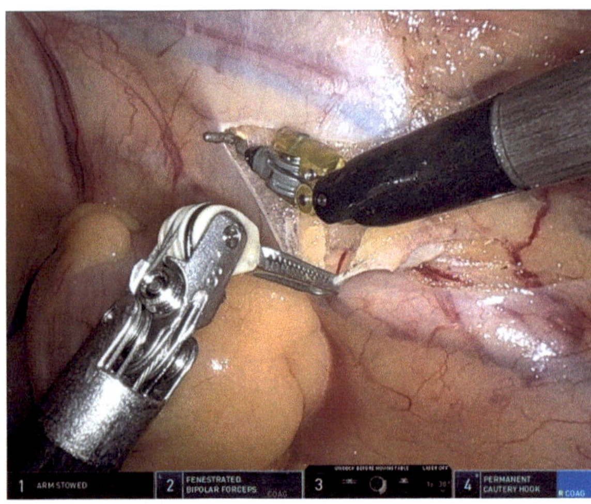

Fig. 6 Peritoneal window creation

lower quadrant, for right side graft implantation (Fig. 1). The patient is positioned in a steep Trendelenburg position tilt to the left side. Patient cart is docked again.

Initially, the cecum and the ascending colon are mobilized, the peritoneum at the right iliac fossa is incised and the retroperitoneum is exposed (Fig. 6). External iliac artery is identified and dissected first followed by the careful dissection of the iliac vein. For vascular dissection electric Hook or scissors can be used. Gonadal vessels and native ureter are carefully preserved.

A vessel loop is used to help for proper retraction of the External iliac artery (EIA) and exposure of the External iliac vein (EIV) (Fig. 7).

As per the usual approach, venous anastomosis is done first. EIV is clamped proximally and distally with robotic bulldogs and a 15 mm venotomy is made with robotic scissors. The kidney graft is brought into the field by the assistant surgeon

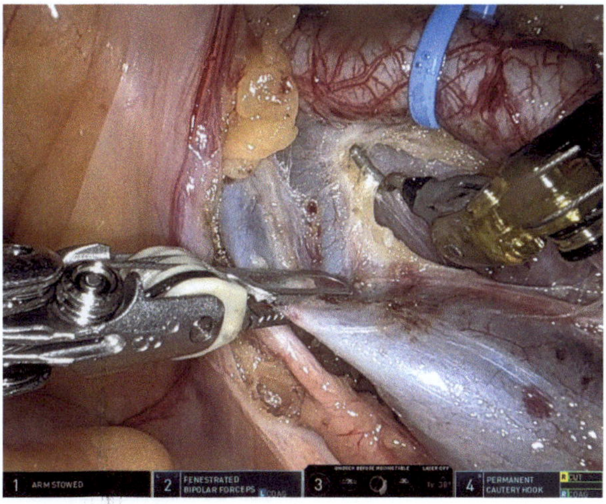

Fig. 7 Iliac vessels dissection

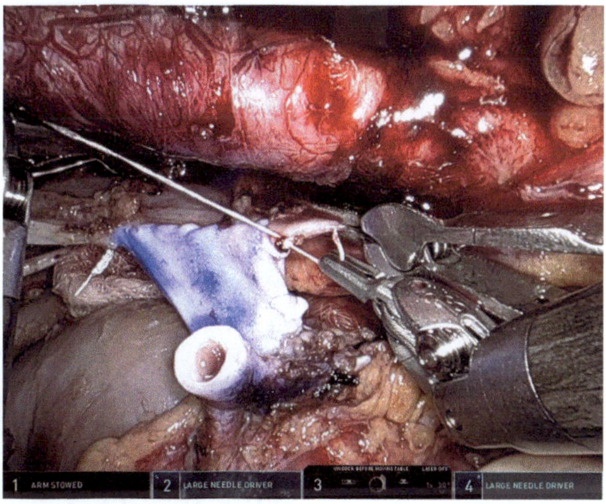

Fig. 8 Venous anastomosis

and properly oriented by hand. If hand assistance is not used, the graft must be properly oriented by instrument handling.

Venous anastomosis is performed between EIV and renal vein usually with 5–0 PTFE in a running fashion (Fig. 8). PTFE is a preferred material because of easier handling with the robotic needle driver but alternatively, anastomosis could be done with a 5.0 or 6.0 Prolene suture.

Following completion of the venous anastomosis, EIA is released from the vessel loop and clamped proximally and distally with robotic bulldog clamps. A 4–8 mm oval-shaped arteriotomy is performed into the anterior wall of the EIA with very sharp robotic scissors or alternatively with a N° 11 blade held with the robotic needle driver. End-to side anastomosis is done between renal artery and EIA with a 6–0 or 5–0 continuous PTFE suture (Fig. 9).

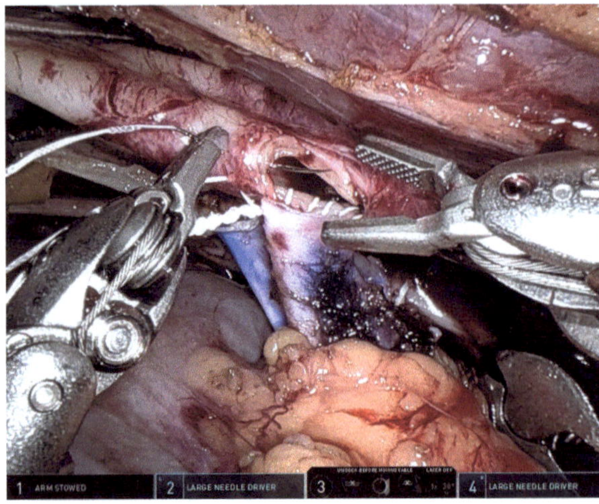

Fig. 9 Arterial anastomosis

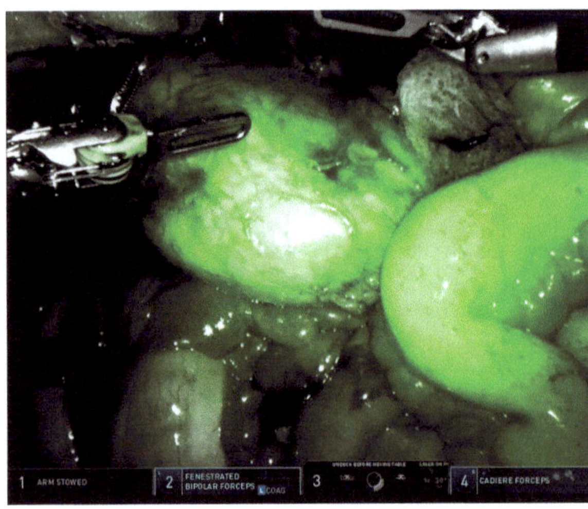

Fig. 10 ICG for perfusion assessment

After completing the vascular anastomosis, the kidney graft is reperfused by unclamping the EIV first and, immediately afterwards, unclamping the EIA. Any possible bleeding is effectively controlled and Doppler probe along with Indocyanine Green (ICG) with Firefly Fluorescence Camera is used to confirm the perfusion of the kidney graft (Fig. 10). After reperfusion, the pneumoperitoneum is decreased below 10 mm Hg, preferably.

To facilitate identification of the urinary bladder, between 100 and 150 ml of methylene blue solution is instilled through the Foley catheter at this stage. At the last step, ureteroneocystostomy is performed over a double-J stent. This anastomosis is performed with a 5.0 running PDS suture and anti-reflux flap from the muscular layer of the urinary bladder is created with three interrupted stiches (Figs. 11 and 12).

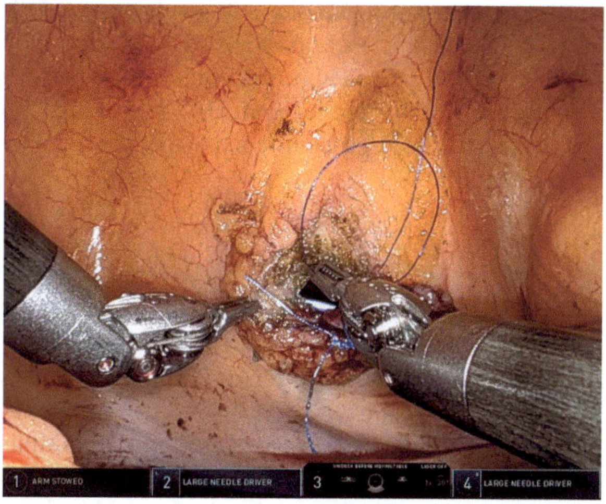

Fig. 11 Ureteroneocystostomy with double-J stent

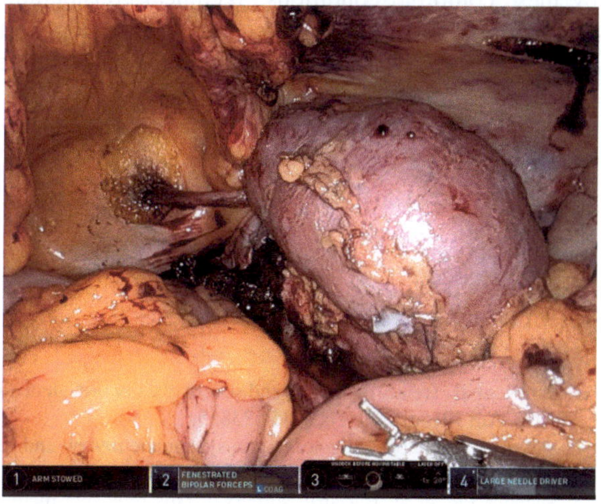

Fig. 12 Completed kidney transplant

After completion, the area is copiously irrigated and properly examined to control any possible bleeding. Finally, the robotic instruments are removed, and the abdominal incisions are closed.

Using Endo-close® device for port incisions closing is highly recommended.

Post Operative Care

The patient is transferred to the critical care or step-down unit for strict follow-up and is started on a clear liquid diet the same day of surgery. Over the course of 6 weeks, the diet is gradually progressed under strict supervision of a nutritionist, starting from a clear liquid diet, soft diet to a general diet. The post-operative follow up is conducted at 2 weeks postoperatively with the surgical team.

This combined surgical procedure is ideally performed with LD but can also be done with a deceased kidney graft [10]. In that scenario, full collaboration between bariatric and transplant team remains extremely important to achieve comparable results.

Conclusions

The feasibility of combining robotic sleeve gastrectomy and kidney transplantation as a dual surgical approach for managing chronic kidney disease and morbid obesity represents a significant advancement in multidisciplinary treatment. The robotic platform offers enhanced precision, reduced tissue trauma, and improved postoperative outcomes, which are critical when addressing the unique challenges posed by these comorbid conditions. Technical considerations, such as careful patient selection, optimal timing of procedures, and perioperative management strategies, are pivotal to ensure the success of this complex intervention. Furthermore, the combined approach minimizes the cumulative risks associated with separate surgeries, accelerates recovery, and maximizes the benefits of weight loss for renal graft survival and overall health. This integrative strategy has redefined care paradigms, offering hope to a challenging patient population with dual burdens of disease.

References

1. Fan K, et al. Trends in obesity and severe obesity prevalence in the United States from 1999 to 2018. Am J Hum Biol. 2023;35:e23855.
2. Padwal R, et al. Bariatric surgery: a systematic review and network meta-analysis of randomized trials. Obes Rev. 2011;12:602–21.
3. Schauer PR, et al. Bariatric surgery versus intensive medical therapy for diabetes – 5-year outcomes. N Engl J Med. 2017;376:641–51.
4. Gastrointestinal surgery for severe obesity: National Institutes of Health consensus development conference statement. Am J Clin Nutr. 1992;55:615S–9S.
5. Segev DL, et al. Obesity impacts access to kidney transplantation. J Am Soc Nephrol. 2008;19:349–55.
6. Spaggiari M, et al. Simultaneous robotic kidney transplantation and bariatric surgery for morbidly obese patients with end-stage renal failure. Am J Transplant. 2021;21:1525–34.
7. Tzvetanov IG, et al. Robotic kidney transplantation in the obese patient: 10-year experience from a single center. Am J Transplant. 2020;20:430–40.
8. Spaggiari M, et al. Timing considerations for sleeve gastrectomy in kidney transplant patients: a single Center evaluation. Transpl Int. 2024;37:12690.
9. Castillo-Larios R, Gunturu NS, Elli EF. Outcomes of bariatric surgery before, during, and after solid organ transplantation. Obes Surg. 2022;32:3821–9.
10. Frontiers Publishing Partnerships | Timing Considerations for Sleeve Gastrectomy in Kidney Transplant Patients: A Single Center Evaluation. https://www.frontierspartnerships.org/journals/transplant-international/articles/10.3389/ti.2024.12690/full.

Gastroesophageal Reflux Disease

Endoscopic Transoral Incisionless Fundoplication (TIF)

Diego Camacho and Diego L. Lima

Abstract Gastroesophageal reflux disease (GERD) is a common condition that affects patients quality of life. Typical symptoms of GERD are heartburn, regurgitation and bloating. GERD results from the loss of an effective anti-reflux valve in the stomach. Transoral incisionless fundoplication (TIF) is an endoscopic fundoplication technique safe for a selected group of patients with typical GERD symptoms.

Keywords Obesity · Gastroesophageal reflux disease · Fundoplication · Endoscopy · TIF

Introduction

Gastroesophageal reflux disease is common worldwide, with significant socioeconomic burden and impaired quality of life for patients. The prevalence of the disease ranges from 18 to 27% in North America. Heartburn and regurgitation are common symptoms of GERD caused by reflux of stomach contents into the esophagus. There are several different treatment options for GERD: pharmacologic with proton pump inhibitors (PPI), lifestyle changes and, ultimately, surgery.

Laparoscopic anti-reflux fundoplication is the current gold standard surgical technique for the treatment of GERD in patients with refractory symptoms or patients who do not want to take medicine for the rest of their lives. There are different surgical techniques, with Nissen (360°) and Toupet (partial 270°) as the two most common surgical techniques. Despite its high efficacy, surgical fundoplication is not free of complications and recurrence of symptoms.

Transoral incisionless fundoplication (TIF) is an endoscopic anti-refux procedure that has been used as a primary GERD intervention in selected patients with

D. Camacho (✉) · D. L. Lima
Department of Surgery, Montefiore Medical Center, Bronx, NY, USA
e-mail: dicamach@montefiore.org

F. Schlottmann, M. A. Masrur (eds.), *Endoscopic, Laparoscopic and Robotic Techniques for Foregut Disorders*, https://doi.org/10.1007/978-3-032-00811-4_15

hiatal hernias length ≤2 cm and Hill grade 1–2. TIF was introduced in 2005 as a new endoscopic fundoplication technique, and it has evolved over the years. Recent studies have showed that TIF is a safe alternative for selected patients with GERD [1–4].

Indications of TIF

All patients should undergo pre-procedural endoscopy and ambulatory pH reflux testing. Indications for the procedure are as follows: Reflux diagnosed during pH testing (mean acid exposure time >4%), endoscopic evidence of Grade C or D esophagitis or Barrett's esophagus and hiatal hernia <3 cm or no hiatal hernia present.

Procedure Description

Proton Pump inhibitors (PPI) and IV antibiotics are administered preoperatively to prevent bleeding and infection since the plication is transmurally. Anti-emetics are also administered to prevent aspiration. The patient is placed in standard position for upper GI endoscopy.

TIF is performed under general endotracheal anesthesia and a complete diaphragm relaxation is needed for the procedure. A preoperative endoscopy is performed aiming to determine the distance between the incisor teeth and the diaphragmatic hiatus and the greatest transverse dimension of the hiatus at the GEJ under gastric distention. The procedure is performed with TIF 2.0 technique using the EsophyX device (EndoGastric Solutions, Inc., Redmond, Wash, USA) with the goal to restore the valve at the gastroesophageal junction (GEJ). It is anatomically and functionally similar to a surgical fundoplication.

A retroflexed view with full gastric distention demonstrates the edges of the crura impinging on the GEJ. Patients with the transverse size of the hiatus <3 cm can easily have the TIF procedure performed (Fig. 1).

The stomach is insufflated with CO_2 once the device is introduced. The scope is placed in retroflexion and the view of the 12 o'clock position is defined as the location of the lesser curvature. The 6 o'clock position faces the great curvature of the stomach (Fig. 2).

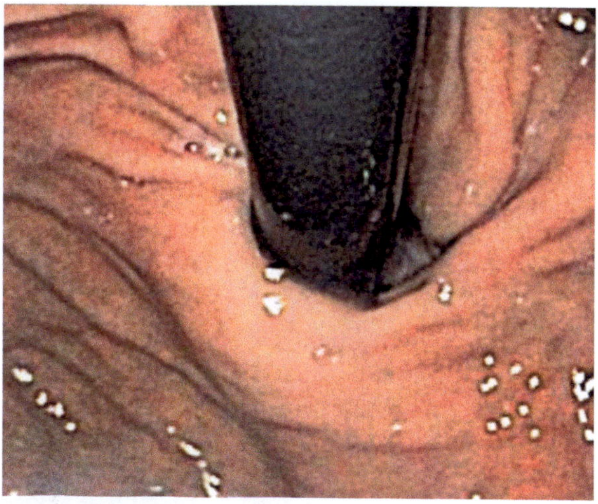

Fig. 1 Retroflexion view of the GEJ

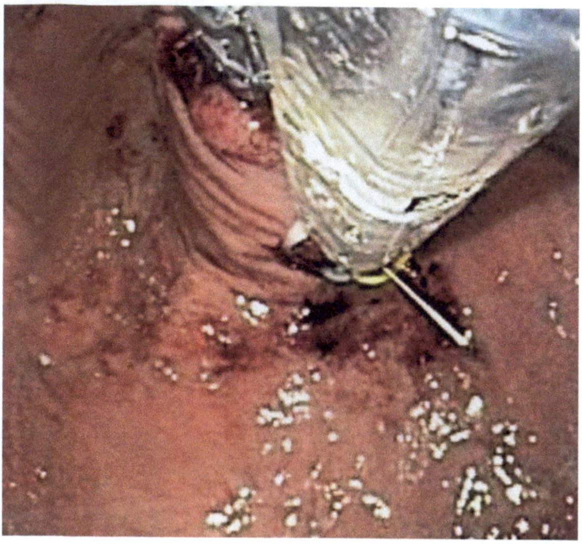

Fig. 2 TIF device

The device uses cartridges with 20 fasteners each. The objective of this technique is to deploy all 20 fasteners as 10 plication sets: 3 anterior rotational sets toward 1 o'clock; 3 posterior rotational sets toward 11 o'clock; 2 anterior longitudinal sets between 12 o'clock and 2 o'clock; and 1 longitudinal at 6 o'clock; the remaining 1 plication is set at 6 o'clock or as a "cleanup" fixation where the fastener may not have deployed well the first time (Fig. 3).

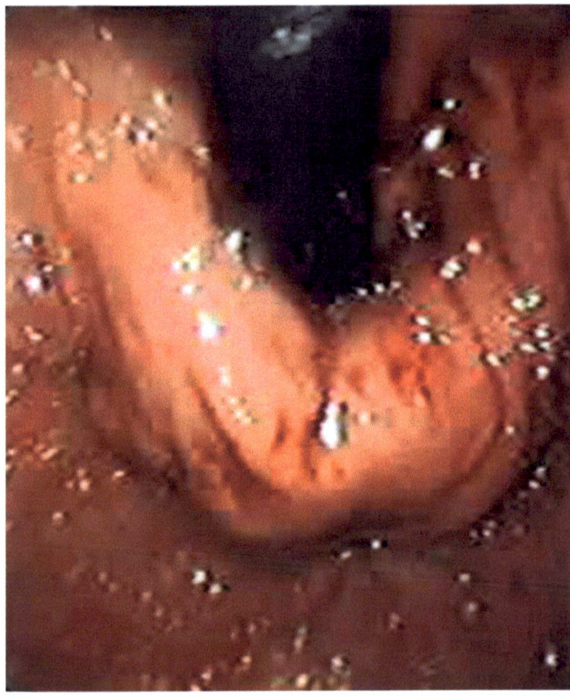

Fig. 3 Post-procedural retroflexion view

Conclusions

The endoscopic fundoplication technique using TIF 2.0 is effective and safe. TIF has the potential to be an important treatment option for selected patients with GERD that do not want a more invasive surgical procedure.

Conflict of Interest Diego Camacho and Diego Lima declare that they have no conflicts of interest.

References

1. Huang X, Chen S, Zhao H, Zeng X, Lian J, Tseng Y, Chen J. Efficacy of transoral incisionless fundoplication (TIF) for the treatment of GERD: a systematic review with meta-analysis. Surg Endosc. 2017;31(3):1032–44. https://doi.org/10.1007/s00464-016-5111-7.
2. Bell RC, Cadière GB. Transoral rotational esophagogastric fundoplication: technical, anatomical, and safety considerations. Surg Endosc. 2011;25(7):2387–99. https://doi.org/10.1007/s00464-010-1528-6.

3. Haseeb M, Brown JRG, Hayat U, Bay C, Bain PA, Jirapinyo P, Thompson CC. Impact of second-generation transoral incisionless fundoplication on atypical GERD symptoms: a systematic review and meta-analysis. Gastrointest Endosc. 2023;97(3):394–406.e2. https://doi.org/10.1016/j.gie.2022.11.002.
4. Ghosh G, Choi AY, Dbouk M, Greenberg J, Zarnegar R, Murray M, Janu P, Thosani N, Dayyeh BKA, Diehl D, Nguyen NT, Chang KJ, Canto MI, Sharaiha R; TIF Research Consortium. Transoral incisionless fundoplication for recurrent symptoms after laparoscopic fundoplication. Surg Endosc. 2023;37(5):3701–9. https://doi.org/10.1007/s00464-023-09880-4.

Endoscopic Ablative Therapies

Sriya S. Muralidharan and Uzma D. Siddiqui

Abstract The treatment of Barrett's esophagus (BE) has been revolutionized by the introduction of radiofrequency ablation (RFA) and cryoablation (CA) therapy. These are subsets of endoscopic eradication therapy for BE, which also includes endoscopic submucosal dissection and endoscopic mucosal resection. In this chapter, we will review the efficacy, safety, and outcomes of RFA and CA use for the treatment of Barrett's esophagus with dysplasia and intramucosal adenocarcinoma.

Keywords Barrett's Esophagus · Radiofrequency ablation · Cryoablation · Cryotherapy

Introduction

Barrett's esophagus (BE) is a disease entity in which intestinal metaplasia has replaced the normal stratified squamous epithelium of the esophagus [1]. Endoscopically, BE is characterized by the "salmon-colored" appearance of the esophageal mucosa. The diagnosis is defined by the presence of ≥1 centimeter of intestinal-type epithelium including the presence of goblet cells.

Greater than or equal to 3 centimeters of circumferential length is classified as "long-segment" BE whereas less than 3 centimeters of circumferential extent is classified as "short-segment" BE [2]. There are also classifications of "ultra-short" and "ultra-long" segments of BE which refer to BE extending <5 mm and ≥ 8 centimeters or more in length [3, 4]. The Prague criteria are used for the characterization of the length and circumferential extent of the Barrett's segment [5]. BE should also be evaluated endoscopically for the presence or absence of nodular mucosa.

S. S. Muralidharan · U. D. Siddiqui (✉)
Center for Endoscopic Research and Therapeutics (CERT), University of Chicago, Chicago, IL, USA
e-mail: usiddiqui@bsd.uchicago.edu

F. Schlottmann, M. A. Masrur (eds.), *Endoscopic, Laparoscopic and Robotic Techniques for Foregut Disorders*, https://doi.org/10.1007/978-3-032-00811-4_16

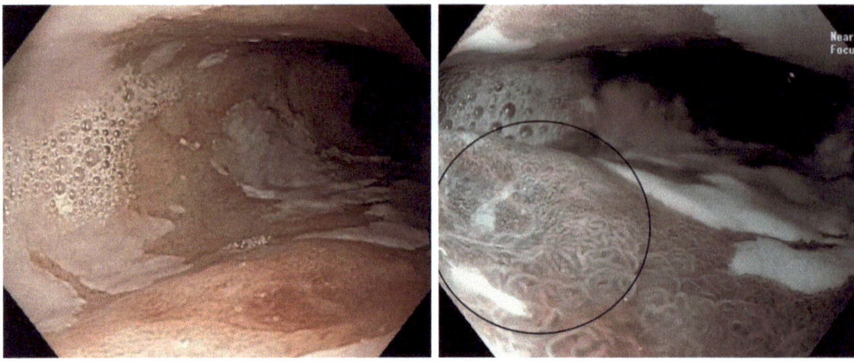

Fig. 1 Narrow Band Imaging (NBI) of Barrett's with high grade dysplasia

Nodular mucosa refers to raised lesions or irregularity in the esophageal mucosal surface that may suggest the presence of cellular dysplasia or adenocarcinoma [6] (Fig. 1).

The presence of dysplastic cells is a pre-malignant condition preceding the development of esophageal adenocarcinoma. The degree of dysplasia is categorized into low-grade and high-grade dysplasia. Governing bodies including the American College of Gastroenterology, the American Society for GI Endoscopy, and the American Gastroenterology Association all recommend the use of endoscopic-eradication therapies for the treatment of recurrent low-grade dysplasia and any occurrence of high-grade dysplasia [1, 7, 8].

Procedure Description

Previous Treatment Options and their Limitations

The pathogenesis of BE begins with esophageal injury from gastroesophageal reflux [9, 10]. Some abnormalities in patients with GERD that predispose to BE include hypotension of the lower esophageal sphincter, esophageal hypomotility, hypersecretion of gastric acid, and proposed decreased salivary secretion of epidermal growth factor (EGF) [11, 12]. Ultimately, it is thought that molecular changes lead to the transformation of esophageal squamous epithelial cells into columnar cells [13, 14].

When an endoscopist identifies mucosa suggestive of BE during an upper endoscopy, biopsies are obtained using the Seattle protocol. The Seattle protocol involves taking cold-forceps biopsies in four quadrants every one to two centimeters along the length of the abnormal appearing segment [5]. Pathology can then determine with immunohistochemical staining if the segment demonstrates normal squamous mucosa, non-dysplastic intestinal metaplasia, low-grade dysplasia, high-grade dysplasia, or adenocarcinoma. Additional imaging adjuncts can improve the diagnostic rate [15, 16].

The likelihood of BE being present in all upper endoscopies has been reported between 5% and 15% [17]. The risk of low-grade dysplasia progressing to high-grade dysplasia is increased with the presence of p53 and ki67, which can be evaluated with staining [18, 19]. The annual risk of malignant conversion from intestinal metaplasia is approximately 0.3%, while the risk of malignant conversion from low-grade dysplasia is 0.5% and from high-grade dysplasia is 6% [20].

The medical treatment of BE includes acid suppression with proton pump inhibitors usually for the duration of the patient's lifetime [21]. The new class of medications termed potassium competitive acid blockers (PCABs) are being investigated for use in BE [22].

Endoscopic ablative methods were first introduced to BE in the late 1990s. Prior to the development and widespread use of endoscopic resection and ablation techniques, the presence of high-grade dysplasia resulted in more frequent surveillance and sometimes esophagectomy. The presence of adenocarcinoma would typically lead to esophagectomy regardless of stage [23]. The combination of BE screening and ablative methods are aimed at decreasing the incidence of esophageal adenocarcinoma and the need for invasive treatments. Endoscopic ultrasound is now widely used to stage adenocarcinoma [24]. Both high-grade dysplasia (stage 0) and esophageal adenocarcinoma that has invaded only to the mucosa, termed intramucosal adenocarcinoma (stage 1a), can potentially respond to endoscopic ablative therapies if accurately staged initially [25]. It is imperative to have a detailed and thorough initial exam to ensure there is no invasive cancer present prior initiating ablative therapies for Barrett's esophagus.

Radiofrequency Ablation

Radiofrequency (RF) ablation was first introduced to the medical field in the form of the Bovie knife in 1982. RFA has since been adapted for use in multiple specialties. RFA was first applied to the esophagus using a porcine and human esophageal model in the 1970s [26]. Then RFA was approved for use endoscopically by the Food and Drug Administration in 2005.

Radiofrequency is the range on the electromagnetic spectrum from 3 hertz to 300 megahertz [27]. When applied as a high-frequency current, it is converted into thermal energy that causes coagulative necrosis of the tissue. As with electrosurgical platforms, a pulsed current at radiofrequency causes cauterization of tissue, while a continuous current allows for cutting of tissue [27, 28].

The components of all RFA application include a generator for the current, a transmitter such as a needle or a catheter probe, and the tissue itself. Mechanistically, this means the tip of the RFA transmitter does not become hot. Rather, the transmitter and tip are part of the delivery mechanism of the radiofrequency waves to the tissue molecules. The tissue molecules then become agitated and conduct the thermal energy. Similarly to electrocautery, the current can be applied through a bipolar or a monopolar probe, changing the depth and area of tissue exposure.

Currently, Barrx (Medtronic, Minneapolis, MN, USA) is the only manufacturer of RFA catheters. The catheters are either inserted through the accessory channel of the endoscope (through the scope device), attached to the tip of the endoscope (focal catheter) (Fig. 2), or over a guidewire independent from the scope (balloon catheter). The balloon design, called the Halo-360, allows for circumferential RF application, while the focal and through the scope designs allows for targeted application of smaller areas with RFA [29]. There is a newer Halo 360 "express" catheter that has a "self-adjusting" balloon that sizes to the patient's esophageal lumen to make administration simpler [30]. Each cycle of RF lasts approximately 1–2 s.

During the procedure, the target area is first defined by visualization of the proximal to distal extents. These can be better visualized with the use of narrow-band imaging to visualize the mucosa. The esophagus is also examined for irregularity of the mucosa as well as for strictures or other anatomic limitations to RFA application.

The dosing of RFA is based on several factors. These include the energy setting itself, the treatment area, total number of applications, and the tissue appearance in response. The energy settings for RFA are reported in joules per centimeter squared (J/cm^2). The settings are generally pre-determined by the manufacturer for safety purposes, but most commonly is 12 J/cm^2 for treating dysplasia. Typically, treatment begins distally and moves proximally to treat the entire visible Barrett's segment. The depth of effect with each treatment is 500 micrometers [31]. The depth of low and high-grade dysplasia is generally limited to the mucosa, which is approximately 1000 micrometers in depth. As a result, the catheter tip—whether it is the balloon or focal design—should be well-apposed to the mucosa to offer sufficient effect.

After the first session, RFA is re-applied 8–12 weeks after the initial application, and can be repeated every 2–3 months thereafter until BE is eradicated. In the

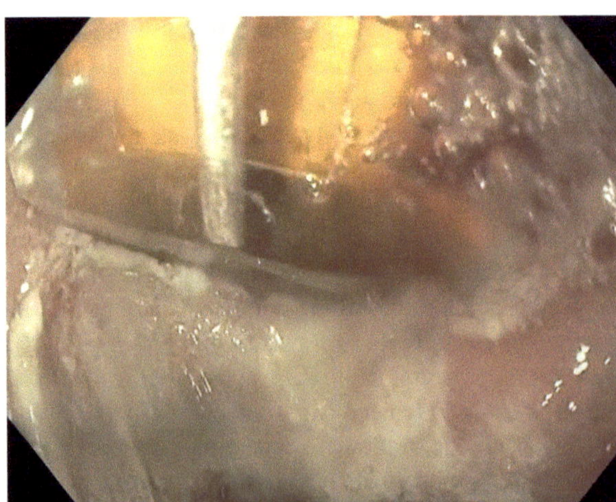

Fig. 2 Focal RFA

landmark randomized controlled trial of RFA in BE with dysplasia (AIM Dysplasia Trial, Shaheen et al), 127 patients with low-grade dysplasia or high-grade dysplasia received up to 4 treatments in 1 year, at 0, 2, 4, and 9 months [32]. Regardless of dysplasia, this study found that 77.4% who received ablation achieved complete eradication of intestinal metaplasia. Furthermore, in patients with low-grade dysplasia, complete eradication of dysplasia was seen in 90.5% and in patients with high-grade dysplasia, complete eradication of dysplasia was achieved in 81.0% [33]. Disease progression after 1 year was also assessed as a secondary outcome. The study found that in patients with high-grade dysplasia, 2.4% of patients receiving RFA had progression to adenocarcinoma. They also found that in the control group of patients with high-grade dysplasia who did not receive RFA, 19.0% (or 4 patients) had progression to adenocarcinoma (primarily intramucosal).

Cryoablation

Cryoablation is a form of cryotherapy that has been applied to BE eradication. Cryotherapy was first investigated as an oncologic treatment in the nineteenth century and has since been applied through both surgical and percutaneous techniques [34, 35]. The principle of cryotherapy involves freezing the esophageal epithelium using a liquefied gas. Nitrous oxide or carbon dioxide are typically used to induce extra and intra-cellular ice formation. This exposure stimulates apoptosis of the lesion, and at a later phase, leads to an unfavorable milieu for tissue regeneration due to reperfusion injury in the post-thaw period [36, 37].

There are two FDA-approved endoscopic cryoablation systems currently available. One is a spray that utilizes liquid nitrogen in a spray formulation, and the other applies nitrous oxide in a balloon design. Both devices can be passed through the accessory channel of a standard endoscope. The spray formulation, called the truFreeze system (Steris, Cleveland, OH, USA), is applied through a catheter without requiring direct contact of the catheter to the tissue (Fig. 3). This allows for both focal and more diffuse application of cryotherapy (Cryospray). Notably, as the liquefied nitrogen evaporates, there is a risk of perforation [38, 39]. This is mitigated using an orogastric decompression tube and careful monitoring. The balloon design is called the C2 CryoBalloon Focal Ablation System (Pentax, Montvale, NJ, USA) (Fig. 4). As the name suggests, the CryoBalloon system allows for focal application of cryotherapy using nitrous oxide for BE. No decompression tube is needed with this device.

Compared to RFA, there are overall less data on the efficacy of cryoablation for BE and dysplasia eradication as this has not gained as widespread usage. Cryospray therapy was first studied prospectively as a primary therapy for BE with dysplasia through the National Cryospray Registry [40]. In a multicenter prospective study, spray cryotherapy was applied in 2–3 cycles of twenty seconds or four cycles of 10-second freezes. This was repeated every two to three months until there was endoscopic eradication of BE, as well as no histologic dysplasia. The study found

Fig. 3 Cryospray

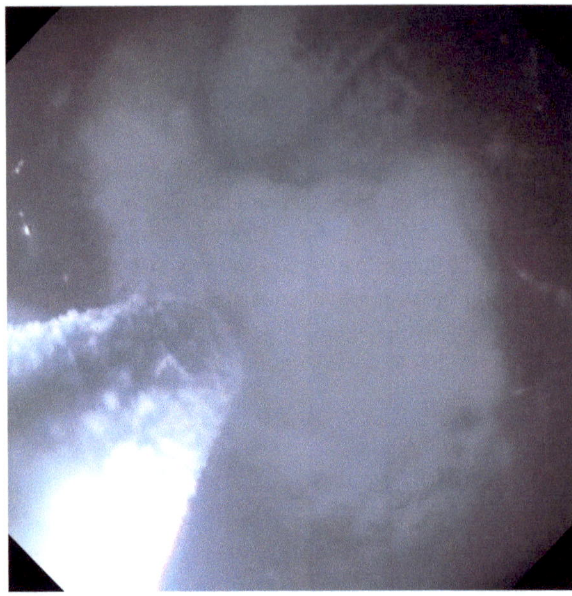

Fig. 4 Cryoballoon

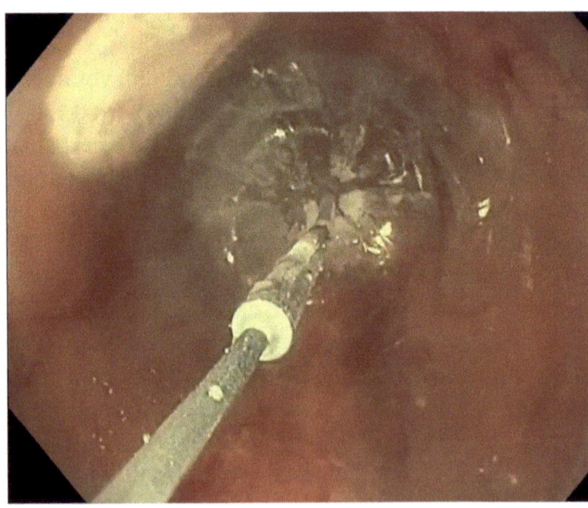

that of patients with low-grade dysplasia, with an average of 2.9 Cryospray sessions, 91% had eradication of dysplasia, and 68% had eradication of intestinal metaplasia. Those with high-grade dysplasia received an average of 3.5 Cryospray sessions, and 81% had eradication of dysplasia and 65% had eradication of intestinal metaplasia.

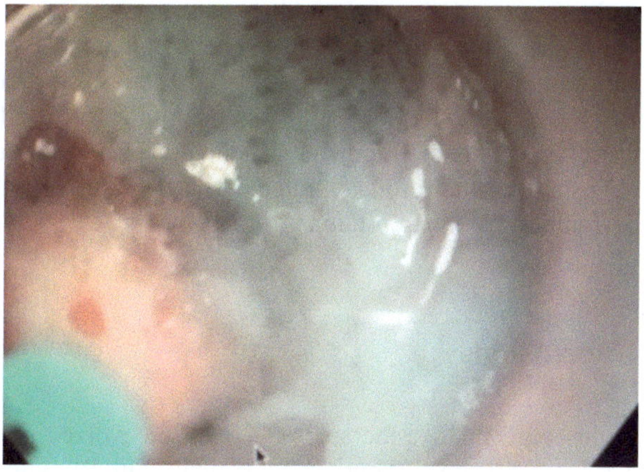

Fig. 5 Hybrid APC

Hybrid Argon Plasma Coagulation (Hybrid APC)

Hybrid APC involves performing a submucosal injection and then applying APC to the Barrett's mucosa (Fig. 5). The submucosal lifting is done to reduce the risk of injury to the muscle layer of the esophageal wall. There is limited data on this technique but one small study of 50 patients showed efficacy in eradicating residual BE after endoscopic mucosal resection of early cancer. This study showed a complete endoscopic remission in 96% and histological eradication in 78% [41]. More long-term data on safety and efficacy are needed before this modality gains widespread use.

Complications and Contraindications with Endoscopic Ablation Techniques

Adverse events associated with all types of endoscopic ablation used to treat BE includes strictures (5%), chest pain (20%), and less commonly bleeding or perforation (<1%) [1]. Risk factors for complications include ablation of longer Barrett's segments and circumferential application. Typically, chest pain is the most common symptom after ablation and resolves within 24–48 h. Post procedure, the patients are advised to adjust their diets for a few days to liquid or soft consistency and given medications (i.e. carafate and vicious lidocaine). If dysphagia persists more than 2 weeks post procedure, then repeat endoscopy with dilation usually resolves any structuring.

There are no absolute contraindications to RFA of BE. However, there are a few relative contraindications to consider. Prior radiation therapy could lead to greater risk of stricture formation and is associated with poor healing [42]. RFA should not be used on raised or nodular mucosa because there could potentially be underlying malignancy and therefore endoscopic mucosal resection to create a more even mucosal surface [41]. RFA alone is not recommended in the presence of esophageal varices that have not previously been treated. Contraindications to cryotherapy of BE include stricture preventing passage of the CryoBalloon device, active gastrointestinal bleeding or significant esophagitis [43]. Caution must be taken when using Cryospray in the setting of altered anatomy due to a theoretical increased risk of perforation from barotrauma [44].

Conclusions

Endoscopic ablative therapies for BE have evolved significantly over recent years. There are now myriad options for patients with BE with dysplasia and even intramucosal adenocarcinoma that are less invasive than esophagectomy. Further comparative studies are being done to discern optimal strategies for utilizing these new therapies, particularly in specific populations.

References

1. Shaheen NJ, Falk GW, Iyer PG, Souza RF, Yadlapati RH, Sauer BG, et al. Diagnosis and management of Barrett's esophagus: an updated ACG guideline. Am J Gastroenterol. 2022;117(4):559–87.
2. Hamade N, Vennelaganti S, Parasa S, Vennalaganti P, Gaddam S, Spaander MCW, et al. Lower annual rate of progression of short-segment vs long-segment Barrett's Esophagus to Esophageal adenocarcinoma. Clin Gastroenterol Hepatol. 2019;17(5):864.
3. Anand O, Wani S, Sharma P. When and how to grade Barrett's columnar metaplasia: the Prague system. Best Pract Res Clin Gastroenterol. 2008;22(4):661–9.
4. Dulai PS, Pohl H, Levenick JM, Gordon SR, MacKenzie TA, Rothstein RI. Radiofrequency ablation for long- and ultralong-segment Barrett's esophagus: a comparative long-term follow-up study. Gastrointest Endosc. 2013;77(4):534–41.
5. Muthusamy VR, Wani S, Gyawali CP, Komanduri S, Bergman J, Canto MI, et al. AGA clinical Practice update on new technology and innovation for surveillance and screening in Barrett's Esophagus: expert review. Clin Gastroenterol Hepatol. 2022;20(12):2696.
6. Draganov PV, Wang AY, Othman MO, Fukami N. AGA institute clinical Practice update: endoscopic submucosal dissection in the United States. Clin Gastroenterol Hepatol. 2019;17(1):16–25.e1.
7. Qumseya B, Sultan S, Bain P, Jamil L, Jacobson B, Anandasabapathy S, et al. ASGE guideline on screening and surveillance of Barrett's esophagus. Prepared by: ASGE Standards of Practice Committee. Gastrointest Endosc. 2019;90(3):335–359.e2.
8. Rubenstein JH, Sawas T, Wani S, Eluri S, Singh S, Chandar AK, et al. AGA clinical practice guideline on endoscopic eradication therapy of Barrett's esophagus and related neoplasia. Gastroenterology. 2024;166(6):1020–55.
9. Souza RF. Reflux esophagitis and its role in the pathogenesis of Barrett's metaplasia. J Gastroenterol. 2017;52(7):767–76.
10. Que J, Garman KS, Souza RF, Spechler SJ. Pathogenesis and cells of origin of Barrett's Esophagus. Gastroenterology. 2019;157(2):349.

11. Martinucci I, Bortoli N de, Giacchino M, Bodini G, Marabotto E, Marchi S, et al. Esophageal motility abnormalities in gastroesophageal reflux disease. World J Gastrointest Pharmacol Ther 2014;5(2):86.
12. Saha B, Vantanasiri K, Mohan BP, Goyal R, Garg N, Gerberi D, et al. Prevalence of Barrett's Esophagus and Esophageal adenocarcinoma with and without gastroesophageal reflux: a systematic review and meta-analysis. Clin Gastroenterol Hepatol. 2024;22(7):1381–1394.e7.
13. Aichler M, Walch A. In brief: the (molecular) pathogenesis of Barrett's oesophagus. J Pathol. 2014;232(4):383–5.
14. Vithayathil M, Modolell I, Ortiz-Fernandez-Sordo J, Oukrif D, Pappas A, Januszewicz W, et al. Image-enhanced endoscopy and molecular biomarkers vs Seattle protocol to diagnose dysplasia in Barrett's esophagus. Clin Gastroenterol Hepatol. 2022;20(11):2514–2523.e3.
15. Kolb JM, Wani S. Barrett's esophagus: current standards in advanced imaging. Transl. Gastroenterol Hepatol. 2021:6.
16. Meinikheim M, Messmann H, Ebigbo A. Role of artificial intelligence in diagnosing Barrett's esophagus-related neoplasia. Clin Endosc. 2023;56(1):14–22.
17. Lewis JD. Barrett's esophagus: the long and the short of it. Gastroenterology. 2000;119(4):1165–6.
18. Skacel M, Petras RE, Gramlich TL, Sigel JE, Richter JE, Goldblum JR. The diagnosis of low-grade dysplasia in Barrett's esophagus and its implications for disease progression. Am J Gastroenterol. 2000;95(12):3383–7.
19. Weston AP, Banerjee SK, Sharma P, Tran TM, Richards R, Cherian R. p53 protein overexpression in low grade dysplasia (LGD) in Barrett's esophagus: immunohistochemical marker predictive of progression. Am J Gastroenterol. 2001;96(5):1355–62.
20. Rastogi A, Puli S, El-Serag HB, Bansal A, Wani S, Sharma P. Incidence of esophageal adenocarcinoma in patients with Barrett's esophagus and high-grade dysplasia: a meta-analysis. Gastrointest Endosc. 2008;67(3):394–8.
21. Haag S, Nandurkar S, Talley NJ. Regression of Barrett's esophagus: the role of acid suppression, surgery, and ablative methods. Gastrointest Endosc. 1999;50(2):229–40.
22. Wong N, Reddy A, Patel A. Potassium-competitive acid blockers: present and potential utility in the armamentarium for acid peptic disorders. Gastroenterol Hepatol (N Y). 2022;18(12):693.
23. Avery KNL, Metcalfe C, Berrisford R, Barham CP, Donovan JL, Elliott J, et al. The feasibility of a randomized controlled trial of esophagectomy for esophageal cancer–the ROMIO (Randomized Oesophagectomy: Minimally Invasive or Open) study: protocol for a randomized controlled trial. Trials. 2014;15(1):200.
24. Weusten BLAM, Bisschops R, Dinis-Ribeiro M, di Pietro M, Pech O, Spaander MCW, et al. Diagnosis and management of Barrett esophagus: European Society of Gastrointestinal Endoscopy (ESGE) guideline. Endoscopy. 2023;55(12):1124–46.
25. Radlinski M, Shami VM. Role of endoscopic ultrasound in esophageal cancer. World J Gastrointest Endosc. 2022;14(4):205–14.
26. Ganz RA, Utley DS, Stern RA, Jackson J, Batts KP, Termin P. Complete ablation of esophageal epithelium with a balloon-based bipolar electrode: a phased evaluation in the porcine and in the human esophagus. Gastrointest Endosc. 2004;60(6):1002–10.
27. Hong K, Georgiades C. Radiofrequency ablation: mechanism of action and devices. J Vasc Interv Radiol. 2010;21(8):S179–86.
28. Chaudhary S, Sun SY. Endoscopic ultrasound-guided radiofrequency ablation in gastroenterology: new horizons in search. World J Gastroenterol. 2017;23(27):4892.
29. Fleischer DE, Sharma VK. Endoscopic ablation of Barrett's Esophagus using the halo® system. Dig Dis. 2009;26(4):280.
30. Phoa KN, Van Vilsteren FGI, Weusten BLAM, Bisschops R, Schoon EJ, Ragunath K, et al. Radiofrequency ablation vs endoscopic surveillance for patients with Barrett esophagus and low-grade dysplasia: a randomized clinical trial. JAMA. 2014;311(12):1209–17.

31. Levink IJM, Tearney GJ, Erler NS, Wolfsen HC, Siersema PD, Wallace MB. Barrett's epithelial thickness, assessed by volumetric laser endomicroscopy, is associated with response to radiofrequency ablation. Clin Gastroenterol Hepatol. 2021;19(6):1160–1169.e2.
32. Shaheen NJ, Sharma P, Overholt BF, Wolfsen HC, Sampliner RE, Wang KK, et al. Radiofrequency ablation in Barrett's esophagus with dysplasia. N Engl J Med. 2009;360(22):2277–88.
33. Shaheen NJ, Overholt BF, Sampliner RE, Wolfsen HC, Wang KK, Fleischer DE, et al. Durability of radiofrequency ablation in Barrett's esophagus with dysplasia. Gastroenterology. 2011;141(2):460–8.
34. Hui GC, Tuncali K, Tatli S, Morrison PR, Silverman SG. Comparison of percutaneous and surgical approaches to renal tumor ablation: metaanalysis of effectiveness and complication rates. J Vasc Interv Radiol. 2008;19(9):1311–20.
35. Arnott J. Practical illustrations of the remedial efficacy of a very low or anæsthetic temperature.—I. In cancer. Lancet. 1850 Aug 31;56(1409):257–9.
36. Freund S, Probst A, Messmann H. Update on ablative therapy for Barrett's related dysplasia. Annals of Esophagus 2023;6(0).
37. Vantanasiri K, Iyer PG. State-of-the-art management of dysplastic Barrett's esophagus. Gastroenterol Rep (Oxf). 2022:10.
38. Lal P, Thota PN. Cryotherapy in the management of premalignant and malignant conditions of the esophagus. World J Gastroenterol. 2018;24(43):4862.
39. Greenwald BD, Dumot JA, Abrams JA, Lightdale CJ, David DS, Nishioka NS, et al. Endoscopic spray cryotherapy for esophageal cancer: safety and efficacy. Gastrointest Endosc. 2010;71(4):686–93.
40. Ghorbani S, Tsai FC, Greenwald BD, Jang S, Dumot JA, Mckinley MJ, et al. Safety and efficacy of endoscopic spray cryotherapy for Barrett's dysplasia: results of the National Cryospray Registry. Dis Esophagus. 2016;29(3):241–7.
41. Manner H, May A, Kouti I, et al. Efficacy and safety of hybrid APC for the ablation of Barrett's esophagus. Surg Endosc. 2016;30(4):1364–70. https://doi.org/10.1007/s00464-015-4336-1.
42. Rouphael C, Anil Kumar M, Sanaka MR, Thota PN. Indications, contraindications and limitations of endoscopic therapy for Barrett's esophagus and early esophageal adenocarcinoma. Ther Adv Gastroenterol. 2020:13.
43. Alzoubaidi D, Hussein M, Sehgal V, Makahamadze C, Magee CG, Everson M, et al. Cryoballoon ablation for treatment of patients with refractory esophageal neoplasia after first line endoscopic eradication therapy. Endosc Int Open. 2020;8(7):E891.
44. Parsi MA, Trindade AJ, Bhutani MS, Melson J, Navaneethan U, Thosani N, et al. Cryotherapy in gastrointestinal endoscopy VideoGIE 2017;2(5):89.

Anti-Reflux Mucosectomy (ARMS)

Derrius Anderson and Michael B. Ujiki

Abstract Gastroesophageal Reflux Disease (GERD) impacts approximately 20% of the population in the western world. Mainstays for treatment include proton pump inhibitors (PPIs) and anti-reflux interventions. Anti-Reflux Mucosectomy (ARMS) has emerged as a promising endoscopic anti-reflux procedure. In this chapter, we describe each surgical step of the endoscopic ARMS procedure.

Keywords Gastroesophageal reflux disease · Endoscopic surgery · Anti-reflux mucosectomy · Anti-reflux surgery

Introduction

Gastroesophageal Reflux Disease (GERD) affects approximately 20% of the population in the western world [1]. Standard treatment for GERD includes antiacid medical therapy or surgical intervention to reinforce the gastroesophageal junction (GEJ) to prevent reflux. Anti-reflux interventions have been proven as durable long-term interventions for improving patient symptoms and quality of life [2–4].

In 2003, Inoue et al. published a case study where a patient who underwent endoscopic mucosal resection (EMR) for Barrett's Esophagus at the GEJ had subjective improvement of their acid reflux symptoms [5]. From there the procedure was refined and the first case series was published in 2014. Ten patients underwent an

D. Anderson
Department of Surgery, Endeavor Health, Evanston, IL, USA

M. B. Ujiki (✉)
Department of Surgery, Endeavor Health, Evanston, IL, USA

Department of Surgery, NorthShore University Health System, Evanston, IL, USA
e-mail: MUjiki@northshore.org

F. Schlottmann, M. A. Masrur (eds.), *Endoscopic, Laparoscopic and Robotic Techniques for Foregut Disorders*, https://doi.org/10.1007/978-3-032-00811-4_17

Anti-Reflux Mucosectomy (ARMS) procedure and were found to have improved subjective GERD symptoms and DeMeester scores following their endoscopic intervention [6]. Within this chapter, we discuss the procedural steps for successful completion of the ARMS procedure.

Procedure Description

Pre-operative Evaluation

Indications for undergoing an ARMS procedure include patients who have failed medical management of GERD or patients who are unable to tolerate proton pump inhibitors due to side effects or medication interactions. If a patient is considered a candidate for ARMS, they must undergo a comprehensive pre-operative evaluation. This includes upper endoscopy, manometry, and pH testing. If a patient has a hiatal hernia larger than 2 cm or a hill grade score of 4, they should not be offered an ARMS procedure. Of note, this intervention has been shown to be feasible in patients who have undergone previous fundoplication or sleeve gastrectomy.

Patient Positioning

The patient is placed in supine position on the operating room table. No preoperative antibiotics are given for this procedure. Sequential compression devices are placed for mechanical venous thromboembolism prophylaxis. Once endotracheal intubation is achieved, arms are secured at the patient's side. The endotracheal tube should be positioned along of the right side of the patient's oropharynx and secured along the patient's right with the operator at the patient's left. An endoscopic bite block should be in place to protect the lips from injury between the teeth and endoscope.

Pre-procedure Endoscopy

Prior to undergoing the ARMS procedure all patients should undergo endoscopy to carefully inspect the GEJ including in retroflexion to ensure the absence of a hiatal hernia, ulcerations, or masses. Currently, we recommend the use of impedance planimetry of the GEJ for post procedural comparison.

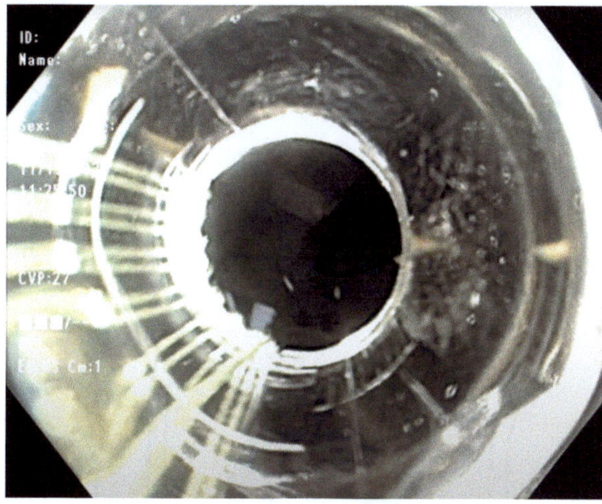

Fig. 1 CaptivatorTM EMR device affixed to GIF HQ190 endoscope. Please note the bands are located at the 7 o clock position for ease of positioning and firing around mucosal tissue

Preparation of Endoscopic Mucosal Resection (EMR) Kit

Once initial endoscopic assessment is completed, and the decision is made to proceed with a mucosectomy a CaptivatorTM EMR device (Boston Scientific, Marlborough, MA) is fixed onto a GIF HQ190 upper endoscope (Olympus, Tokyo, Japan) (Fig. 1). The bands from the EMR kit are positioned at 7 o clock to allow for easy deployment from the working channel. There are typically 6 bands included in the EMR kit with three bands fired along the anterior gastric cardia and three bands fired along the posterior gastric cardia. This butterfly pattern allows bridges of intact mucosa along the greater and lesser curve (Fig. 2). This is divergent from what was originally reported, where only the greater curve was spared. By sparing the greater and lesser curve of the stomach, there is a decreased rate of postoperative dysphagia.

Mucosal Lift and Resection

In retroflexion, the anterior and posterior gastric cardia are marked with electrocautery sparing a 1 cm bridge along the greater and lesser curve (Fig. 2). The resection begins along the anterior surface of the stomach 2 cm from the lesser curve, and proceeds in a counterclockwise fashion around the GEJ, sparing a bridge at the greater curve and lesser curve. An injector needle is passed through the working channel and the mucosa of the gastric cardia is raised with a solution of saline and indigo carmine (1 ml in 500 ml saline). To achieve mucosal lift, the needle tip must be in the submucosa and typically requires 2–3 cc of the indigo carmine solution for appropriate lift (Fig. 3). The needle is removed from the working channel, and the mucosa is suctioned into the EMR cap (Fig. 4). The band is fired when the mucosa

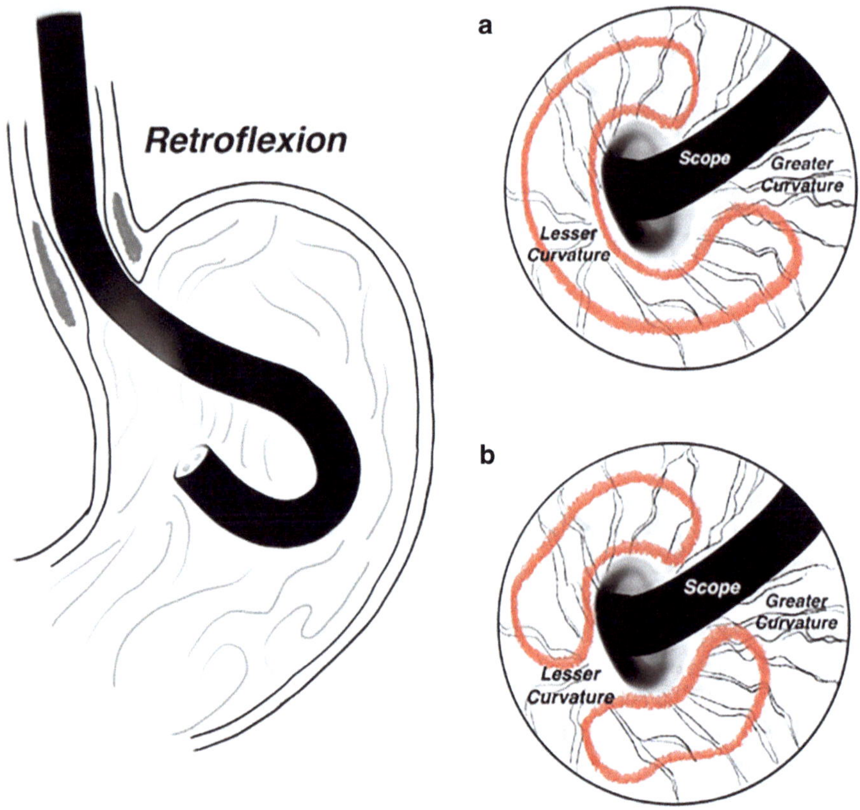

Fig. 2 Retroflexed endoscope with areas of resection outlined in red. (**a**) Depicts the original procedure with sparing of only the greater curvature. (**b**) Depicts the modified technique with sparing of the greater and lesser curvature to decrease rate of postoperative dysphagia requiring dilation. (Used with permission from: Wong et al. [7])

abuts the endoscope camera lens (Fig. 5). With the use of a snare the banded tissue is transected using forced coagulation (effect 2, max W 40) (Fig. 6).

After the tissue is transected, the submucosa is inspected for bleeding. Visible vessels or bleeding are coagulated with soft coagulation (effect 5, max W 80). The steps of lifting, snaring, and transecting the mucosa are repeated until an adequate resection is achieved along the anterior and posterior gastric cardia. The bands of mucosa will typically collect in the gastric fundus and can be retrieved by a Roth net at the conclusion of the case or allowed to pass into the gastrointestinal tract (Fig. 7).

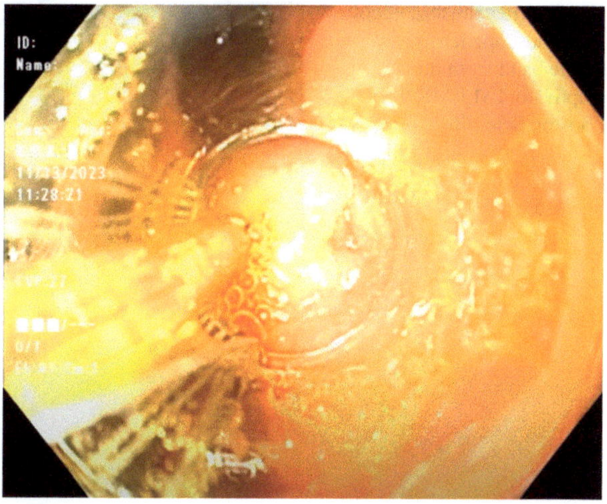

Fig. 3 Injector needle entering mucosa from the working channel at 7 o clock to lift mucosa from submucosa in preparation for mucosectomy

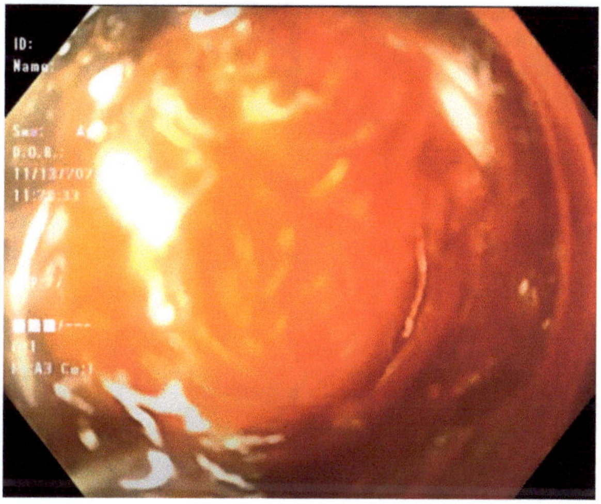

Fig. 4 Suctioning of lifted mucosa into the CaptivatorTM EMR device (Boston Scientific, Marlborough, MA) cap until it abuts the endoscope lens

Postoperative Care

Post operatively it is crucial that patients tolerate oral intake to have the ability to remain hydrated once discharged home. The post operative diet is limited to a soft pureed diet for 2 weeks post procedure. Proton pump inhibitors can be discontinued immediately following the procedure or weaned over a few weeks post operatively; this decision is made via surgeon preference. Acetaminophen and NSAIDs are

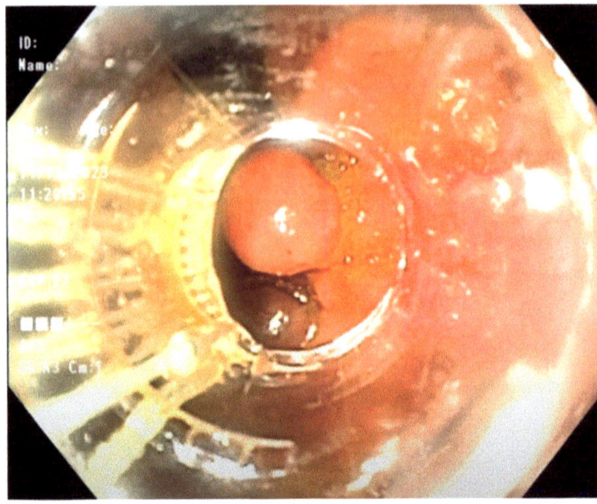

Fig. 5 After mucosa abuts the endoscope lens, a single band from the CaptivatorTM EMR device (Boston Scientific, Marlborough, MA) is fired to encompass the lifted mucosa

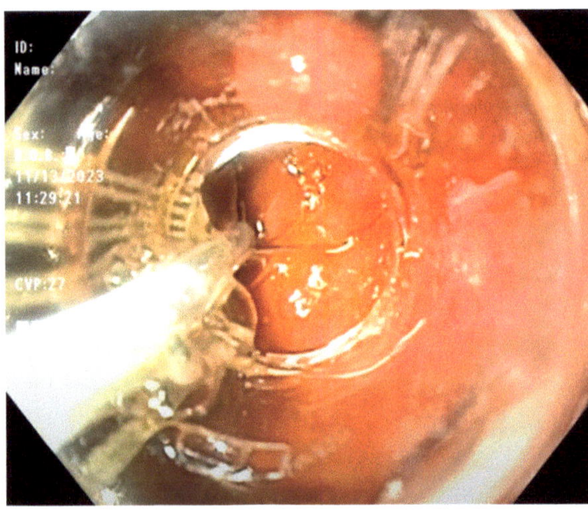

Fig. 6 Snaring of the banded mucosal tissue for resection

routinely adequate for pain control post procedure. A weak narcotic can be prescribed if necessary for discomfort not controlled with acetaminophen or NSAIDs. The most common post procedure complication is typically dysphagia, which is usually managed with diet (full liquid or soft diet) and lifestyle modifications. Patients are encouraged to drink plenty of water with meals to aid in swallowing. Balloon dilation is typically employed for dysphagia lasting beyond 6 weeks.

Conflict of Interest Michael B. Ujiki and Derrius Anderson declare that they have no conflicts of interest.

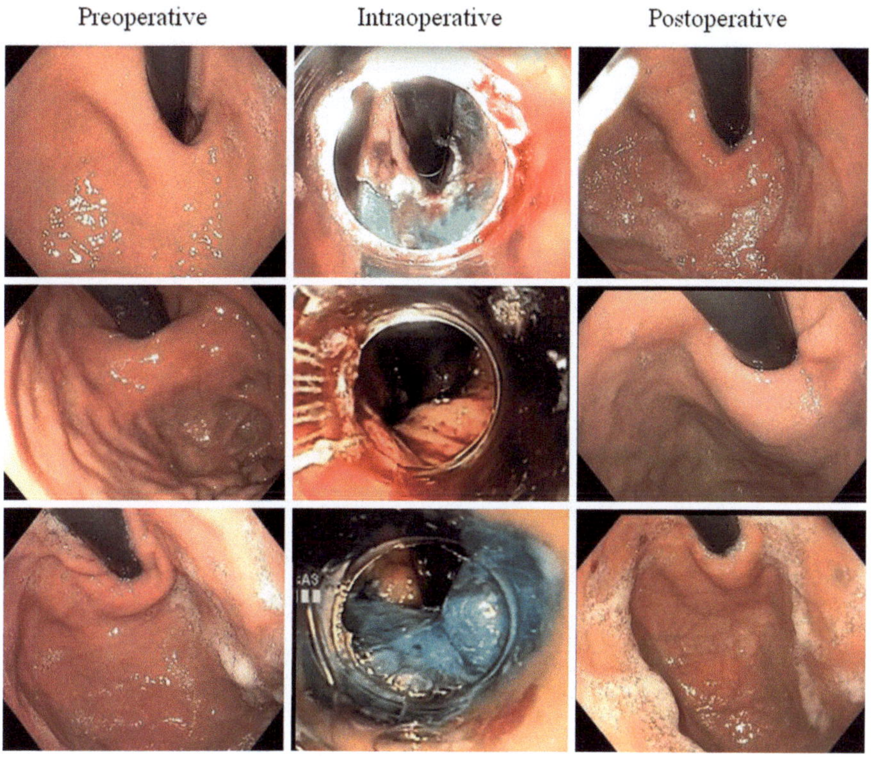

Fig. 7 Overview of the anti-reflux mucosectomy procedure

References

1. Maret-Ouda J, Markar SR, Lagergren J. Gastroesophageal reflux disease. JAMA. 2020;324(24):2565. https://doi.org/10.1001/jama.2020.21573.
2. Lee YS, Kim JH, Yon DK, Yoo IK. Short and long term effect of anti-reflux mucosectomy with cap-assisted endoscopic mucosal resection for refractory gastroesophageal disease. Surg Endosc. 2024;38(4):2180–7. https://doi.org/10.1007/s00464-024-10766-2.
3. Sadowitz BD, Luberice K, Bowman TA, et al. A single institution's first 100 patients undergoing laparoscopic anti-reflux fundoplications: where are they 20 years later?: the American surgeon. Am Surg. 2015;81(8):791–7.
4. Salvador R, Vittori A, Capovilla G, et al. Antireflux surgery's lifespan: 20 years after laparoscopic fundoplication. J Gastrointest Surg. 2023;27(11):2325–35. https://doi.org/10.1007/s11605-023-05797-4.
5. Satodate H, Inoue H, Yoshida T, et al. Circumferential EMR of carcinoma arising in Barrett's esophagus: case report. Gastrointest Endosc. 2003;58(2):288–92. https://doi.org/10.1067/mge.2003.361.
6. Inoue H, Ito H, Ikeda H, et al. Anti-reflux mucosectomy for gastroesophageal reflux disease in the absence of hiatus hernia: a pilot study. Ann Gastroenterol Q Publ Hell Soc Gastroenterol. 2014;27(4):346–51.
7. Wong HJ, Su B, Attaar M, et al. Anti-reflux mucosectomy (ARMS) results in improved recovery and similar reflux quality of life outcomes compared to laparoscopic Nissen fundoplication. Surg Endosc. 2021;35:7174–82. https://doi.org/10.1007/s00464-020-08144-9.

Magnetic Sphincter Augmentation

Katie M. Galvin and Caitlin Houghton

Abstract Gastroesophageal reflux disease (GERD) is prevalent condition associated with heartburn, dysphagia, and regurgitation. It arises from a malfunctioning lower esophageal sphincter (LES) and an abnormal esophageal hiatus or hiatal hernia. The magnetic sphincter augmentation (MSA) device (LINX Reflux Management System, Ethicon, Johnson & Johnson) offers an effective alternative to traditional gastric fundoplication of the esophagus for treating GERD. In addition to serving as an alternative to Nissen fundoplication, the MSA device is particularly valuable for patients who have previously undergone sleeve gastrectomy—a group for whom fundoplication is typically not viable due to the lack of a sufficient gastric fundus. The MSA presents several advantages over the Nissen procedure for the right candidates, including shorter operative and recovery times, the preservation of the ability to belch or vomit, and the reversibility of the device, which can be easily removed without altering gastric anatomy.

Keywords Gastroesophageal reflux disease (GERD) · Lower esophageal sphincter (LES) · Magnetic sphincter augmentation (MSA) device · Robotic surgery · Sleeve gastrectomy · Barrett's esophagus

K. M. Galvin (✉) · C. Houghton
Department of Surgery, University of Southern California, Keck, Los Angeles, CA, USA
e-mail: Katie.galvin@med.usc.edu

F. Schlottmann, M. A. Masrur (eds.), *Endoscopic, Laparoscopic and Robotic Techniques for Foregut Disorders*, https://doi.org/10.1007/978-3-032-00811-4_18

Introduction

Gastroesophageal reflux disease (GERD) is a common and often chronic condition leading to symptoms such as heartburn, regurgitation, dysphagia, and chest pain. GERD is due to a weakened or dysfunctional lower esophageal sphincter (LES) in conjunction with an abnormal hiatus. Despite the use of acid suppression drugs, the incidence of GERD continues to increase with patients having varying degrees of response to proton pump inhibitors (PPI) therapy.

One innovative surgical option for patients with GERD is the magnetic sphincter augmentation (MSA) device (LINX Reflux Management System, Ethicon, Johnson & Johnson) which provides an equally efficacious alternative to fundoplication. This device offers an effective alternative to traditional fundoplication without altering the anatomical structure of the stomach or gastroesophageal junction. Instead, it works by augmenting the LES, creating a functional barrier to reflux. Following the passage of food, the magnetic beads in the device are drawn back together through magnetic attraction, effectively restoring the integrity of the LES (Fig. 1).

The MSA can be utilized regardless of whether a hiatal hernia is present or if the gastric fundus has been surgically removed, and it is associated with a lower incidence of postoperative complications, such as the inability to belch or vomit, compared to conventional anti-reflux surgical procedures.

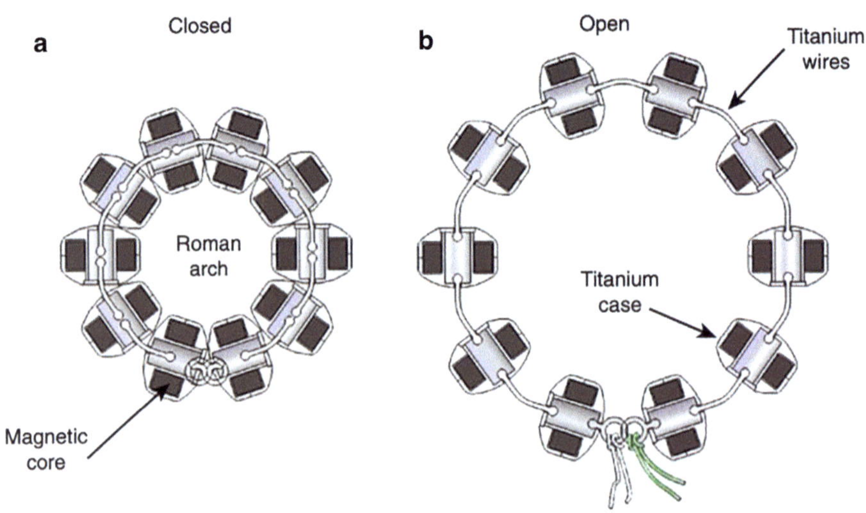

Fig. 1 Magnetic sphincter augmentation device (Linx). The MSA device consists of an expansile bracelet-like ring of magnetic beads to be placed around the distal esophagus. The beads are connected by independently articulating titanium wires, limiting device expansion and maintaining bead spacing. (**a**) At rest the magnetic forces keep the MSA device in the closed configuration without exerting pressure on the wall of the esophagus, maintaining its configuration to Roman arch design. (**b**) Expanded. (Courtesy Ethicon US, LLC.)

Table 1 Contraindication and precautions to the use of the MSA

Contraindications	
	Known or suspected allergy to titanium, nickel, steel, or any ferrous metal
Precautions	
	Scleroderma
	Suspected or confirmed esophageal or gastric cancer
	Prior esophageal or gastric surgery or endoscopic intervention
	Distal esophageal motility <35 mm Hg peristaltic amplitude on wet swallows or <70% (propulsive) peristaltic sequences on high-resolution manometry equivalent, or known motility disorder
	Symptoms of dysphagia more than once/week within the last 3 months
	Esophageal or gastric varices
	Lactating, pregnant, or planning to become pregnant
	Age <21 years
	Los Angeles classification grade C or D esophagitis
	Patients with electrical implants such as pacemaker, defibrillator, or other metallic abdominal implants
Warning	
	Conditional compatibility with MRI imaging; up to 0.7 0.7 T MRI or 1.5 1.5 T, depending on early or late generation MSA device

MRI magnetic resonance imaging, *MSA* magnetic sphincter augmentation device

Indications

The MSA device is indicated in the treatment of any patient with adequate esophageal motility and an appropriate work up confirming a diagnosis of GERD, with several exceptions. The MSA device cannot be implanted in the setting of intraabdominal infection, at the time of violation of an enteric lumen, in patients with a nickel or titanium allergy or in those who have a future need for magnetic resonance imaging greater than 1.5 Tesla. In addition to these contraindications, precautions currently listed by the Food and Drug Administration can be seen in Table 1. Of note, the MSA device precautions by the FDA since approval in 2012 have changed and now can be used in patients with a size of hiatal hernia greater than 3 cm and patients with Barrett's esophagus. In addition, MSA device is now approved for pathologic reflux after sleeve gastrectomy, however the precaution for use after gastric bypass remains in place. Like the Nissen fundoplication, the MSA device is ill advised in patients with abnormal esophageal motility.

Patient Evaluation, Selection, and Exclusion

The evaluation of patients with suspected reflux is the same as it would be in preparation for a fundoplication procedure. Upper endoscopy with biopsy and pH probe must be performed to assess for hiatal hernia, esophagitis, metaplasia, dysplasia, or tumor. The diagnosis of GERD requires the objective documentation of pathologic levels of acid reflux into the esophagus. Adequate motility must be confirmed before offering any surgical anti-reflux procedure. Patients with evidence of inadequate peristalsis are not candidates for MSA.

Surgical Technique

Preparation and Positioning

Laparoscopic Approach

The patient is placed in low lithotomy with arms tucked and legs secured to facilitate steep reverse Trendelenburg positioning. Legs are kept neutral at the hips and spread at an angle to accommodate the surgeon positioned between the patient's legs.

An initial 5-mm optically guided trocar is placed without insufflation into the virgin abdomen, approximately 2 cm superior to the umbilicus and 2 cm to the left of midline. An 8-mm trocar is introduced through the left upper quadrant in midclavicular line 2 cm caudal to the costal margin. This 8-mm trocar facilitates the later introduction of the MSA device, as well as sutures to repair the hiatal hernia. A 5-mm trocar is then placed in the right upper quadrant at the mid clavicular line 2 cm inferior to the costal margin. A Nathanson hook liver retractor is introduced through a trocar stab wound directly below the xiphoid along the midline. An additional 5-mm assistant's port is placed approximately 5 cm caudal and 3 cm lateral to the 8-mm port (Fig. 2).

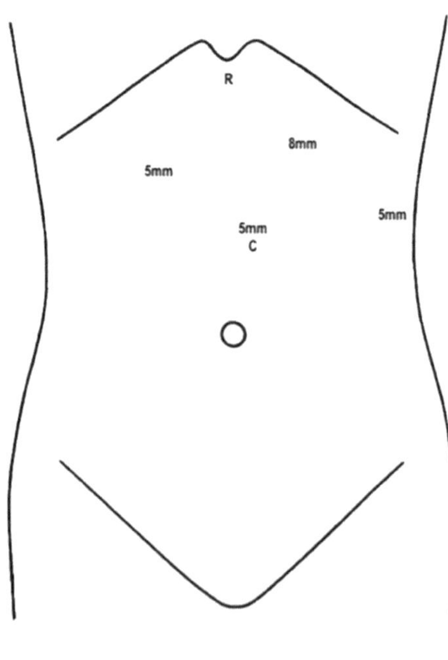

Fig. 2 Laparoscopic port placement. The Nathanson retractor is subxiphoid (R), camera above the umbilicus, with left lateral port as assistant

Preparation and Positioning

Robotic Approach

The patient is placed in the supine position with arms tucked and a foot board to facilitate 27 degrees of steep reverse Trendelenburg positioning.

An initial 5-mm optically guided trocar is placed without insufflation into the virgin abdomen, approximately 2 cm superior to the umbilicus and 2 cm to the left of midline (arm 2, camera port). An 8-mm robotic trocar is introduced through the left upper quadrant in midclavicular line 2 cm caudal to the costal margin (Arm 3, Vessel Sealer Extend). An 8-mm trocar is then placed in the right upper quadrant at the mid clavicular line 2 cm inferior to the costal margin (Arm 1, Fenestrated bipolar). An 8 mm in the left lateral position (Arm 4, Cadiere). A Nathanson hook liver retractor is introduced directly below the xiphoid along the midline. An additional 8-mm assistant's port is between arms 1 and 2 to facilitate the later introduction of the MSA device, as well as sutures to repair the hiatal hernia (Fig. 3).

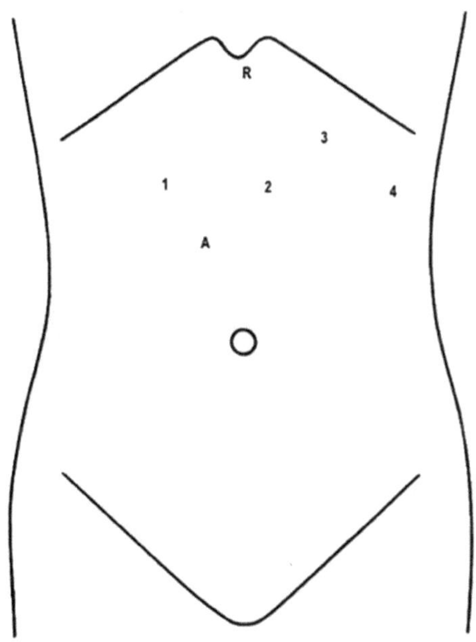

Fig. 3 Robotic port placement. Nathanson retractor subxiphoid, arm 1 is fenestrated bipolar, arm 2 is camera, arm 3 is vessel sealer extend, arm 4 is caudiere, assist port is between arms 1 and 2

Dissection of the Crura and Hiatus

The pars flaccida is opened toward the hiatus, sharp then blunt dissection of peritoneum and phrenoesophageal membrane is carried out in a clockwise fashion around the crura. The stomach is then retracted laterally toward the patient's left, and careful dissection inferior to the esophagus is completed with the creation of a retroesophageal window, through which a Penrose drain is placed. Retraction on the Penrose facilitates exposure and traction of the esophagus allowing completion of the hiatal dissection to the level of the pulmonary veins. A minimum of 3 cm of esophagus should be easily reducible into the abdomen.

Crural Closure

The right and left crura are approximated with two to three figure-of-eight 0-braided absorbable sutures and secured with tie knots to create a snug hiatal opening. Alternatively, if using the robot, a running 2–0 V lock suture from posterior to anterior to close the hiatus is used (Fig. 4).

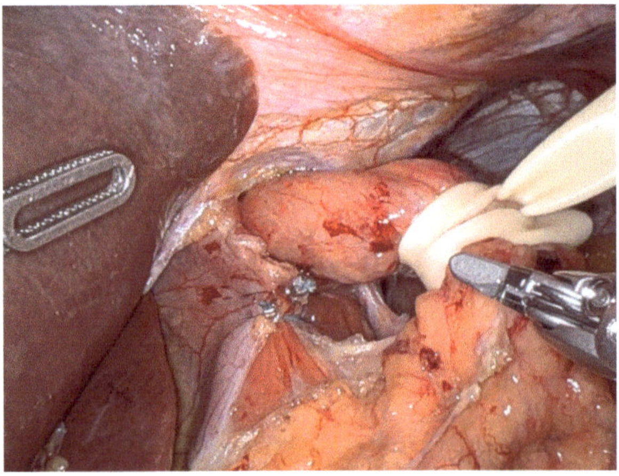

Fig. 4 Closure of the diaphragmatic crura

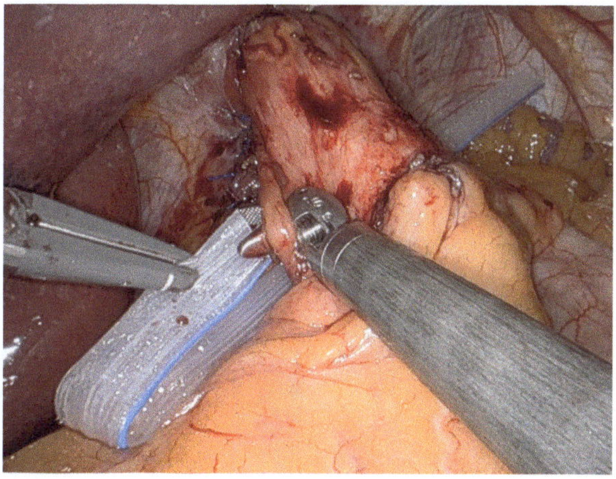

Fig. 5 Dissection of the posterior vagus nerve from the esophageal wall

Identification and Dissection of the Posterior Vagus Nerve

Identify the posterior vagus nerve at a location just proximal to the anatomic GEJ. Gently hook the nerve and pull it away from the esophageal body. Using careful and precise dissection, create a plane between the nerve and the esophagus. Next, pass a grasper between the posterior vagus nerve and the esophagus, moving from medial to lateral through the retroesophageal window. A Penrose drain is placed medially to laterally through the tunnel, anterior to the posterior vagus nerve and around the esophagus (Fig. 5).

Device Sizing

All temperature probe or gastric tubes placed by anesthesia must be removed before sizing. Ethicon Medical offers a proprietary instrument essential for device sizing. This instrument features a magnet-tipped piston that can be extended from a durable hard-plastic housing. The device is positioned along the pathway of the Penrose drain, between the posterior vagus nerve and the esophageal wall. The magnet-tipped piston is then extended and wrapped around the esophagus, securing itself loosely through magnetic attraction, thus forming a loop around the esophagus (Fig. 6).

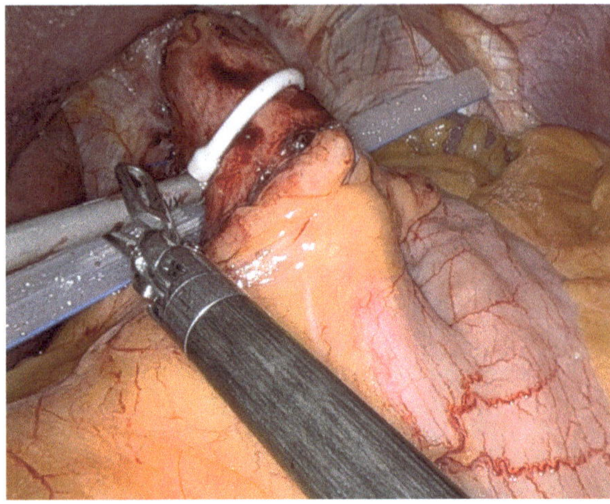

Fig. 6 Insertion of sizing device between the posterior vagus nerve and esophageal wall

The tool features a dial on its handle that, when gently retracted, tightens the sizing loop around the esophagus. Two markers are essential for determining the appropriate size. First, the sizing loop should rest comfortably around the esophagus without compressing the tissue. The sizing loop around the esophagus should still have some sliding mobility. Second, continue ratcheting down the sizing loop until the magnet separates, causing the loop to spring open, and take note of the measurement at this point. The appropriate size is three measurements larger than this loop separation, which should align with the initial visual cue of the sizing loop resting securely around the esophagus without causing compression. If these measurements do not correlate, select the larger size for device selection. A window on the device's handle indicates the size of the esophagus throughout this process. The measuring procedure is repeated twice to ensure correct measurement.

Device Placement

The MSA device is then brought into the abdomen through the 8-mm trocar or robotic assist port. The device is brought from lateral to medial around the esophagus in the same fashion as the Penrose drain was initially placed, using the looped suture on the ends for aid. The Penrose drain should be left in place, with the ends free, during insertion to aid in its passage through the retroesophageal tunnel. The free ends of the MSA device are then brought together, bring one superior and one inferior and then use gentle movements to clasp. The Penrose drain is then removed, and the looped sutures are snipped free from the device, completing the procedure (Fig. 7).

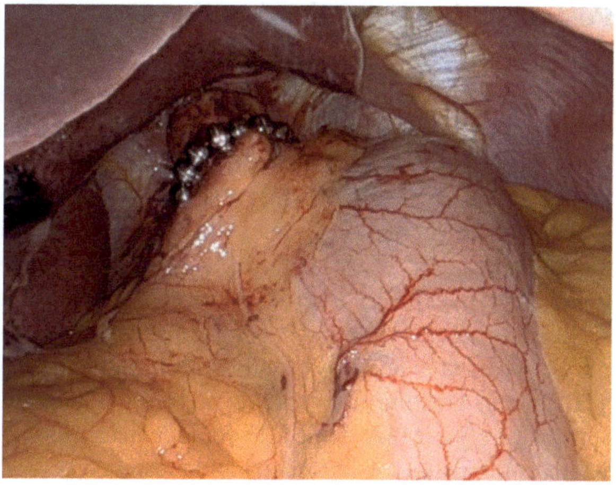

Fig. 7 MSA device placed with clasp secured in its final position, approximately 3 cm caudad to the insertion of the phrenoesophageal ligament on the esophageal wall, in the plane and flush with the diaphragmatic crura

Long-Term Outcomes

Long-term control of GERD symptoms is similar to the results after Nissen fundoplication in series extending nearly a decade since the adoption of the MSA into surgical practice. Early results suggest that the MSA device may affect some regression of Barrett's esophagus at a rate similar to what has been experienced with Nissen fundoplication. Use of Magnetic Sphincter Augmentation for patients with medically intractable GERD after laparoscopic sleeve gastrectomy was evaluated in a multi institution prospective study which showed patients were 80% better symptomatically with 50% improvement in pH parameters.

The 5 year results of the US Food and Drug Administration's approved trial evaluates the MSA device for safety and effectiveness. In terms of side effects, all patients saw marked improvement or resolution of moderate to severe regurgitation, heartburn, and gas bloat. Studies with patients with larger hiatal hernias have shown a lower recurrence rate of 6.3% when compared to Nissen recurrence rate at 30–59%, which is likely due to the adhesive inflammatory response generated at the diaphragmatic hiatus after implantation.

The 10-year follow up data provided reasonable assurance that the risk of MSA complications does not increase with longer implant duration. The MSA device does not replace fundoplication, however it provides a safe, durable alternative with a lesser side effect profile without significant safety issues after 12 years of follow up. It has also been shown to control reflux in patients with large hiatal hernias with an acceptably low recurrence rate [1–8].

Postoperative Complications

Immediate postoperative dysphagia is the most common side effect of MSA placement. Incidence and speed of resolution is reduced in patients who can take multiple small meals per day for the first 6 weeks after surgery. If patients are unable to tolerate solid foods and are struggling with oral intake, a short course of steroids usually will help them get back to eating solid food. Failure to induce frequent expansion of the MSA device with swallowing results in the MSA device becoming encapsulated in the contracted position, resulting in persistent dysphagia.

Erosion occurs in 0.3–0.4% of patients. Erosions present with new-onset dysphagia 1–3 years after surgery, usually with 1 or 2 beads having eroded into the esophageal lumen, creating a contained perforation of the esophagus into the capsule surrounding the MSA device. Eroded devices can be removed endoscopically or with a combination of endoscopy and laparoscopy.

Conflict of Interest Katie Galvin and Caitlin Houghton declare that they have no conflicts of interest.

References

1. Alicuben E, Tatum J, Bildzukewiczet N, et al. Regression of intestinal metaplasia following magnetic sphincter augmentation device placement. Surg Endosc. 2019;33(2):576–9.
2. Bonavina L, DeMeester T, Fockens P, Dunn D, Saino G, Bona D, Lipham J, Bemelman W, Ganz RA. Laparoscopic sphincter augmentation device eliminates reflux symptoms and normalizes esophageal acid exposure—one and 2 year results of a feasibility trial. Ann Surg. 2010;252:857–62.
3. Bonavina L, Saino GI, Bona D, Lipham J, Ganz RA, Dunn D, DeMeester T. Magnetic augmentation of the lower esophageal sphincter: results of a feasibility clinical trial. J Gastrointest Surg. 2008;12:2133–40.
4. Bonavina L, Saino G, Lipham JC, DeMeester TR. LINX reflux management system in chronic gastroesophageal reflux: a novel effective technology for restoring the natural barrier to reflux. Therap Adv Gastroenterol. 2013;6:261–8.
5. Bell R, Lipham J, Louie B, et al. Laparoscopic magnetic sphincter augmentation versus double-dose proton pump inhibitors for management of moderate-to-severe regurgitation in GERD: a randomized controlled trial. Gastrointest Endosc. 2019;89(1):14–22.e1.
6. Ferrari D, Asti E, Lazzari V, Siboni S, Bernardi D, Bonavina L. Six to 12-year outcomes of magnetic sphincter augmentation for gastroesophageal reflux disease. Sci Rep. 2020;10(1):13753.
7. Ganz R, Edmundowicz S, P T, et al. Long-term outcomes of patients receiving magnetic sphincter augmentation device for gastroesophageal reflux. Clin Gastroenterol Hepatol. 2016;14:671–7.
8. Khaitan L, Hill M, Michel M, Chiasson P, Woodworth P, Bell R, Sadek R, Hoffman A, Loing K, Veldhuis P, Petraiuolo W, Anciano C. Feasibility and efficacy of magnetic sphincter augmentation for the management of gastroesophageal reflux disease post-sleeve gastrectomy for obesity. Obes Surg. 2022;33(1):387–96.

Laparoscopic Antireflux Surgery

Francisco Schlottmann, Sofia Bertona, Mario A. Masrur, and Rudolf Buxhoeveden

Abstract Although most patients with gastroesophageal reflux disease have adequate symptom control with lifestyle modifications and medical therapy, some will eventually need anti-reflux surgery. A careful patient selection, a thorough preoperative work-up, and a properly executed operation are critical for the success of the operation. In this chapter, we present a detailed step-by-step description of the surgical technique of laparoscopic antireflux surgery.

Keywords Gastroesophageal reflux disease · Antireflux surgery · Nissen fundoplication · Hiatal hernia · Laparoscopy

Introduction

Gastroesophageal reflux disease (GERD) is a very common gastrointestinal disorder. It is estimated that around 20% of adult individuals are affected by GERD in Western countries. Although most patients have adequate symptom control with lifestyle modifications and medical therapy, some will eventually need anti-reflux

F. Schlottmann (✉)
Department of Surgery, Hospital Alemán of Buenos Aires, Buenos Aires, Argentina

Department of Surgery, University of Illinois at Chicago, Chicago, IL, USA

S. Bertona · R. Buxhoeveden
Department of Surgery, Hospital Alemán of Buenos Aires, Buenos Aires, Argentina
e-mail: sbertona@hospitalaleman.com; rbuxhoeveden@hospitalaleman.com

M. A. Masrur
Department of Surgery, University of Illinois at Chicago, Chicago, IL, USA
e-mail: mmasrur@uic.edu

F. Schlottmann, M. A. Masrur (eds.), *Endoscopic, Laparoscopic and Robotic Techniques for Foregut Disorders*, https://doi.org/10.1007/978-3-032-00811-4_19

surgery. An operation should be considered for the following patients: persistence of symptoms despite the use of medication (e.g., frequent regurgitation), presence of large hiatal hernia, poor compliance to medication, refusal to take medication for a long time, or side effects related to medical therapy.

Diagnosis of GERD solely based on symptoms is commonly wrong due to an heterogenous clinical presentation which overlaps with many other gastrointestinal disorders. For this reason, we suggest performing the following tests before an anti-reflux operation: upper endoscopy, barium esophagogram, high-resolution manometry, and pH monitoring.

A careful patient selection, a thorough preoperative work-up, and a properly executed operation are critical for the success of anti-reflux surgery [1–5].

Procedure Description

Patient Positioning and Trocar Placement

The patient should be in low lithotomy position with the lower extremities extended on stirrups and with the knees flexed around 20–30°. We strongly suggest the use of pneumatic compression devices for legs to reduce the risk of deep vein thrombosis. During the entire operation, the surgeon stands between the patient's legs. A total of five laparoscopic ports (two 10 mm and three 5 mm) are commonly used for the operation (Fig. 1).

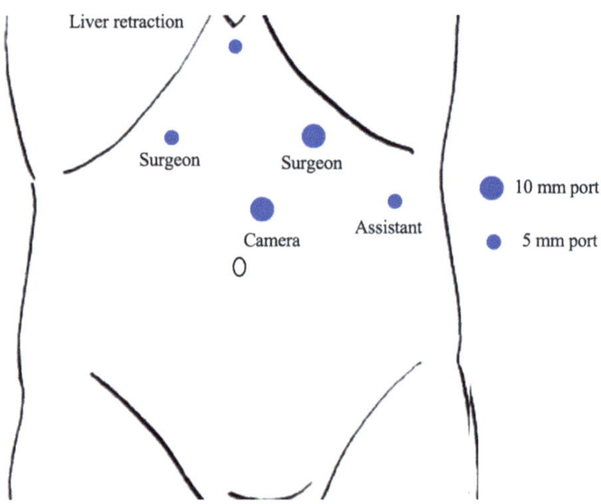

Fig. 1 Ports placement for laparoscopic antireflux surgery. (1) camera, (2) surgeon, (3) surgeon, (4) liver retractor (could be replaced for a subxiphoid port for Nathanson retractor), (5) assistant port

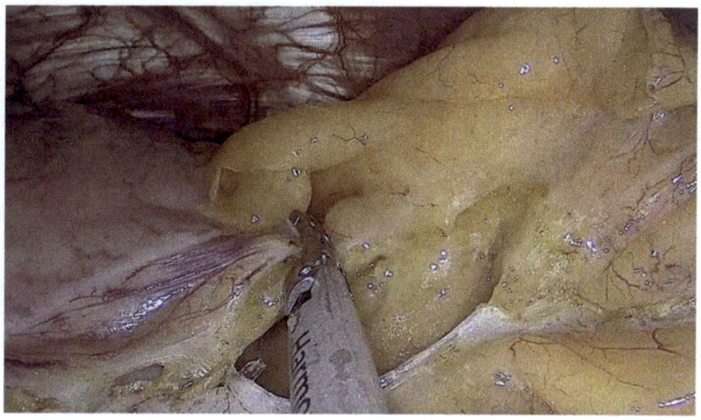

Fig. 2 Division of short gastric vessels

Division of Short Gastric Vessels

We use a vessel sealing instrument to divide the short gastric vessels starting from a point midway along the greater curvature of the stomach towards the fundus. The division of the vessels continues all the way up until de left pillar of the crus. This step of the operation will help obtaining a tension-free fundoplication afterwards (Fig. 2).

Division of the Phrenoesophageal Membrane

Once the left pillar is completely dissected, we continue dividing the phrenoesophageal membrane just above the esophagus (Fig. 3). The anterior vagus should be carefully identified and left attached to the esophageal wall to avoid its injury. At this point, we can do blunt maneuvers to separate the esophagus from anterior mediastinal attachments and the left crus.

Division of the Gastrohepatic Ligament

The gastrohepatic ligament is divided with electrocautery or harmonic device starting just above the caudate lobe of the liver. The division continues all the way up until the right pillar of the crus (Fig. 4). The right crus is then dissected all the way down towards the junction with the left crus (Fig. 5). The esophagus can now be separated from the right crus and posterior attachments with blunt maneuvers. The posterior vagus nerve is identified and preserved during this step of the operation.

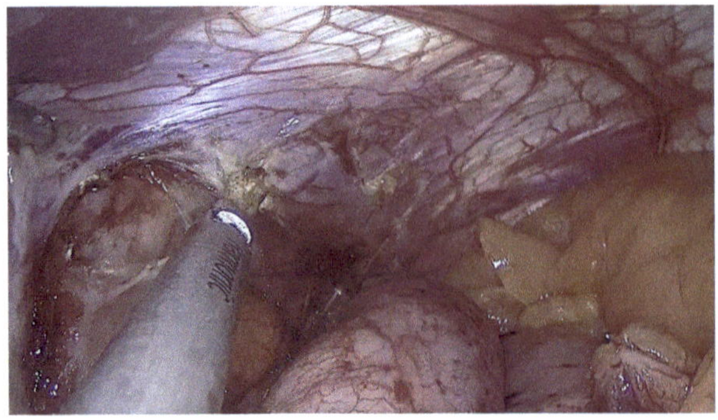

Fig. 3 Division of the phrenoesophageal membrane

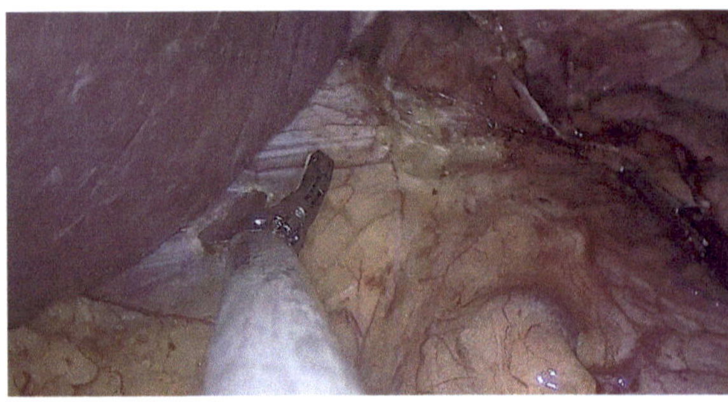

Fig. 4 Division of the gastrohepatic ligament

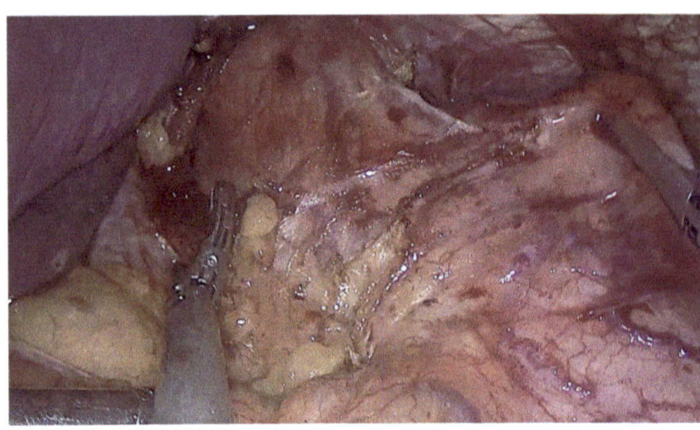

Fig. 5 Dissection of the right crus

Mediastinal Dissection

Once the esophagus is completely detached from the right and left crus, we open a posterior window under the esophagus with blunt dissection (Fig. 6). The window should be enlarged to pass a Penrose drain or umbilical tape around the esophagus. The Penrose drain is secured with a large clip or hem-o-lok and the esophagus is retracted away from the hiatus. This maneuver is extremely helpful to perform an extensive mediastinal dissection of the distal esophagus (Fig. 7). The esophagus should be circumferentially dissected in the mediastinum in order to obtain at least 3 cm of esophagus under the diaphragm (Fig. 8).

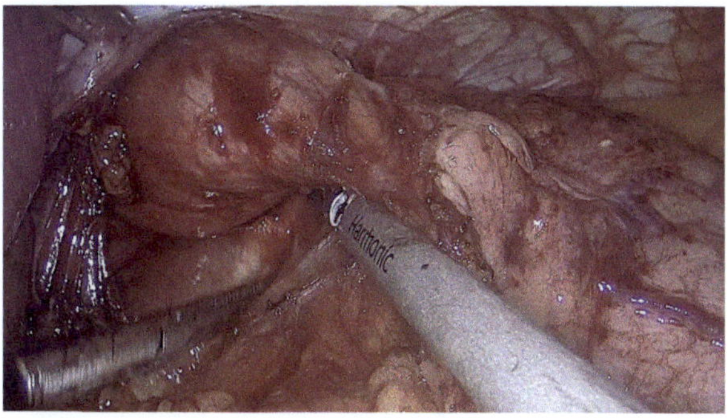

Fig. 6 Posterior window under the esophagus

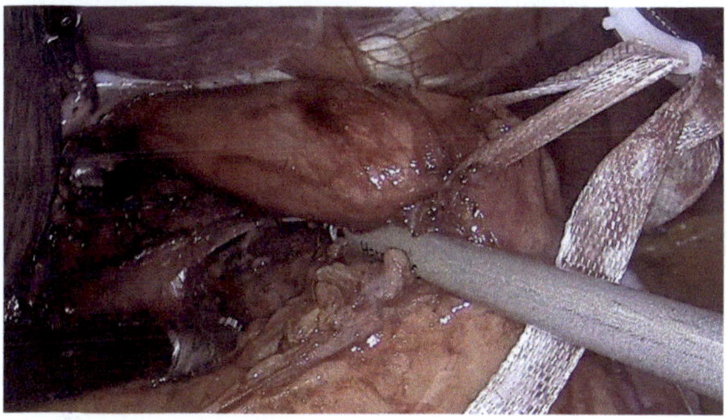

Fig. 7 Umbilical tape around the esophagus for retraction

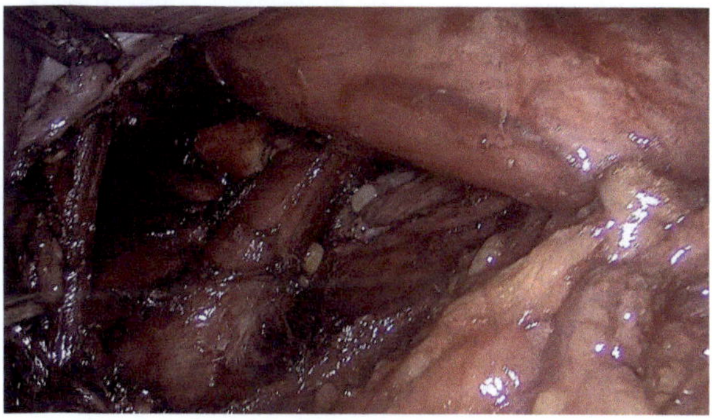

Fig. 8 Complete mediastinal dissection with at least 3 cm of esophagus under the diaphragm

Closure of the Esophageal Hiatus

The hiatus is completely exposed by retracting the esophagus upwards and towards the left. The crura is closed with interrupted non-absorbable sutures (e.g. 2–0 silk or polyester). The first stitch is placed just above the junction of the right and left pillars. Additional stitches are then placed superiorly 1 cm apart. The closure of the crura should not be too tight to avoid postoperative dysphagia (a closed grasper should slide easily between the esophagus and the last stich at the crura) (Figs. 9 and 10).

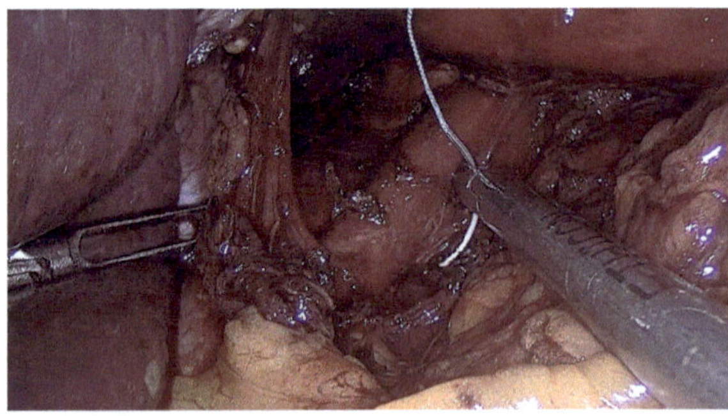

Fig. 9 Closure of the hiatus with interrupted non-absorbable sutures

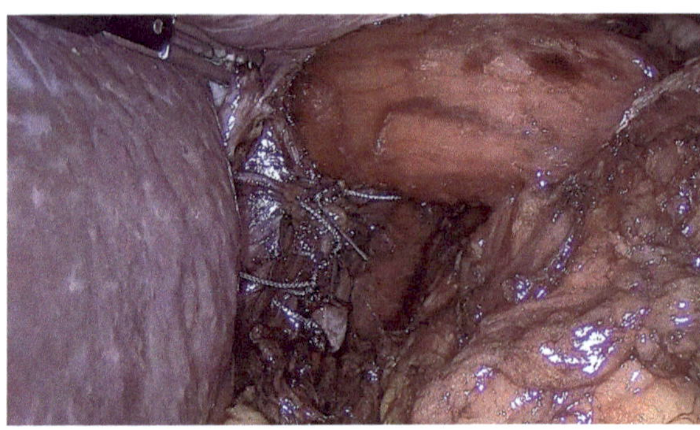

Fig. 10 The hiatus is adequately closed

Fundoplication

Once the hiatus is adequately closed, the fundus of the stomach is passed behind the esophagus and a "shoe-shine" maneuver is performed to verify sufficient fundic mobilization. We usually do a total 360° fundoplication (Nissen fundoplication). A bougie is preferably inserted into the esophagus before doing the fundoplication to prevent postoperative dysphagia. It is very helpful to hold the left and right sides of the fundus with a grasper above the gastroesophageal junction during the placement of the first stitch. We usually use only 3 stitches at 1 cm intervals to approximate the right and left sides of the fundoplication. The result should be a short (about 2 cm in length) and floppy fundoplication (Figs. 11 and 12).

In patients with severe esophageal dysmotility, a partial fundoplication is recommended.

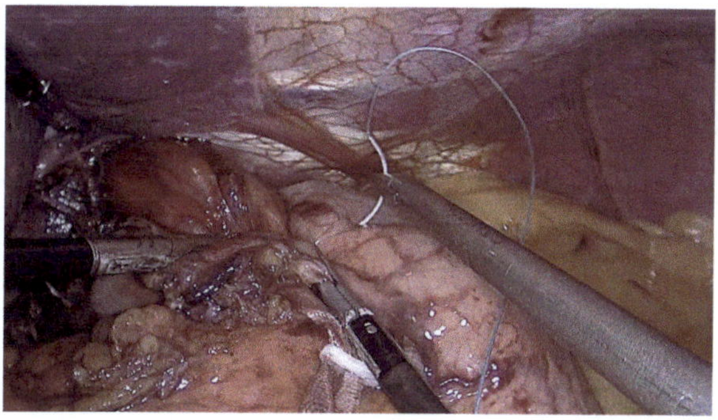

Fig. 11 First stitch of the Nissen fundoplication

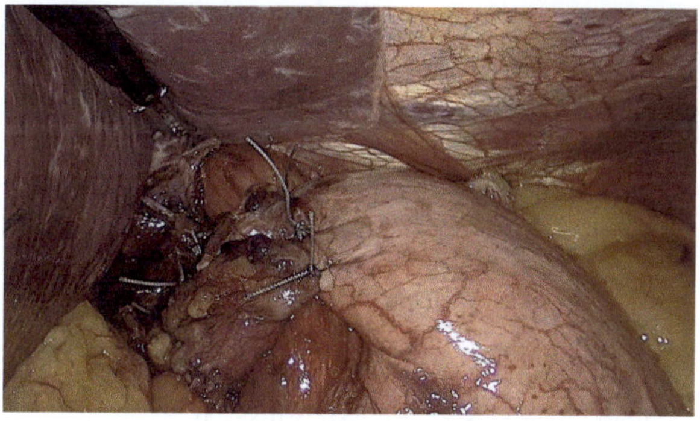

Fig. 12 Completed Nissen fundoplication

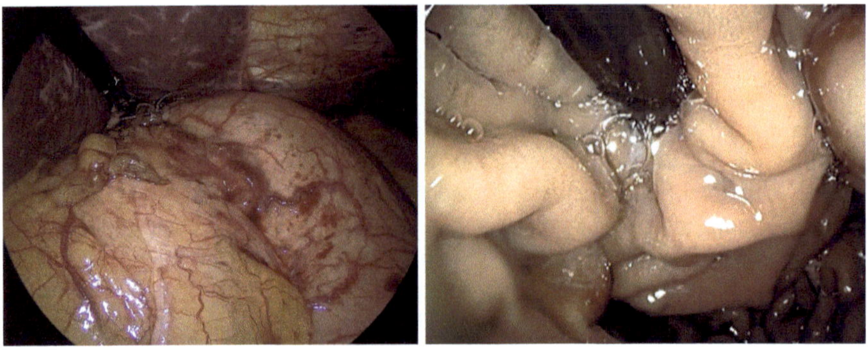

Fig. 13 Intraoperative endoscopy evaluating the wrap from the inside

Final Inspection

The bougie is removed from the esophagus by the anesthesiologist and the Penrose drain is cut and removed. We usually perform an upper endoscopy to double check that the esophagogastric junction is not too tight and to evaluate the wrap from the inside (Fig. 13). We then remove all trocars under direct vision and check for adequate hemostasis. The fascia of the 10–12 mm ports should be closed.

Postoperative Care

Patients can start with clear liquids the day of the operation, and then advance to soft diet as per tolerance. Most patients are discharged within 48 hours of the operation. Anti-reflux medications are commonly discontinued after 4 weeks.

Conflicts of Interest The authors have no conflicts of interest.

References

1. El-Serag HN, Sweet S, Winchester CC, et al. Update on the epidemiology of gastro-esophageal reflux disease: a systematic review. Gut. 2014;63:871–80.
2. Schlottmann F, Herbella FA, Allaix ME, et al. Surgical treatment of gastroesophageal reflux disease. World J Surg. 2017;41(7):1685–90.
3. Schlottmann F, Strassle PD, Patti MG. Antireflux surgery in the USA: influence of surgical volume on perioperative outcomes and costs – time for centralization? World J Surg. 2018;42(7):2183–9.
4. Patti MG, Schlottmann F, Farrell TM. Fundoplication for gastroesophageal reflux disease: tips for success. J Laparoendosc Adv Surg Tech A. 2017;27(1):1–5.
5. Patti MG, Schlottmann F. Recurrence of reflux after laparoscopic antireflux surgery. JAMA. 2018;319(1):82–3.

Robotic Antireflux Surgery

Lorna A. Evans and E. Fernando Elli

Abstract Gastroesophageal reflux disease (GERD) is a globally high-prevalence disease, affecting up to 27% of the North American population. Anti-reflux surgery is an effective option for patients who are refractory to pharmacological treatment. This chapter will describe the technical aspects of different anti-reflux techniques and their robotic-assisted approach.

Keywords GERD · Anti-reflux surgery · Robotic surgery · Fundoplication

Introduction

Gastroesophageal reflux disease (GERD) is a globally high-prevalence disease, affecting up to 27% of the North American population [1]. It is characterized by a range of symptoms and complications resulting from the movement of gastric contents into the esophagus. The dysfunction of the lower esophageal sphincter (LES) plays a leading role in this pathology along with other risk factors such as smoking, anxiety, insufficient physical activity, and a high body mass index (BMI) [2]. The most prevalent symptoms of GERD include heartburn, dysphagia, regurgitation, and chest pain. Extraesophageal symptoms may include cough, laryngeal hoarseness, dysphonia, pulmonary fibrosis, asthma, dental erosions, sinus, and ear disease [3].

L. A. Evans
Department of Surgery, Mayo Clinic Florida, Jacksonville, FL, USA

E. F. Elli (✉)
Department of Surgery, Mayo Clinic Florida, Jacksonville, FL, USA

Division of Advanced Gastrointestinal and Bariatric Surgery, Mayo Clinic, Jacksonville, FL, USA
e-mail: Elli.enrique@mayo.edu

F. Schlottmann, M. A. Masrur (eds.), *Endoscopic, Laparoscopic and Robotic Techniques for Foregut Disorders*, https://doi.org/10.1007/978-3-032-00811-4_20

The diagnosis does not rely on a single gold standard method, rather, it requires a comprehensive clinical evaluation [4]. Imaging studies include esophagogastroduodenoscopy (EGD), upper gastrointestinal series (UGI), and esophageal manometry. Furthermore, functional studies such as the Bravo pH study and 24-hour pH-impedance test are performed to evaluate acid and bile exposure and reflux events [5].

The first-line treatment for this condition typically involves the use of proton pump inhibitors (PPI) [6]. However, anti-reflux surgery is an effective option for those patients who are refractory to the pharmacological treatment [7]. This chapter outlines the surgical technique of robotic anti-reflux surgery.

Procedure Description

Patient Positioning and Trocar Placement

Following the induction of general anesthesia, the patient is positioned supine. Trocar placement begins with an 8 mm trocar in the upper quadrant using the OptiView technique. A pneumoperitoneum is then established at 12 mmHg to allow for initial exploration and direct vision placement of the remaining ports.

The additional trocars include an 8 mm robotic trocar placed above the umbilicus on the left side and another 8 mm robotic trocar positioned in the right upper quadrant. An extra 8 mm robotic trocar is placed in the left upper quadrant, and an assistant trocar is positioned in the left lower quadrant. A Nathanson liver retractor is inserted in the epigastrium to expose the hiatus. At this point, the docking of the robotic platform can proceed (Fig. 1).

Initial Dissection

A vessel sealer device is employed to dissect the short gastric vessels from the mid-portion of the spleen up to the gastroesophageal (GE) junction. The left crus is dissected, and the gastroesophageal membrane is opened.

Attention is then directed to the right side, where the pars flaccida is incised to expose the right crus. Electrocautery is then used to separate the crus from the esophagus. The dissection proceeds inferiorly to create a retroesophageal window, which facilitates the placement of a Penrose drain. Gentle traction is applied to circumferentially dissect the esophagus up to the level of the inferior pulmonary vein (Fig. 2).

During this procedure, the anterior and posterior vagus nerves are carefully identified and preserved. Subsequently, the posterior aspect of the stomach is mobilized from the right side, ensuring the complete division of the posterior short gastric vessels.

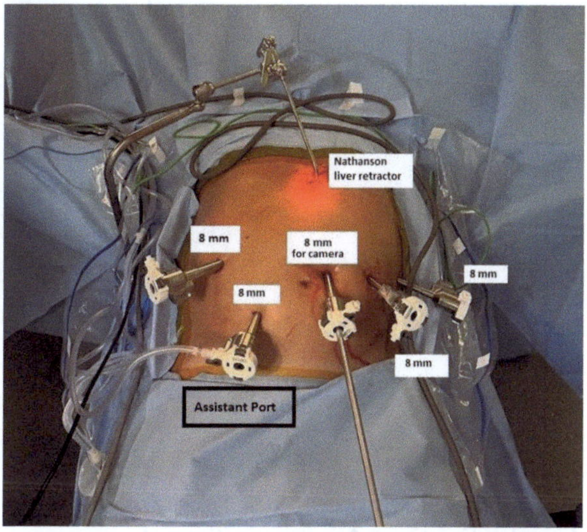

Fig. 1 Trocar placement

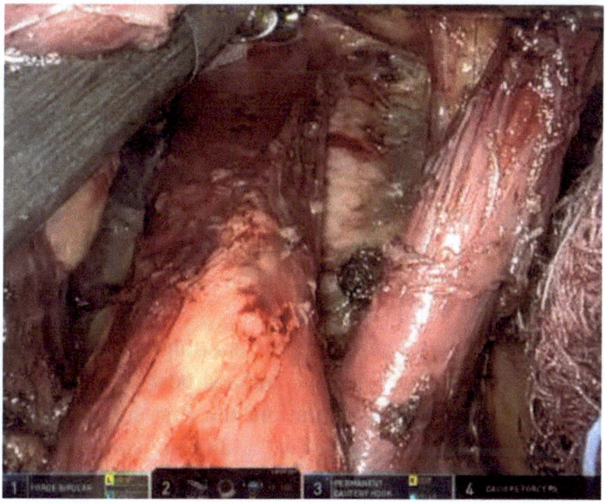

Fig. 2 Hiatal dissection

Hiatal Repair

After achieving complete esophageal mobilization, at least 3 cm of intra-abdominal esophagus is obtained. The hiatal hernia repair involves placing posterior and anterior interrupted 0 nonabsorbable polyester sutures (Fig. 3). During the Nissen fundoplication, a 48–56 Fr bougie, (depending on the patient's weight) is then introduced into the patient's oropharynx and advanced through the esophagus into the stomach.

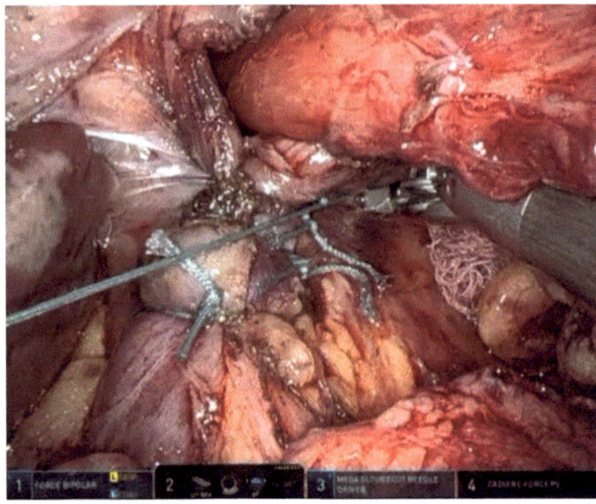

Fig. 3 Hiatal repair

Fundoplication: Nissen or Toupet

The Toupet fundoplication, also known as a posterior partial fundoplication, involves wrapping the stomach around the esophagus in a manner that covers approximately 270° of the esophageal circumference. This fundoplication is usually considered for patients with ineffective esophageal motility and concomitant GERD. The Nissen fundoplication is a complete (360°) stomach wrap around the lower esophagus. This configuration of the wrap increases pressure at the lower esophageal sphincter, effectively preventing acid reflux. While highly effective for controlling reflux symptoms, it can sometimes lead to dysphagia and gas-bloat syndrome due to a tight wrap.

Once the hiatal hernia repair is completed, the stomach is maneuvered through the retroesophageal window, and a shoeshine maneuver is performed. (Fig. 4).

In the Toupet fundoplication, the first suture is placed between the esophagus, the crus, and the stomach. Two additional sutures are then placed between the right side of the wrap and the esophagus. The left side of the wrap is constructed similarly, incorporating the stomach, diaphragm, and esophagus. Finally, two more interrupted sutures are placed between the stomach and the esophagus to complete the fundoplication (Figs. 5 and 6).

To perform a Nissen fundoplication, three anterior gastrogastric sutures are placed. The final two sutures also engage the anterior aspect of the esophagus. As previously noted, the fundoplication is adjusted during the procedure using a 48–56 Fr bougie, depending on the patient's size. Once the Nissen fundoplication is constructed, the bougie is removed (Figs. 7 and 8).

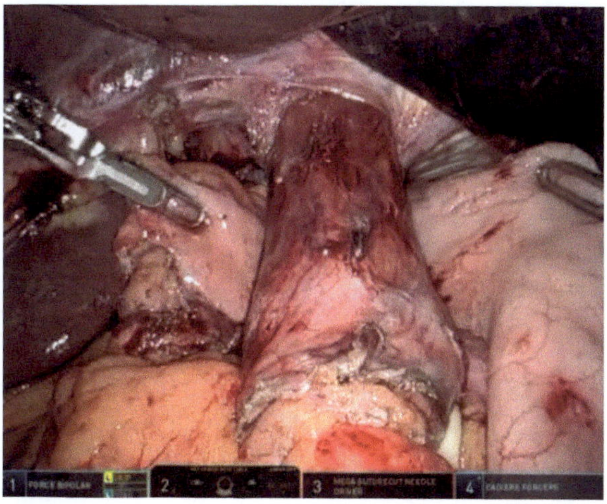

Fig. 4 Shoeshine maneuver

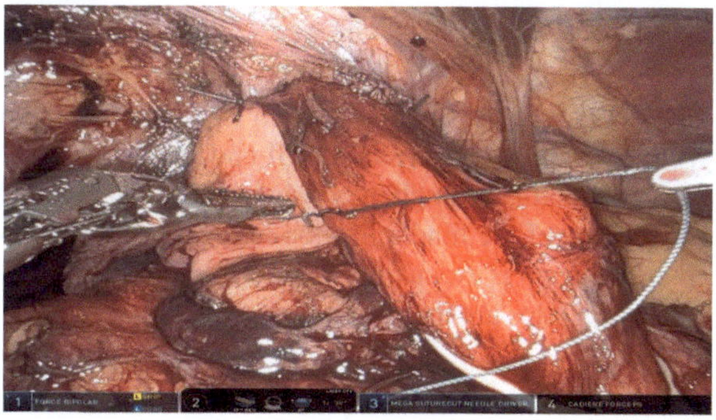

Fig. 5 Right-side stitches of Toupet fundoplication

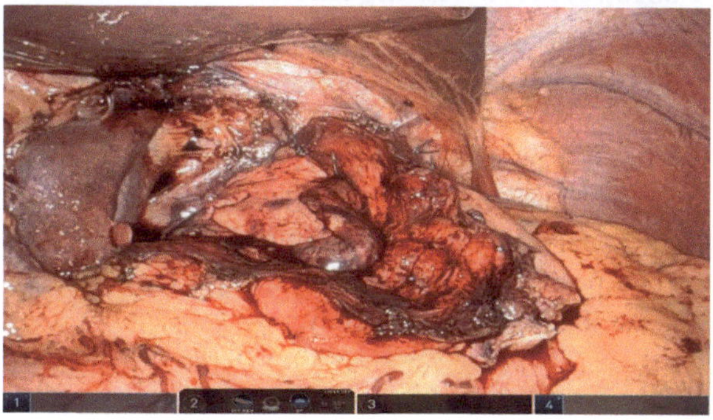

Fig. 6 Completed Toupet fundoplication

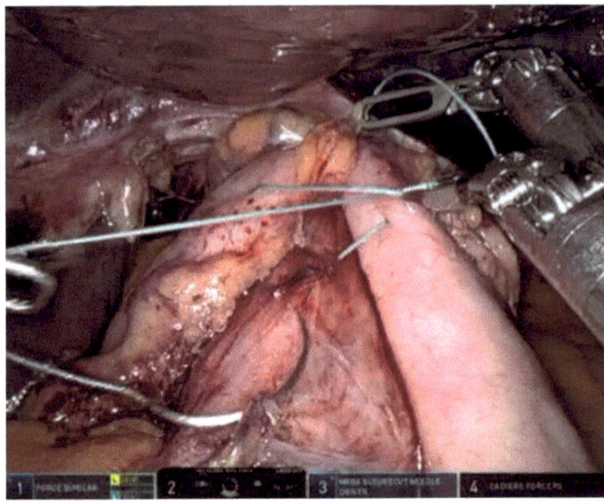

Fig. 7 Nissen fundoplication

Final Aspects

The tightness of the fundoplication is assessed manually with laparoscopic instruments. An intraoperative upper GI endoscopy is conducted to verify that the scope passes smoothly through the GE junction, without tension, and to confirm the proper positioning of the fundoplication in the retroversion view. Subsequently, the pneumoperitoneum is evacuated, and the trocars are removed under direct visualization. The trocar sites are then closed.

Postoperative Management

On the day of surgery (postoperative day 0), patients should begin a blenderized diet to facilitate easy swallowing and minimize food impaction, dysphagia and strain on the surgical site. Depending on individual recovery and health status, some patients may be discharged on the same day or require a short 23-hour observation period in the hospital to monitor for any immediate postoperative complications. Additionally, certain patients experiencing dysphagia may need a swallow study to assess and address this issue appropriately.

Conclusions

Robotic anti-reflux surgery is a highly effective intervention for patients requiring pharmacological treatment or for whom medical treatment is ineffective. This surgical approach is distinguished by its low complication rate and its precision. The

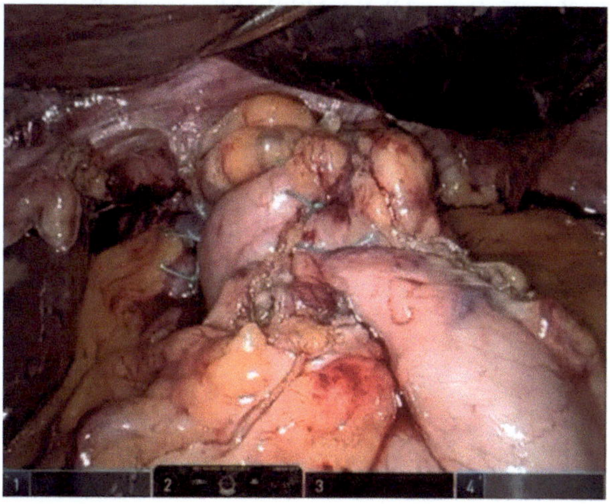

Fig. 8 Completed Nissen fundoplication

robotic platform offers several advantages, including enhanced mediastinal dissection, greater dexterity, and improved visualization. These features enable superior suturing capabilities, particularly in confined anatomical spaces. The range of available fundoplication techniques, though fundamentally based on similar surgical principles, varies in their specific applications. A thorough assessment of each patient's individual needs and clinical circumstances is crucial for selecting the most appropriate technique. Tailoring the surgical approach enhances the potential for successful outcomes and highlights the importance of personalized care in managing gastroesophageal reflux disease.

Conflict of Interest Lorna A. Evans and E. Fernando Elli declare that they have no conflicts of interest.

References

1. El-Serag HB, Sweet S, Winchester CC, Dent J. Update on the epidemiology of gastro-oesophageal reflux disease: a systematic review. Gut. 2014;63:871–80.
2. Chhabra P, Ingole N. Gastroesophageal reflux disease (GERD): highlighting diagnosis, treatment, and lifestyle changes. Cureus. 2022 Aug 29;14(8):e28563. https://doi.org/10.7759/cureus.28563.
3. Chen JW, Vela MF, Peterson KA, Carlson DA. AGA clinical practice update on the diagnosis and Management of Extraesophageal Gastroesophageal Reflux Disease: expert review. Clin Gastroenterol Hepatol. 2023 Jun;21(6):1414–1421.e3. https://doi.org/10.1016/j.cgh.2023.01.040.
4. Katz PO, Dunbar KB, Schnoll-Sussman FH, et al. ACG clinical guideline for the diagnosis and management of gastroesophageal reflux disease. Am J Gastroenterol. 2022;117:27–56.
5. Evans LA, Castillo-Larios R, Cornejo J, Elli EF. Challenges of Revisional metabolic and bariatric surgery: a comprehensive guide to unraveling the complexities and solutions of Revisional bariatric procedures. J Clin Med. 2024;13(11):3104. https://doi.org/10.3390/jcm13113104.

6. Katz PO, Gerson LB, Vela MF. Guidelines for the diagnosis and management of gastroesophageal reflux disease. Am J Gastroenterol. 2013;108:308–28.
7. Lee J, Lee I, Oh Y, Kim JW, Kwon Y, Alromi A, Eledreesi M, Khalid A, Aljarbou W, Park S. Current status of anti-reflux surgery as a treatment for GERD. Medicina (Kaunas). 2024;60(3):518. https://doi.org/10.3390/medicina60030518.

Robotic Paraoesophageal Hernia Repair

Emiliano G. Manueli Laos, Francisco Schlottmann, and Mario A. Masrur

Abstract Hiatal hernia (HH) is a common condition characterized by the abnormal displacement of the stomach into the thoracic cavity. While laparoscopic repair has been the standard approach, robotic surgery offers several advantages, including enhanced visualization, precision, and dexterity. This chapter provides a detailed description of the surgical technique for robotic paraoesophageal hernia repair (Type II, II and IV). The careful dissection of the herniated stomach and surrounding structures allows for a precise repair of these defects. By following the steps described in this chapter, robotic paraoesophageal repair can be safely and effectively performed, leading to improved patient outcomes and reduced postoperative complications.

Keywords Robotic surgery · Anti-reflux procedures · Mesh · Hiatal hernia

Introduction

Hiatal hernia (HH) is a condition characterized by the abnormal displacement of the upper portion of the stomach through the esophageal hiatus of the diaphragm, resulting in its entry into the thoracic cavity. HH are commonly related to gastro-esophageal reflux disease and dysphagia. There are 4 types of HH (Fig. 1):

E. G. Manueli Laos · M. A. Masrur (✉)
Department of Surgery, University of Illinois, Chicago, IL, USA
e-mail: mmasrur@uic.edu

F. Schlottmann
Department of Surgery, University of Illinois, Chicago, IL, USA

Department of Surgery, Hospital Alemán of Buenos, Aires, Argentina

F. Schlottmann, M. A. Masrur (eds.), *Endoscopic, Laparoscopic and Robotic Techniques for Foregut Disorders*, https://doi.org/10.1007/978-3-032-00811-4_21

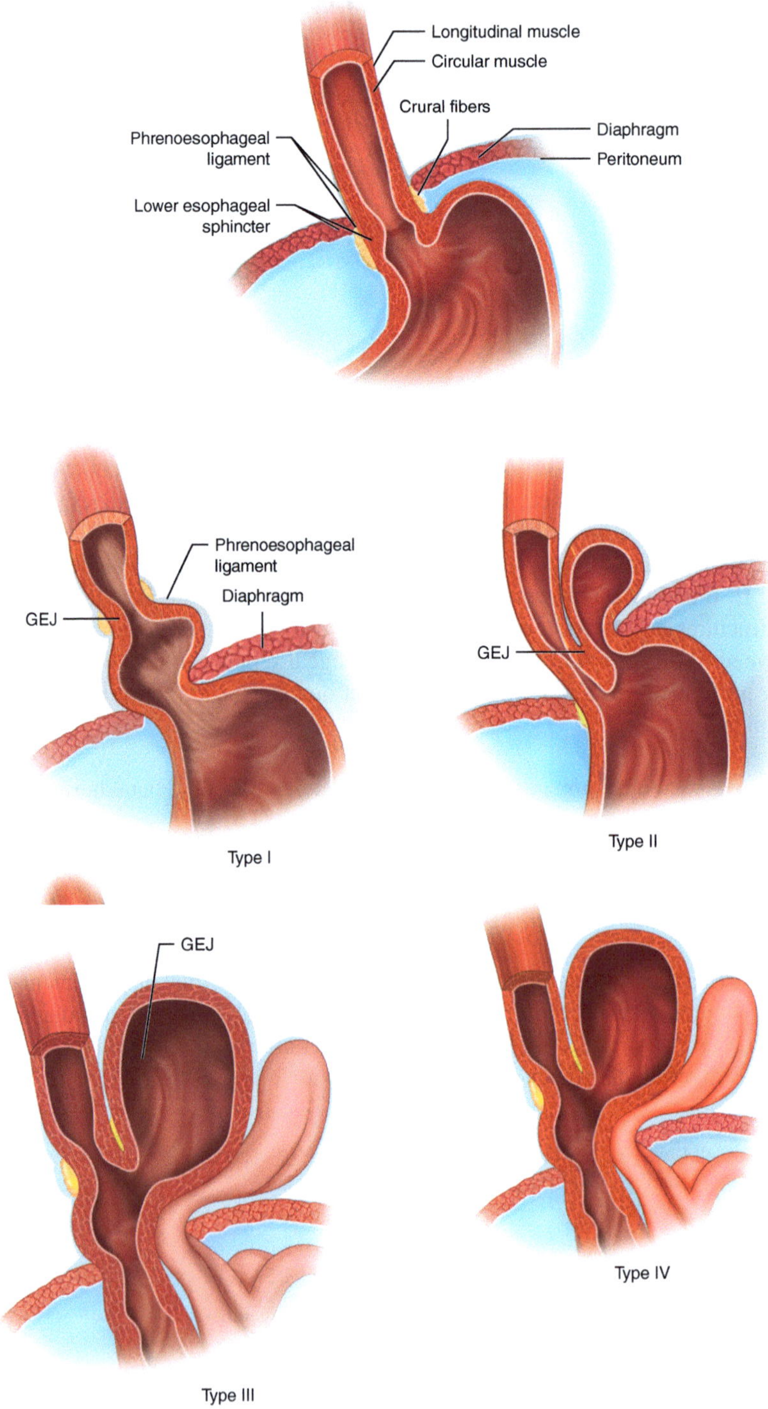

Fig. 1 Types of hiatal hernias

Type I: the proximal portion of the stomach protrudes to the thorax. Also called sliding hernias, these represents 95% of the HH.
Type II: the fundus of the stomach herniates parallel to the esophagus while the esophagogastric junction (EGJ) stays in place.
Type III: consists of a combination of both type I and type II hernias, where both fundus and EGJ are displaced to the mediastinum
Type IV: an abdominal organ other than the stomach herniates through the defect (e.g.: colon, spleen, pancreas, omentum, etc.)

Although there is not clear consensus, in the surgical environment type II, III and IV are considered true paraoesophageal hernias [1]. Some groups define it, as more than 30% of stomach herniated, others at least 50% of the stomach.

Robotic surgery has demonstrated several advantages over laparoscopy, including lower length of stay and complications rate [2]. Additionally, the better range of motion of the robotic platform allows the surgeon to perform a neat procedure. In this chapter, the surgical approach and technique of robotic paraoesophageal hernia repair will be described.

Procedure Description

The procedure is done under general anesthesia. The patient is positioned in dorsal decubitus, at 45° in reverse Trendelenburg. Pneumatic compression of lower limbs is applied, and antibiotic prophylaxis is used for optimal perioperative outcomes.

Under aseptic and antiseptic draping technique of the abdomen, a Veress needle is inserted in the Palmer's point and the abdomen is insufflated until reaching an intrabdominal pressure of 15 mmHg. A 5 mm optic trocar is placed in the left flank, which will be used for diagnostic laparoscopy and direct view for placement of the remaining trocars.

The robotic ports are placed in a straight line, approximately 5 cm above the transverse umbilical line. A Nathanson liver retractor is also placed subxiphoid. An additional 8–10 mm assistance port can be placed on the right-flank (Fig. 2).

Operative Technique

Diagnostic Evaluation and Reduction of Hernia Content

After docking of the robot, the procedure starts with identification of the hernia and content. The herniated content is reduced gently using robotic forceps. The assistant can hold the reduced stomach using laparoscopic grasper, avoiding excessive forces to minimize the risk of serosal injury (Figs. 3 and 4).

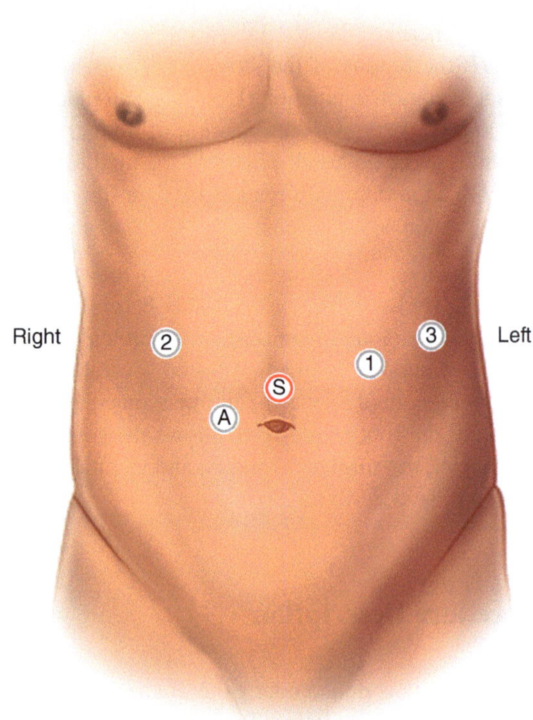

Fig. 2 Patient positioning and port placement. N: Nathanson liver retractor; A: assistant port; S: scope port; 1, 2 and 3: robotic 8 mm ports

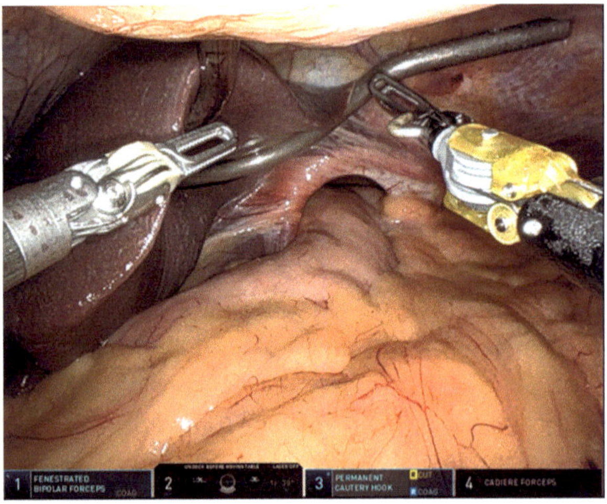

Fig. 3 Assessment of anatomy and Hiatal defect

Hiatus Dissection

The next step consists of dissecting the diaphragm hiatus and the resection of the short gastric vessels. Using the robotic monopolar hook, the dissection is most commonly performed from the left crus to the right where there are less chances of injury important anatomical structures (Fig. 5). It can also be done right-to-left, depending on the visualization and accessibility of the structures (Fig. 6). Neurovascular structures running in the lesser curve, as the vagus nerve branches and gastric vascularization, should be preserved in order to guarantee optimal stomach functionality. Once the whole hiatus has been completely exposed, a robotic vessel sealer is used to transect the short gastric vessels (Fig. 7).

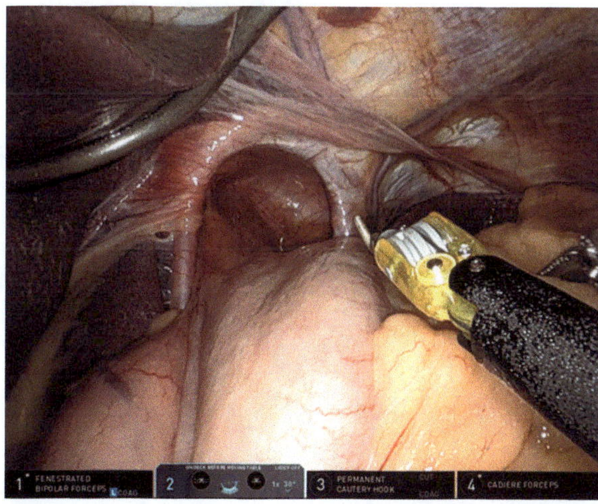

Fig. 4 Reduction of hernia content

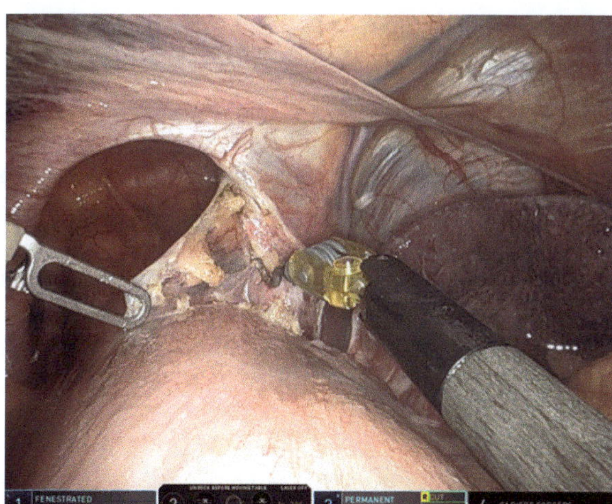

Fig. 5 Dissection of left crus

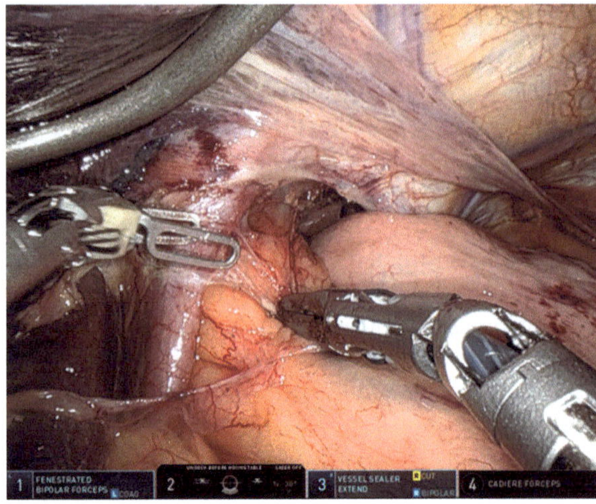

Fig. 6 Dissection of right crus

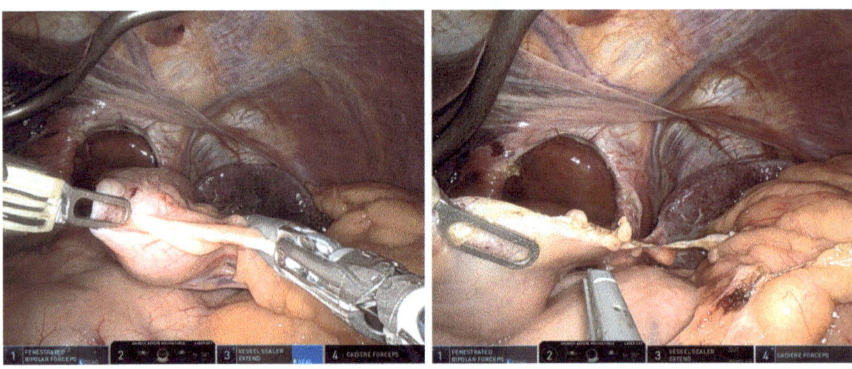

Fig. 7 Transection of short gastric vessels

Hernia Sac Dissection

It is recommended to fully dissect the hernia sac away from the mediastinal structures (Figs. 8 and 9), given that simple reduction is connected to higher recurrence rate. In patients with very large defects and colon or spleen in the hernia (Type IV HH), a partial sac excision should be attempted [3, 4].

A complete disconnection of the sac from the mediastinal structure is necessary to prevent early recurrences, allowing a complete 360 mobilization of the esophagus and at least 3 cm of the intra-abdominal esophagus (Fig. 10).

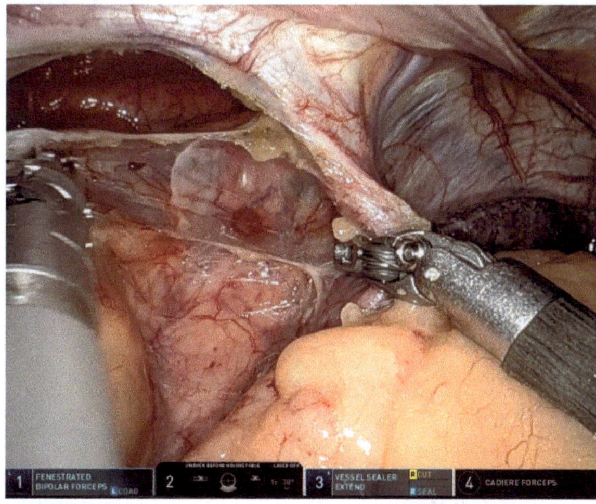

Fig. 8 Dissection of the hernia sac

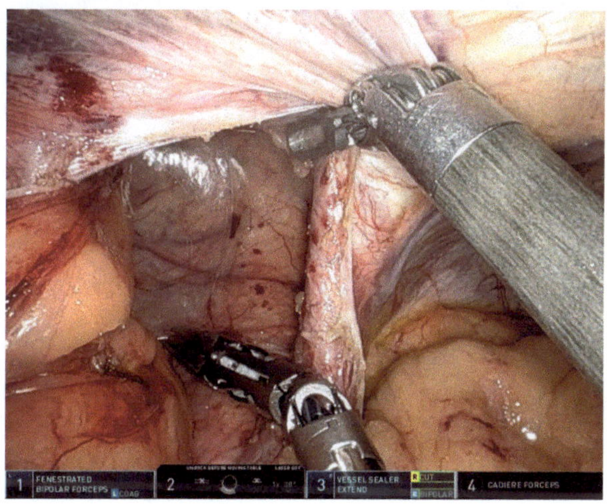

Fig. 9 Dissection of the hernia sac away from the mediastinal structures on the left side

Mediastinal Dissection

A Penrose drain is placed in the retroesophageal window to allow better mobilization.

Dissection of the mediastinal structures is done carefully using a combination of both energy and blunt maneuvers, avoiding violation of the visceral pleura. When the pleura is accidentally entered a capnothorax occurs. Most of the time this transit without major repercussion, but in the event of hypertensive iatrogenic capnothorax

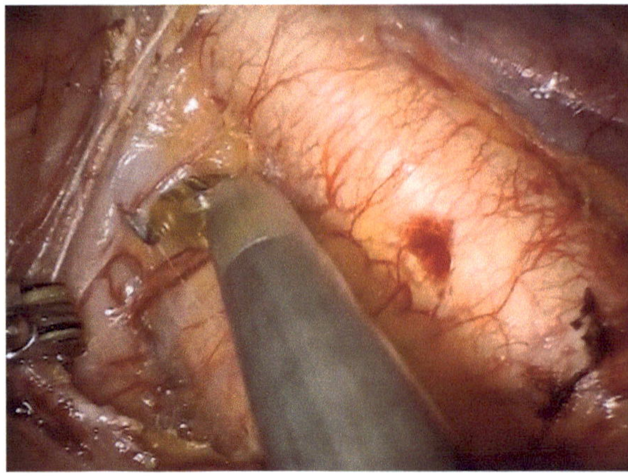

Fig. 10 Intra-mediastinum hernia sac disconnection

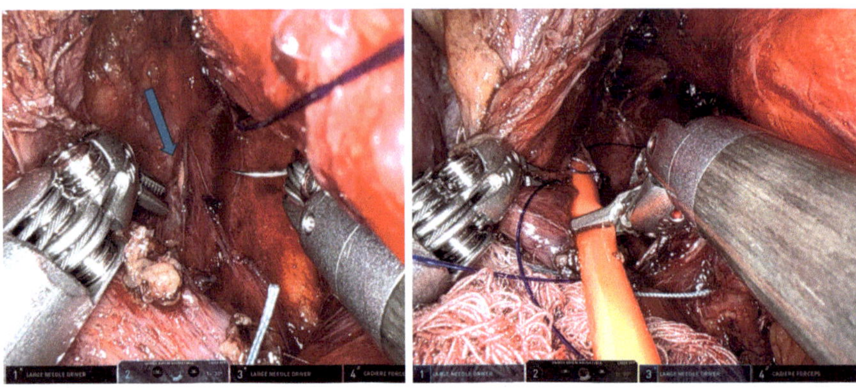

Fig. 11 Drainage of capnothorax and closure of pleural injury using Red-rubber catheter aspiration. The blue arrow indicates the location of the iatrogenic lesion

with cardiovascular repercussion to the patient, a red rubber catheter should be quickly introduced in the pleura cavity trans-mediastinal to evacuate the CO2. In coordination with the anesthesia team, inspiratory maneuvers (Valsalva maneuver) holding expanded lung in combination with aspiration through the red-rubber catheter should be conducted, followed by suture closure of the injured pleura (Fig. 11).

Once a complete mobilization of the esophagus has been performed, at least 3 cm of intra-abominal esophagus should be achieved without tension (Fig. 12).

Cruroplasty

The next step is to perform a cruroplasty or hiatoplasty. Both diaphragmatic pillars are approximated using 3–4 interrupted unabsorbable stitches, preferably 2-0 polyester sutures (Fig. 13). Other suture material are optional in this step including:

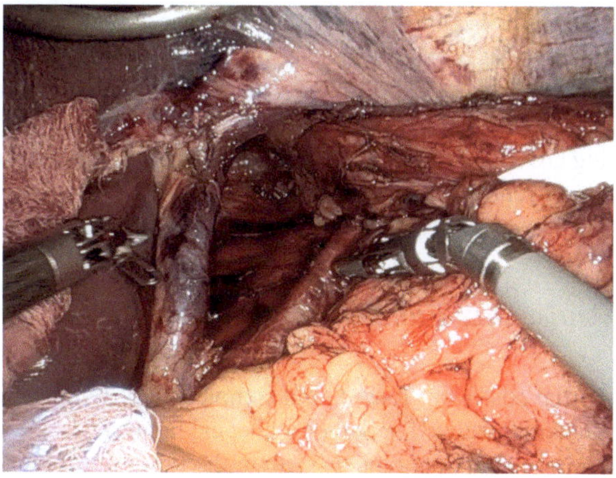

Fig. 12 Complete exposure of the hiatus achieving at least 2–3 cm of intra-abdominal esophagus

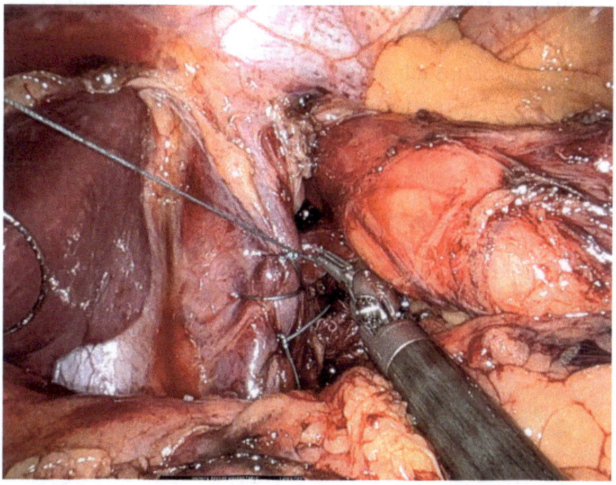

Fig. 13 Cruroplasty or hiatoplasty

pledged stitched of Polypropylene sutures, unabsorbable V-Loc™ braided sutures. Careful consideration must be given to avoid excessive tightness, as increased pressure in the hiatus may induce dysphagia. When excessive tension is applied to the closure of the pilar, relaxing incisions can be performed in the diaphragm next to the pilar, but it's not of common practice.

Mesh Reinforcement

Mesh reinforcement continues to be controversial when repairing a Hiatal hernia [5] It is of common acceptance that the use of mesh is associated to lower recurrence rates post-hiatoplasty. In general, mesh should be placed in large hiatal defects or with poor muscular hiatal strength. Despite the past trend of using unabsorbable materials, it is now recommended the use of partially absorbable or biological mesh, which have proven beneficial both in short and long terms including lower recurrence rates [6, 7]. Biological mesh once very popular use in the US, had now decreased it used due to increased cost. The slow absorbable synthetic mesh including GORE® BIO-A® and Phasix™ ST (BD- NJ-USA) are both preferable for hiatoplasty reinforcement (Fig. 14).

Anti-reflux Fundoplication

Partial posterior (Toupet) and complete 360° (Nissen) are the most common fundoplications utilized in paraoesophageal hernias.

For the Toupet fundoplication, the lower portion of the esophagus is posteriorly by the fundus of the stomach leaving an anterior gap. Both sides of the fundus are sutured to the esophageal wall using unabsorbable interrupted stitches (Fig. 15).

For the Nissen fundoplication, the esophagus is wrapped 360° suturing the fundus of the stomach antero-medial to the esophagus. To avoid twisting and/or wrap sliding, the plication can be sutured to the hiatal pillars to anchor the wrap intra-abdominally (Fig. 16).

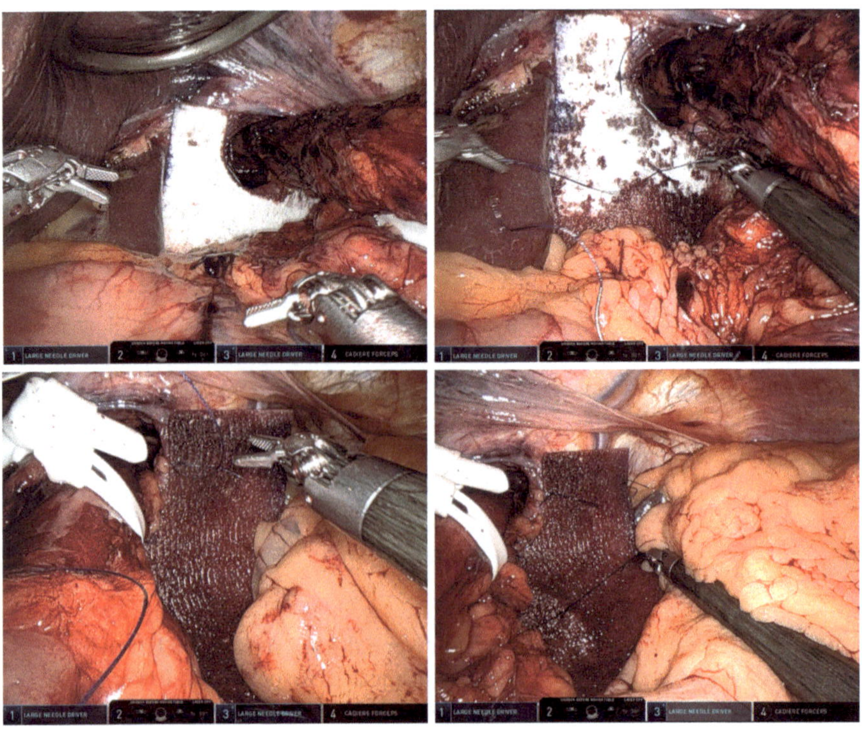

Fig. 14 Mesh hiatoplasty reinforcement using GORE® BIO-A®

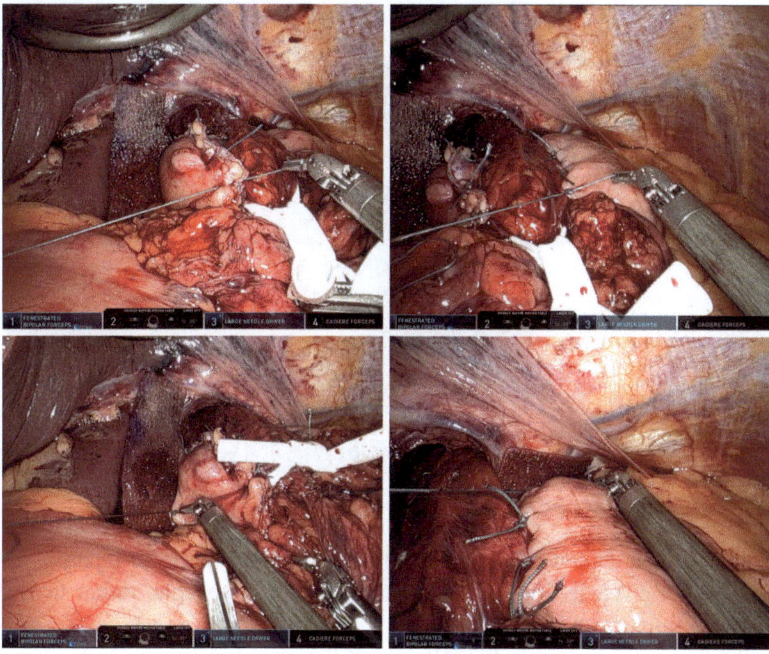

Fig. 15 Anti-reflux fundoplication: toupet fundoplication

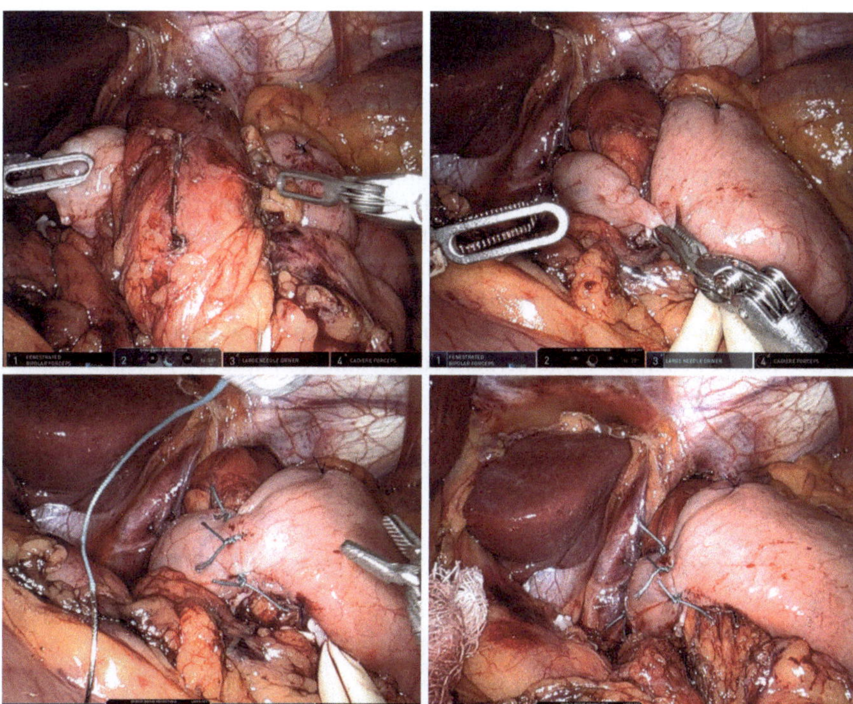

Fig. 16 Anti-reflux fundoplication: Nissen fundoplication

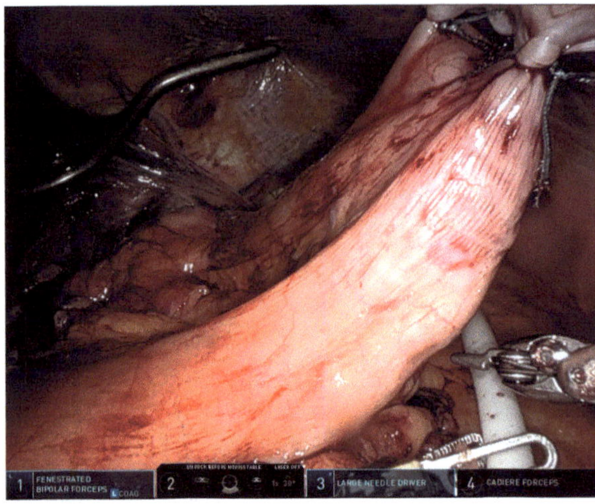

Fig. 17 Gastropexy. The body of the stomach is sutured anchored to the abdominal wall

There is now a tendency in the foregut community to perform a partial Toupet fundoplication, given its lower risk of postoperative dysphagia, rather than a full wrap Nissen fundoplication.

Lastly, a gastric fixation to the left side of the abdominal wall can be done particularly when a large portion of stomach has been herniated into the chest to avoid early recurrence, although there is no clear literature to favor this step (Fig. 17).

Conclusions

The robotic approach to hiatal hernia repair, particularly for large paraoesophageal hernias (Types II, III, and IV), offers significant advantages over traditional laparoscopic techniques. The enhanced dexterity and range of motion provided by the robotic platform allow surgeons to perform complex maneuvers with greater precision, ultimately reducing complications and minimizing patient recovery time. As robotic systems continue to evolve, they may establish a new standard in the surgical treatment of complex hiatal hernias, contributing to improved patient outcomes and efficiency in operative techniques.

Conflict of Interest Authors declare no conflict of interest to disclose.

References

1. Dean C, Etienne D, Carpentier B, Gielecki J, Tubbs RS, Loukas M. Hiatal hernias. Surg Radiol Anat. 2012;34(4):291–9. https://doi.org/10.1007/s00276-011-0904-9.
2. Powell C, DeGregorio A, Bews K, Wigle D, Habermann E. Perioperative outcomes of robotic versus laparoscopic paraesophageal hernia repair: a NSQIP analysis. Surg Endosc. 2024;38(10):5851–7. https://doi.org/10.1007/s00464-024-11158-2.
3. Frantzides CT, Madan AK, Carlson MA, Stavropoulos GP. A prospective, randomized trial of laparoscopic polytetrafluoroethylene (PTFE) patch repair vs simple cruroplasty for large hiatal hernia. Arch Surg. 2002;137(6):649–52. https://doi.org/10.1001/archsurg.137.6.649.
4. Granderath FA, Schweiger UM, Kamolz T, Asche KU, Pointner R. Laparoscopic Nissen fundoplication with prosthetic hiatal closure reduces postoperative intrathoracic wrap herniation: preliminary results of a prospective randomized functional and clinical study. Arch Surg. 2005;140(1):40–8. https://doi.org/10.1001/archsurg.140.1.40.
5. Angeramo CA, Schlottmann F. Laparoscopic paraesophageal hernia repair: to mesh or not to mesh. Systematic review and meta-analysis. Ann Surg. 2022;275(1):67–72. https://doi.org/10.1097/SLA.0000000000004913.
6. Olson MT, Mittal SK, Bremner RM. A collective review of gore bio-A absorbable synthetic mesh in cruroplasty reinforcement. J Laparoendosc Adv Surg Tech A. 2021;31(1):61–70. https://doi.org/10.1089/lap.2020.0343.
7. Panici Tonucci T, Asti E, Sironi A, Ferrari D, Bonavina L. Safety and efficacy of crura augmentation with phasix ST mesh for large hiatal hernia: 3-year single-center experience. J Laparoendosc Adv Surg Tech A. 2020;30(4):369–72. https://doi.org/10.1089/lap.2019.0726.

Achalasia

Endoscopic Botulinum Toxin Injection

Daniel Ludi and Anna M. Lipowska

Abstract Achalasia is a rare esophageal motility disorder that causes difficulty swallowing due to failure of peristalsis and inability to relax the lower esophageal sphincter. Botulinum toxin injection is a treatment option for achalasia that relaxes the lower esophageal sphincter, allowing improved emptying of the esophagus. This chapter describes each endoscopic botulinum toxin injection step with representative images.

Keywords Achalasia · Esophagogastroduodenoscopy · Botulinum toxin

Introduction

Achalasia is a rare esophageal motility disorder that causes difficulty swallowing due to failure of peristalsis and inability to relax the lower esophageal sphincter (LES). Myotomy, where the muscles of the LES are cut, is the mainstay therapy that can provide definitive treatment of achalasia symptoms. This can be performed in a variety of ways including a surgical heller myotomy, pneumatic dilation, or peroral endoscopic myotomy. For patients who are not good candidates for more definitive therapy or require initial bridging to other therapies, botulinum toxin (Botox) injection is a valuable treatment modality. Botox relaxes the lower esophageal sphincter, allowing improved emptying of the esophagus. This therapy overall has a good safety profile, though carries with it the likely need for repeat treatments and concerns that may make future myotomy more difficult [1].

In this chapter, the endoscopic botulinum toxin injection procedure with representative images is described.

D. Ludi · A. M. Lipowska (✉)
Division of Gastroenterology and Hepatology, Department of Medicine, University of Illinois at Chicago, Chicago, IL, USA
e-mail: lipowska@uic.edu

F. Schlottmann, M. A. Masrur (eds.), *Endoscopic, Laparoscopic and Robotic Techniques for Foregut Disorders*, https://doi.org/10.1007/978-3-032-00811-4_22

Procedure Description

Lower esophageal sphincter botox injection is performed via esophagogastroduodenoscopy (EGD). The standard protocol for an EGD is for the patient to be fasting after midnight on the day of the procedure. However, patients with achalasia are at greater risk of retained food content in the esophagus and aspiration. Thus, as a precautionary measure, it may be considered to have patients on a clear liquid diet the day before the endoscopy procedure and then nil per os (NPO) after midnight [2]. Anticoagulant or antiplatelet therapy should be held in concordance with guidelines for other endoscopic procedures.

Patient Positioning

To perform an EGD, the patient should be positioned on their left side in the left lateral decubitus position. The patient's head should be in a comfortable, neutral position. The bed height is determined by the endoscopist with the goal of performing the procedure in a neutral ergonomically optimized pose. This endoscopic procedure can be done under moderate sedation or with anesthesia support. Once sedation begins, a bite block is placed to protect the patient's teeth during the procedure and the endoscope is advanced into the patient's mouth.

Procedure Description

Initial Evaluation of Upper Gastrointestinal Tract

The endoscopist will insert the tip of the endoscope over the tongue, carefully advancing the scope through direct visualization under the epiglottis and cricoarytenoid cartilage to intubate the esophagus. Before intervention in the distal esophagus, the whole of the esophagus, stomach, and first and second portions of the duodenum are examined for significant pathology. It will also be essential to suction any retained contents in the esophagus or stomach.

Inspection of the Lower Esophageal Sphincter

The LES is examined on both forward and retroflexed views. On forward view, landmarks to be noted include the squamocolumnar junction ("z-line"), the diaphragmatic pinch, and the top of the gastric folds. Significant pathology to evaluate includes hiatal hernia, esophagitis, stricture, and any mass or nodules at the

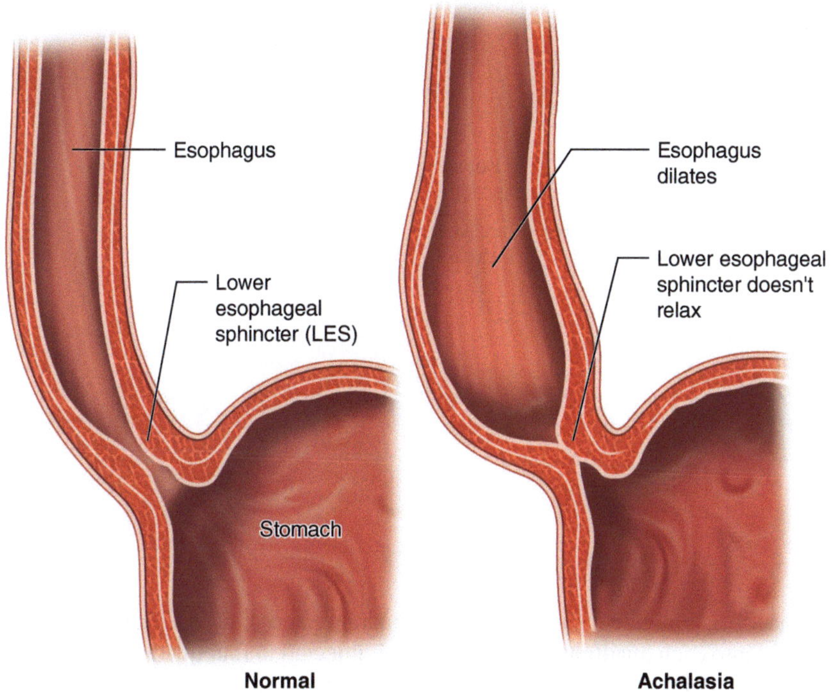

Fig. 1 Puckering gastroesophageal junction and dilated esophagus

gastroesophageal junction. In the case of more advanced achalasia, a hypertonic puckered LES and/or a dilated esophagus can be present (Fig. 1).

Injection of Botulinum Toxin

Once satisfied with the inspection of the anatomy, preparation for injection of botulinum toxin can commence. Using a Botox vial containing 100 units of powder, the vial is diluted in 4 mL of normal saline to yield a solution containing 25 U/mL. The reconstituted solution in a sterile syringe is then connected to the injection catheter. The sclerotherapy needle catheter is passed through the gastroscope until visualized just outside the scope. Once the endoscopist and endoscopy nurse are ready, the needle can be advanced out of the catheter and then pushed into the lower esophageal sphincter (Fig. 2). Generally the LES injection target is located 1 to 2 centimeters proximal to the squamocolumnar junction. It is essential for there to be strong closed-loop communication between the endoscopist and the endoscopy nurse in advancing the needle in and out of the catheter as there is the risk of mucosal damage from the exposed needle.

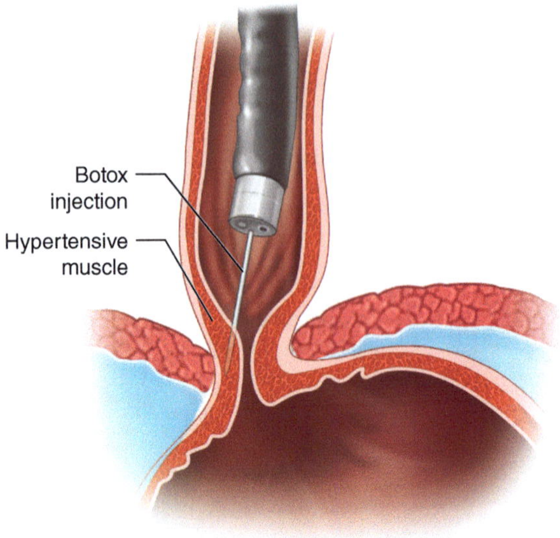

Fig. 2 Botox needle injection

The LES is divided into four equal quadrants and 1 mL of Botox solution is injected into each quadrant for a total of 4 mL injected in four quadrants. The needle should be maintained perpendicular to the esophageal wall and buried into the mucosa to avoid Botox spilling into the lumen. Care should also be taken to avoid injection outside the esophageal wall or creation of visible blebs. As the injection catheter holds 1 mL of fluid, the last injection is done by flushing the catheter with 1 mL of normal saline. The needle is then drawn back into the catheter.

Final Inspection and Discharge

Prior to removing the gastroscope, fluid is removed from the gastric body and a final inspection of the esophagus is done. Patients typically can go home after routine criteria for sedation recovery are met.

Conclusions

Botulinum toxin injection is a minimally invasive approach that offers an alternative to more invasive myotomy procedures, particularly in patients who may be unfit for such interventions due to comorbidities. Caution should be taken in patients under consideration for definitive myotomy treatment. Overall, Botox injection in achalasia management can provide symptomatic relief and improve the quality of life for affected individuals, serving as an effective bridge to more definitive treatments when necessary.

Conflict of Interest Daniel Ludi and Anna Lipowska declare that they have no conflicts of interest.

References

1. Zaninotto G, Annese V, Costantini M, Del Genio A, Costantino M, Epifani M, Gatto G, D'onofrio V, Benini L, Contini S, Molena D, Battaglia G, Tardio B, Andriulli A, Ancona E. Randomized controlled trial of botulinum toxin versus laparoscopic heller myotomy for esophageal achalasia. Ann Surg. 2004;239(3):364–70. https://doi.org/10.1097/01.sla.0000114217.52941.c5. PMID: 15075653; PMCID: PMC1356234.
2. Löser B, Recio Ariza O, Saugel B, Reuter DA, Zöllner C, Werner YB, Rösch T, Petzoldt M. Anesthesia for patients undergoing peroral endoscopic myotomy procedures: a review of the literature. Anesth Analg. 2020;130(5):1331–40. https://doi.org/10.1213/ANE.0000000000004420.

Selected Readings

3. Khashab MA, Vela MF, Thosani N, et al. ASGE guideline on the management of achalasia. Gastrointest Endosc. 2020;91(2):213–227.e6. https://doi.org/10.1016/j.gie.2019.04.231.
4. Shim CS. Endoscopic botulinum toxin injection: benefit and limitation. Gastrointest Interv. 2014;3(1):19–23. https://doi.org/10.1016/j.gii.2014.03.001.
5. Ramzan Z, Nassri AB. The role of botulinum toxin injection in the management of achalasia. Curr Opin Gastroenterol. 2013;29(4):468–73. https://doi.org/10.1097/MOG.0b013e328362292a.

Pneumatic Dilation

Brian R. Boulay

Abstract Pneumatic dilation (PD) has been used for decades as a treatment for symptoms of achalasia. The procedure works by inflating a noncompliant balloon across the gastroesophageal junction to disrupt the muscle fibers of the lower esophageal sphincter. PD can be performed on an outpatient basis and with minimal specialized equipment. PD remains an effective option for achalasia treatment and should be included as a therapeutic option for patients who prefer less invasive treatment options, though repeat treatment may be necessary for recurrent symptoms.

Keywords Pneumatic dilation · Achalasia · Dysphagia · Lower esophageal sphincter · Per oral endoscopic myotomy (POEM)

Introduction

Achalasia is a disorder of esophageal motility in which the lower esophageal sphincter (LES) fails to relax, resulting in dysphagia as well as impaired peristalsis within the esophageal body. Therapy for achalasia has traditionally been surgical in nature, via use of a myotomy of the lower esophageal sphincter muscles. The current version of surgical therapy is the laparoscopic Heller myotomy (LHM), typically performed with the addition of an antireflux surgery to counteract the reduced tone of the LES and prevent symptomatic gastroesophageal reflux disease (GERD) symptoms [1].

Endoscopic injection of botulinum toxin into the muscles of the LES is also effective, but has a limited duration of effect (typically weeks or months) and is reserved for patients unfit for surgery. The past decade has seen a rise in the use of

B. R. Boulay (✉)
Department of Medicine, Division of Gastroenterology & Hepatology, University of Illinois, Chicago, IL, USA
e-mail: bboulay@uic.edu

F. Schlottmann, M. A. Masrur (eds.), *Endoscopic, Laparoscopic and Robotic Techniques for Foregut Disorders*, https://doi.org/10.1007/978-3-032-00811-4_23

per-oral endoscopic myotomy (POEM) to achieve a myotomy of the lower esophageal sphincter via a submucosal tunnel in the esophagus. First perfomed by Inoue in 2010, POEM has now become a widely accepted therapy for POEM and its adoption throughout the world has been rapid [2].

Pneumatic balloon dilation is another effective therapy for achalasia. The premise of pneumatic dilation is to use a large-bore balloon to stretch and disrupt the muscle fibers of the lower esophageal sphincter. This improves dysphagia symptoms by lowering the tone of the LES and allowing passage of food and liquids. The concept of dilation to relieve dysphagia attributed to achalasia dates back to the late seventeenth century, and the use of a water-filled balloon was first reported in 1921 and remained the standard of care for decades [3]. Success of treatment in relieving symptoms can be quantified by the Eckardt score. This score is a sum of symptom scores for dysphagia, regurgitation, chest pain, and weight loss [4]. A post-treatment score of <3 is typically used in clinical studies to indicate successful relief of symptoms.

Within the past decade several subtypes of achalasia have been recognized and described by use of high-resolution manometry. The Chicago Classification recognizes three types of achalasia [5, 6]. Type I and type II achalasia share similar properties on manometry with impaired LES relaxation as well as absent peristalsis within the esophageal body; however, in type I achalasia there is normal esophageal pressure while in type II achalasia there is increased pan-esophageal pressure. It is thought that type II is an earlier phase of the disease and progresses to type I achalasia, which includes the classic radiologic findings of a dilated esophagus with "bird's beak" tapering at the LES. The three subtypes have differing prognoses and responses to treatment, with type II patients having the best outcomes regardless of treatment and type III patients being the most difficult to treat, with the need for a longer myotomy uniquely suited to POEM treatment.

Procedure Description

The treatment of achalasia with PD requires little specialized equipment other than the dilation balloon itself and a manometer to ensure that the balloon is inflated with enough pressure to create an effective myotomy. Prior to the procedure, the endoscopist must choose a balloon size. Balloons are 8–10 cm in length and available in 30 mm, 35 mm, and 40 mm diameter, mounted on a 75–90 mm catheter which can be advanced over a wire. The balloons are designed with fluoroscopic markers at the proximal and distal extent to assist in appropriate positioning across the lower esophageal sphincter. Some balloons may have additional markers at the midline to assist in positioning across the LES (Fig. 1).

A manometer is attached to the balloon catheter to measure the pressure during inflation. Whereas high compliance balloons were once available for purposes of PD, currently available balloons have low compliance so that their maximal intended

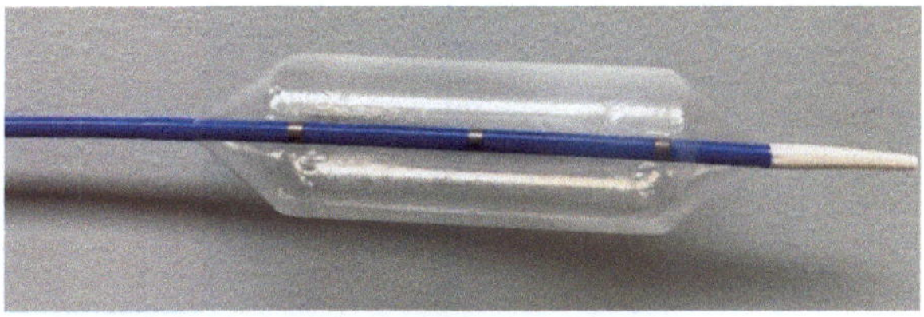

Fig. 1 A 35 mm low compliance pneumatic dilation balloon is pictured, with fluoroscopic markers at each end of the balloon as well as the midpoint. The balloon catheter may be advanced over a wire to the gastroesophageal junction and positioned under fluoroscopic guidance. (Cook Endoscopy, Winston-Salem NC, USA)

diameters are not exceeded even in cases of overinflation. Guidelines from the American College of Gastroenterology recommend initial dilation with a 30 mm balloon, followed by assessment of symptoms 4–6 weeks later [7]. If the response is incomplete, then the next largest size of dilation balloon may be used. European guidelines likewise recommend initial treatment with a 30 mm balloon to decrease the risk of perforation [8].

The procedure should be performed with the patient under general anesthesia, as the dilated esophagus often contains a significant volume of liquid or even solid food due to the underlying disordered motility, and aspiration is a significant risk without airway protection. An upper endoscope with a large caliber (3.2 mm) therapeutic channel should be used to allow for brisk suctioning of fluid through the scope. Clearance of the esophagus may also require removal of solid food debris. This can be performed with use of foreign body retrieval tools such as graspers, baskets, or nets.

Once the esophagus is clear of debris, the scope may be advanced to the stomach. Measurements are taken of the site of the GE junction, which is marked so that the balloon may be placed accurately across the LES. A radiopaque marker such as a paperclip may be placed externally on the patient as a fluoroscopic marker of the level of this critical landmark. Alternatively, 1–2 mL of contrast may be injected into the submucosa at the GE junction as an internal fluoroscopic marker [9]. A stiff guidewire (typically an 0.035 inch flexible wire) is then deployed into the stomach and allowed to coil, and the scope is withdrawn from the esophagus while leaving the wire in place under fluoroscopic guidance. The balloon is then advanced over the wire into the esophagus and across the GE junction. It is important to ensure that the balloon's midpoint lines up with the marker denoting the GE junction, so that the balloon exerts its radial force upon the muscle fibers of the lower esophageal sphincter.

Inflation is performed, using traction on the catheter to prevent the balloon from slipping into the stomach. During inflation there should initially be a visible waist in the midpoint of the balloon, representing the LES. The balloon is inflated until the waist is effaced on fluoroscopy and the pressure within the balloon (as measured by the manometer) matches the required amount to fully inflate the balloon per manufacturer instructions (Fig. 2). Dilation can also be performed under endoscopic

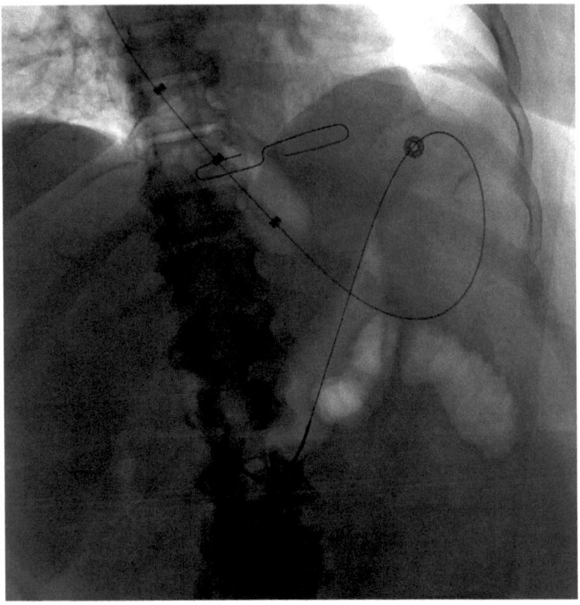

Fig. 2 A 30 mm pneumatic balloon is inflated across the lower esophageal sphincter under fluoroscopic guidance. The midline fluoroscopic marker is aligned with an externally placed paperclip, and the distal segment of the balloon is inferior to the diaphragm and extending into the proximal stomach. The midline waist of the balloon has been completely effaced in this image, indicating successful dilation

guidance with an endoscope passed alongside the balloon catheter to ensure proper location of the balloon [10].

After deflation of the balloon, it may be withdrawn from the mouth along with the guidewire. Successful dilation is often confirmed by the presence of blood on the balloon. The esophagus can then be evaluated for evidence of perforation. This can be performed endoscopically or fluoroscopically. Endoscopic evaluation can be performed to examine the mucosal tear and assess for full thickness perforation. Alternatively, the patient may undergo a gastrograffin esophagram either intraprocedurally or once awake following the procedure. There is not universal agreement as to whether routine contrast study is necessary after achalasia.

A retrospective study of 119 PD procedures in which 49 patients underwent routine esophagram and 70 were simply observed showed that 12 of the 70 patients developed concerning symptoms and then underwent esophagram based on suspicion of perforation. Three of these actually had perforation, while 0 of 58 patients without esophagram were later found to have a perforation [11]. The authors concluded that esophagram is best used only in cases with a clinical suspicion of perforation, rather than in every patient. Guidelines from the American College of Gastroenterology support this strategy and recommend against routine esophagram after PD [7].

Efficacy

Pneumatic dilation is overall quite effective for treatment of achalasia, with the caveat that repeat treatments may be required for a sustained effect. A systematic review and meta-analysis of 52 uncontrolled studies in 4166 patients showed that clinical success (defined as an Eckardt score ≤3) was achieved in 83% of treated patients over a follow up period of 3–6 months. This included a reduction in average LES pressure from 34.47 mmHg (range 32.82–36.13) to 20.80 mmHg (range 12.11–29.49) on manometry after treatment, a difference which was statistically significant ($P < .01$) [12]. It was noted that some of these trials included only a single dilation rather than graded dilation with larger balloons after initial treatment failure. Thus, efficacy in clinical practice may be even higher when using a graded dilation strategy beginning with a 30 mm balloon and increasing if needed based on patient response.

The evidence for ongoing use of PD as a primary therapy for achalasia stems largely from The European Achalasia Trial, a multicenter randomized controlled trial of 201 patients comparing laparoscopic Heller myotomy (LHM) to PD [13]. In this protocol, for the patients in the PD group two dilation procedures were performed using a 30 and 35 mm balloons 1–3 weeks apart. Symptoms were then assessed by Eckardt score. The patients were followed for a median of 43 months, and a third round of dilation was allowed if symptoms recurred after 2 years (without declaring failure of the PD treatment). The primary outcome of the trial was improvement in symptoms as measured by Eckardt score ≤3. PD and LHM success rates were comparable at 1 year (90% vs. 93%) and 2 years (86% vs. 90%). This study has been revisited at 5 year follow-up in which the success rates of PD and LHM were again comparable (84% vs. 82%), though it was noted that 25% of the PD patients required retreatment during the follow-up period [14]. Ten year follow up of this trial has also been reported with similar efficacy (74% vs. 74%) [15]. The authors have proposed that both PD and LHM can be considered as first line modalities for achalasia treatment, though patients in the PD group often required repeat dilation over time to match the more durable results of the initial LHM.

Efficacy of PD has also been studied in comparison to POEM. In a randomized controlled trial of PD versus POEM in treatment-naïve patients, the PD group was initially treated with 30 mm dilation, followed by 35 mm dilation 3 weeks later if needed. Those 66 patients receiving PD were compared to 64 POEM patients. In this study, repeat sessions of PD other than the initial 1–2 were not included and recurrent symptoms were considered a failure of PD therapy. Treatment success (measured as Eckardt score <3, absence of retreatment, and lack of complications) was 92% for POEM compared to 54% for PD over 2 years of follow up [16]. Follow up was extended to 5 years with similar results, with the POEM group having 81% treatment success compared to 40% in the PD group. The reasons for treatment failure included recurrent symptoms in 11 of 62 POEM patients and 25 of 63 PD patients [17]. As this protocol did not allow for repeat dilation sessions among patients with recurrent symptoms over time, PD was less effective as definitive treatment. Whether the need for repeat PD sessions over long-term follow-up truly represents a treatment failure is a matter of perspective, given the improved results for PD when repeat dilations are performed for recurrent symptoms.

Predictors of Response

The subtype of achalasia appears to have an impact on the therapeutic value of treatment. In particular, pneumatic dilation may perform poorly in type III achalasia (also known as spastic achalasia) relative to other treatments such as POEM. Patients with type III achalasia have a suboptimal response to therapies that address only the LES as there is also spastic contraction of a length of the distal esophagus. This was demonstrated by a meta-analysis of 1575 patients who underwent treatment for achalasia and were then grouped by achalasia subtype [18]. In this analysis the success rate of PD for type II achalasia was 84%, which was lower than the 92% for LHM and 97% for POEM but overall deemed acceptable. However, for patients with type III achalasia the success rate of PD was only 31% compared to 71% in the LHM group and 93% in the POEM group. For type I achalasia the success rate for PD was 61%, while LHM and POEM had 81% and 95% success rates respectively. The authors concluded that PD remains a competitive treatment modality for type II achalasia, which seems to respond well to any of the three main treatment strategies. For patients with type I or type III achalasia, other treatment options were recommended.

Of note, some studies have shown a more promising response to PD treatment for type I achalasia than the meta-analysis noted above. Torresan and colleagues conducted a retrospective review of 101 patients excluding type III achalasia (27 type I, 74 type II) who underwent a graded protocol for dilation starting with a 30 mm balloon and progressing to larger balloons as needed if symptoms persisted after 2 weeks. Up to 3 dilations were performed. In long-term follow up with a mean time of 56 months, and with allowance for redilation to treat recurrent symptoms, the rate of successful symptom control (defined as Eckardt score <3) was 95.5% in type I achalasia and 90% in type II [19]. Despite the small size of the study, it is illustrative of the importance of repeat treatments over time in maintaining symptom control, and suggests that type I achalasia patients may well respond to PD under such clinical practice. Current guidelines from the American Gastroenterological Association (AGA) and American Society of Gastrointestinal Endoscopy (ASGE) include PD among the comparable therapies for achalasia types I and II, though POEM is preferred for type III [12, 20]. ACG guidelines also recommend tailoring therapy based on manometric subtype, favoring LHM or POEM over PD in patients with type III achalasia [7].

Aside from achalasia subtype, other factors have been shown to influence the patient response to PD. Demographic factors appear to have an impact. Response is more favorable in older patients, with one retrospective study showing >6 months of clinical remission in 85.7% of patients over 40 years old, and only 38.5% in patients under 40 [21]. When considering whether patient gender predicts response, a meta-analysis showed no association in 20 of 23 studies [22]. Among the 3 studies showing an association with gender, younger men had a less predictable response to PD treatment even using multiple dilations with increasing balloon size [23–25]. ACG guidelines for achalasia treatment note the poor response to PD in young men and recommend initial treatment with a 35 mm balloon rather than the standard initial size of 30 mm [7]. Symptoms of achalasia, including severity and duration of symptoms, do not overall appear to predict the response to treatment [22]. Radiologic factors such as esophageal dilation on a timed barium swallow have yielded conflicting results, with most studies showing no association with treatment outcome after PD.

Adverse Events

The use of pneumatic dilation is likely hindered by the feared complication of full thickness perforation. The procedure should be limited to settings in which the endoscopist has appropriate surgical backup or the capability of managing a perforation endoscopically, such as with placement of a fully covered esophageal stent across the site of perforation. Perforation rate was found to be 2.8% (95% CI, 2.3%–3.5%) in the largest meta-analysis [12]. The other significant periprocedural adverse event was bleeding requiring intervention (2%, 95% CI 1%–4%). Initial treatment with a 30 mm balloon is advised in an effort to reduce the perforation rate. Notably, in the European Achalasia trial the initial protocol was to begin with a 35 mm balloon, but four of the first 13 patients suffered perforation and the protocol was thus revised to begin with a 30 mm balloon [13]. In clinical practice, advancing to larger balloon sizes is advised if patients fail to respond to the initial 30 mm dilation.

Management of perforation relies on local expertise as well as the severity of the perforation. Ghoshal et al. reported a single center two-decade experience of PD for achalasia, in which 12 of 433 patients (2.7%) suffered perforation. In 11 of 12 patients, perforation occurred on their first PD treatment. Treatment was variable, with 7 patients undergoing surgery, one managed with a fully covered esophageal stent, and four with a small leak or pneumomediastinum were managed conservatively. No mortality was observed [26]. Other nonsurgical methods for management of perforation have also been described, including closure of the perforation with through-the-scope clips as well as transnasal endoscopic vacuum therapy across the perforation [27]. Surgical repair of perforation after PD can be performed laparoscopically, with primary suturing of the defect followed by myotomy of the contralateral wall and a partial anterior fundoplication [28].

Some patients may experience symptomatic reflux following the procedure (akin to other endoscopic treatment modalities such as POEM in which no antireflux measures are taken) though the rate of GERD appears to be smaller for pneumatic dilation than it is for POEM. The meta-analysis conducted as part of the ASGE guidelines reports that the rate of symptomatic GERD 6 months after pneumatic dilation was found to be 9% (95% CI, 5%–16%) [12]. In the randomized trial of PD versus POEM conducted by Ponds et al., the rate of reflux esophagitis was significantly higher in the POEM group (41% vs. 7%) in short term follow up, though most of these changes were mild in severity [16]. As for long term effect of disruption of the LES without an antireflux procedure, after 5 years the patients from this trial were found to have significantly higher rate of use of proton pump inhibitors if they had undergone POEM (46%) compared to the patients from the PD group (13%). Thus, even without the antireflux procedure afforded by treatment with LHM, patients treated by PD appear to have less GERD than those treated by POEM.

Use of Pneumatic Dilation After Prior Treatment

Any of the treatment modalities for achalasia may fail over time with recurrence of symptoms. In the case of repeat treatment, any of the three main options (PD, LHM, or POEM) may be offered. However, repeat treatment may be complicated by scarring following myotomy of the LES and resulting scarring. PD may offer a convenient option to treat recurring symptoms on an outpatient basis. We have already seen that repeat treatment can be offered during the follow-up period for patients who were initially treated with PD. In fact, the studies in which PD performs most favorably in comparison to LHM and POEM often included repeat dilations as part of the treatment protocol for patients with recurrent symptoms [13]. The efficacy of PD for repeat treatment in patients who have undergone initial achalasia therapy with LHM or POEM has been studied in a meta-analysis of 87 patients who underwent PD a mean time of 4 months after LHM. The success rate of PD treatment was 89% though patients required a mean number of 2.5 PD treatments at a mean interval of 26 months [29].

More recently, a randomized controlled trial was conducted on 90 patients with persistent or recurrent symptoms after LHM who underwent treatment with PD or POEM. The success rate of POEM (28/45 patients, 62.2%) was higher than that of PD (12/45 patients, 26.7%). Rates of reflux esophagitis were higher in POEM but this did not reach statistical significance. Posttreatment measures such as basal lower esophageal sphincter pressure and integrated relaxation pressure on manometry and barium column height after 2 and 5 min were both significantly less in patients treated with POEM [30]. Importantly, the patients in the PD arm of the study underwent 2 planned dilations and were allowed an additional dilation before 12 months before being considered treatment failures with recurrent symptoms. Still, the strikingly low success rate for PD as a treatment in patients with previous LHM was met with some criticism that the balloon pressures used during dilation may have been suboptimal, and that fluoroscopic confirmation of obliteration of the waist of the balloon may have improved the performance of PD in the study [31]. Further randomized controlled studies will be needed to clarify the efficacy of PD following previous treatment with POEM or LHM.

Comparison to Other Treatment Modalities

Pneumatic dilation has been compared to botulinum toxin therapy in numerous studies, with findings of similar initial efficacy but better duration of effect with PD. Leyden at al conducted a systematic review of seven randomized controlled trials involving 178 patients and found no significant difference in remission within 4 weeks, but the remission rates of symptoms at 6 months favored PD (46 of 57 patients) over botulinum (29 of 56 patients) with a risk ratio of 1.57 (95% CI 1.19–2.08). Likewise, the symptomatic remission rates at 12 months were significantly greater in the patients who had undergone PD (55 of 75 patients) compared to patients receiving botulinum injection (27 of 72), with a risk ratio of 1.88 (95% CI 1.35–2.61). Of note, there were no adverse events in the botulinum toxin group, while 3 of 188 patients receiving PD had esophageal perforation [32].

Pneumatic dilation has also been compared to laparoscopic Heller myotomy. The landmark European Achalasia Trial has been discussed earlier in this chapter, showing similar short-term and long-term success when multiple PD sessions are allowed by protocol [13]. The collective experience of PD versus LHM was analyzed by Cheng et al. in a meta-analysis of five randomized controlled trials involving 498 patients. Laparoscopic Heller myotomy showed a higher clinical success rate in short-term follow-up of 3 months (risk ratio 1.16, 95% CI 1.01–1.35, $p = 0.04$) and 1 year (risk ratio 1.14, 95% CI 1.02–1.27, $p = .02$). However, at 2- and 5-year follow-up the clinical success rates were not significantly different. The 2-year risk ratio was 1.05 (95% CI .91–1.22, $p = .49$) and 5 year risk ratio was 1.17 (95% CI .84–1.64, $p = .34$). The authors concluded that given the comparable long-term efficacy, either treatment could be offered as initial treatment for achalasia [33].

Comparison of pneumatic dilation to POEM has been reported. The most notable trial by Ponds and colleagues (discussed earlier) did show superiority of POEM in treatment-naïve patients, but did not allow for repeat PD treatments over time [16]. Ofosu et al. conducted a meta-analysis of clinical trials with 12-month follow-up, including 66 studies (6268 patients) of which 29 studies reported on POEM and 33 studies reported on pneumatic dilation. Only four studies (299 patients) directly compared POEM to pneumatic dilation. In this analysis, clinical success rate with POEM was superior to dilation at 12 months (92.9% vs. 76.9%, $p = 0.001$), 24 months (90.6% vs. 74.8%, $P = 0.004$), and 36 months (92.3% vs. 41.9%, $p = 0.01$). The OR of GERD was significantly higher with POEM (by symptoms: 2.95, $P = 0.02$ and by endoscopic findings: 6.98, $P = 0.001$). Rates of esophageal perforation (0.3% vs. 0.6%, $P = 0.8$) and significant bleeding (0.4% vs. 0.7%, $P = 0.56$) were comparable between the POEM and PD groups [34]. A second meta-analysis was performed by the authors of the most recent ASGE guideline on achalasia, based on only 3 studies on a total of 114 patients treated with POEM and 92 patients treated with PD. Clinical success at 1 year was higher in the POEM group

(93% vs. 72%, RR 1.28, 95% CI 1.14–1.45, p = <.01). There was a trend towards more symptomatic GERD after POEM compared to pneumatic dilation (23% vs. 9%) [12]. While these analyses favor POEM over pneumatic dilation, other authors have cautioned against making strong conclusions in comparing POEM to PD based on the available data. De Heer at al attempted a meta-analysis of six randomized controlled trials and noted differences in PD regimens as well as clinical dysphagia scores across the trials, as well as methodologic limitations that hindered comparative analysis [35]. As we await additional high-quality studies directly comparing PD to POEM, the apparent superiority of POEM must be considered within the context of this limited and heterogeneous data.

Pneumatic Dilation's Current Role in Modern Achalasia Treatment

The role of PD in current management of achalasia has been challenged by the increasing use of POEM as a definitive treatment. A review of achalasia treatment in the US reported a 19-fold increase in the use of POEM between 2010 and 2017, though LHM remains the most common approach [36]. The increasing adoption of POEM will undoubtedly continue to marginalize the use of PD as equipment and expertise improve, and institutions invest effort and resources into training their staff to offer POEM to patients.

The cost-effectiveness of each strategy for achalasia treatment has been analyzed by several authors, illustrating the trade-off between the initial ease of PD (and botulinum toxin) versus the more resource-intensive but definitive therapies of POEM and LHM. Lois and colleagues found the total 1-year health costs associated with PD were significantly lower than those for POEM (mean cost difference, $7674; 95% CI, $657–$14,692) [36]. Miller and colleagues conducted a cost-utility analysis of the endoscopic and surgical treatments for achalasia over a 4 year period. The measure used in this analysis was "cost per cure" which was measured throughout the follow up period. LHM and POEM had the highest initial costs per cure in year one ($11,582 and $12,120) compared to $7175 for PD. However, by year four the PD group had required repeat interventions due to recurrence of symptoms. This shifted the cost per cure to $2329 for PD, comparable to $2896 for LHM and $3030 for POEM, effectively eroding the cost-effectiveness advantage for PD in the short term [37].

The need for reintervention in PD and its impact on cost were also evaluated in a retrospective cohort study of 1061 patients treated by LHM or PD in the United States. LM was associated with an 82% lower rate of re-intervention ($p < 0.01$), 29% lower rate of subsequent diagnostic testing ($p < 0.01$), and 53% lower rate of re-admission ($p < 0.01$). While the initial costs were higher in LHM than for PD ($29,257 versus $5683, $p < 0.01$), the need for subsequent testing and reintervention in the PD group meant that at 1 year there was no difference in mean total costs ($30,110 versus $23,610, $p = 0.66$) [38]. In contrast, an economic evaluation of the

European Achalasia trial (in which PD was found to have comparable success with LHM with repeated dilations) showed a sustained cost advantage to PD even after 5 years [39].

As seen in the comparative trials of PD to LHM and POEM, the efficacy of PD declines over time with return of symptoms in a significant proportion of patients. To maintain a comparable efficacy to other modalities, repeat dilations over time are required. When discussing treatment options with patients, pneumatic dilation may still be presented as a reasonable approach, but patients should be counselled that repeated dilations over time may be required, in contrast to the more definitive options of LHM and POEM. The benefits of PD include its ease of performance and the use of an outpatient setting. Despite the fear of perforation associated with PD, it generally has little morbidity particularly when dilation is begun with the 30 mm balloon. The PD approach seems to have less of an association with postprocedural GERD in comparison with POEM. All of these factors, in addition to institutional expertise and patient preference, should be considered when planning achalasia treatment.

Conclusions

Pneumatic dilation remains an effective option for treatment of achalasia despite the competing methods of laparoscopic Heller myotomy and POEM. Pneumatic dilation can be performed on an outpatient basis and requires little specialized training or dedicated equipment. The rate of severe adverse events such as perforation is quite low using modern technique and equipment, but appropriate surgical backup is advised. Studies comparing the efficacy of PD to other techniques have mixed results, generally indicating that PD has a less durable effect when compared to LHM or POEM. However, when repeat dilations are considered over time, the effect on resolution of symptoms can likely approach these other two techniques. When discussing achalasia treatment with patients, the benefits and risks of repeated treatment with PD over time should be contrasted with the intended definitive use of a more invasive treatment such as LHM or POEM. Patients with type III achalasia are less likely to respond to any treatment and in particular are ill-suited for PD based on current evidence.

References

1. Fisichella PM, Patti MG. From Heller to POEM (1914-2014): a 100-year history of surgery for achalasia. J Gastrointest Surg. 2014;18(10):1870–5. https://doi.org/10.1007/s11605-014-2547-8.
2. Inoue H, Minami H, Kobayashi Y, et al. Peroral endoscopic myotomy (POEM) for esophageal achalasia. Endoscopy. 2010;42(4):265–71. https://doi.org/10.1055/s-0029-1244080.

3. Markar S, Zaninotto G. Endoscopic pneumatic dilation for esophageal achalasia. Am Surg. 2018;84(4):473–6.
4. Eckardt VF. Clinical presentations and complications of achalasia. Gastrointest Endosc Clin N Am. 2001;11(2):281–92, vi
5. Kahrilas PJ, Bredenoord AJ, Fox M, et al. The Chicago classification of esophageal motility disorders, v3.0. Neurogastroenterol Motil. 2015;27(2):160–74. https://doi.org/10.1111/nmo.12477.
6. Yadlapati R, Kahrilas PJ, Fox MR, et al. Esophageal motility disorders on high-resolution manometry: Chicago classification version 4.0©. Neurogastroenterol Motil. 2021;33(1):e14058. https://doi.org/10.1111/nmo.14058.
7. Vaezi MF, Pandolfino JE, Yadlapati RH, Greer KB, Kavitt RT. ACG clinical guidelines: diagnosis and management of achalasia. Am J Gastroenterol. 2020;115(9):1393–411. https://doi.org/10.14309/ajg.0000000000000731.
8. Oude Nijhuis RAB, Zaninotto G, Roman S, et al. European guidelines on achalasia: United European Gastroenterology and European Society of Neurogastroenterology and Motility recommendations. United European Gastroenterol J. 2020;8(1):13–33. https://doi.org/10.1177/2050640620903213.
9. Ajayeoba OO, Diehl DL. Pneumatic dilation for achalasia: new techniques to improve an old procedure. VideoGIE. 2020;5(10):449–50. https://doi.org/10.1016/j.vgie.2020.05.011.
10. Chuah SK, Wu KL, Hu TH, Tai WC, Changchien CS. Endoscope-guided pneumatic dilation for treatment of esophageal achalasia. World J Gastroenterol. 2010;16(4):411–7. https://doi.org/10.3748/wjg.v16.i4.411.
11. Zori AG, Kirtane TS, Gupte AR, et al. Utility of clinical suspicion and endoscopic re-examination for detection of esophagogastric perforation after pneumatic dilation for achalasia. Endoscopy. 2016;48(2):128–33. https://doi.org/10.1055/s-0034-1392860.
12. Khashab MA, Vela MF, Thosani N, et al. ASGE guideline on the management of achalasia. Gastrointest Endosc. 2020;91(2):213–227.e6. https://doi.org/10.1016/j.gie.2019.04.231.
13. Boeckxstaens GE, Annese V, des Varannes SB, et al. Pneumatic dilation versus laparoscopic Heller's myotomy for idiopathic achalasia. N Engl J Med. 2011;364(19):1807–16. https://doi.org/10.1056/NEJMoa1010502.
14. Moonen A, Annese V, Belmans A, et al. Long-term results of the European achalasia trial: a multicentre randomised controlled trial comparing pneumatic dilation versus laparoscopic Heller myotomy. Gut. 2016;65(5):732–9. https://doi.org/10.1136/gutjnl-2015-310602.
15. Boeckxstaens G, Elsen S, Belmans A, et al. 10-year follow-up results of the European achalasia trial: a multicentre randomised controlled trial comparing pneumatic dilation with laparoscopic Heller myotomy. Gut. 2024;73(4):582–9. https://doi.org/10.1136/gutjnl-2023-331374.
16. Ponds FA, Fockens P, Lei A, et al. Effect of peroral endoscopic myotomy vs pneumatic dilation on symptom severity and treatment outcomes among treatment-naive patients with achalasia: a randomized clinical trial. JAMA. 2019;322(2):134–44. https://doi.org/10.1001/jama.2019.8859.
17. Kuipers T, Ponds FA, Fockens P, et al. Peroral endoscopic myotomy versus pneumatic dilation in treatment-naive patients with achalasia: 5-year follow-up of a randomised controlled trial. Lancet Gastroenterol Hepatol. 2022;7(12):1103–11. https://doi.org/10.1016/S2468-1253(22)00300-4.
18. Andolfi C, Fisichella PM. Meta-analysis of clinical outcome after treatment for achalasia based on manometric subtypes. Br J Surg. 2019;106(4):332–41. https://doi.org/10.1002/bjs.11049.
19. Torresan F, Cortellini F, Azzaroli F, et al. Graded pneumatic dilation in subtype I and II achalasia: long-term experience in a single center. Ann Gastroenterol. 2022;35(1):28–33. https://doi.org/10.20524/aog.2021.0683.
20. Kahrilas PJ, Katzka D, Richter JE. Clinical practice update: the use of per-oral endoscopic myotomy in achalasia: expert review and best practice advice from the AGA Institute. Gastroenterology. 2017;153(5):1205–11. https://doi.org/10.1053/j.gastro.2017.10.001.

21. Tanaka Y, Iwakiri K, Kawami N, et al. Predictors of a better outcome of pneumatic dilatation in patients with primary achalasia. J Gastroenterol. 2010;45(2):153–8. https://doi.org/10.1007/s00535-009-0145-4.
22. Oude Nijhuis RAB, Prins LI, Mostafavi N, van Etten-Jamaludin FS, Smout AJPM, Bredenoord AJ. Factors associated with achalasia treatment outcomes: systematic review and meta-analysis. Clin Gastroenterol Hepatol. 2020;18(7):1442–53. https://doi.org/10.1016/j.cgh.2019.10.008.
23. Farhoomand K, Connor JT, Richter JE, Achkar E, Vaezi MF. Predictors of outcome of pneumatic dilation in achalasia. Clin Gastroenterol Hepatol. 2004;2(5):389–94. https://doi.org/10.1016/s1542-3565(04)00123-5.
24. Ghoshal UC, Kumar S, Saraswat VA, Aggarwal R, Misra A, Choudhuri G. Long-term follow-up after pneumatic dilation for achalasia cardia: factors associated with treatment failure and recurrence. Am J Gastroenterol. 2004;99(12):2304–10. https://doi.org/10.1111/j.1572-0241.2004.40099.x.
25. Vela MF, Richter JE, Khandwala F, et al. The long-term efficacy of pneumatic dilatation and Heller myotomy for the treatment of achalasia. Clin Gastroenterol Hepatol. 2006;4(5):580–7. https://doi.org/10.1016/s1542-3565(05)00986-9.
26. Ghoshal UC, Karyampudi A, Verma A, et al. Perforation following pneumatic dilation of achalasia cardia in a university hospital in northern India: a two-decade experience. Indian J Gastroenterol. 2018;37(4):347–52. https://doi.org/10.1007/s12664-018-0874-5.
27. Oude Nijhuis RAB, Bergman JJGHM, Takkenberg RB, Fockens P, Bredenoord AJ. Non-surgical treatment of esophageal perforation after pneumatic dilation for achalasia: a case series. Scand J Gastroenterol. 2020;55(10):1248–52. https://doi.org/10.1080/00365521.2020.1817541.
28. Sánchez-Pernaute A, Aguirre EP, Talavera P, et al. Laparoscopic approach to esophageal perforation secondary to pneumatic dilation for achalasia. Surg Endosc. 2009;23(5):1106–9. https://doi.org/10.1007/s00464-008-0114-7.
29. Fernandez-Ananin S, Fernández AF, Balagué C, Sacoto D, Targarona EM. What to do when Heller's myotomy fails? Pneumatic dilatation, laparoscopic remyotomy or peroral endoscopic myotomy: a systematic review. J Minim Access Surg. 2018;14(3):177–84. https://doi.org/10.4103/jmas.JMAS_94_17.
30. Saleh CMG, Familiari P, Bastiaansen BAJ, et al. The efficacy of peroral endoscopic myotomy vs pneumatic dilation as treatment for patients with achalasia suffering from persistent or recurrent symptoms after laparoscopic Heller myotomy: a randomized clinical trial. Gastroenterology. 2023;164(7):1108–1118.e3. https://doi.org/10.1053/j.gastro.2023.02.048.
31. Vela MF, Vaezi MF. Should POEM be the rescue therapy of choice after failed laparoscopic Heller myotomy? Gastroenterology. 2023;164(7):1053–5. https://doi.org/10.1053/j.gastro.2023.03.225.
32. Leyden JE, Moss AC, MacMathuna P. Endoscopic pneumatic dilation versus botulinum toxin injection in the management of primary achalasia. Cochrane Database Syst Rev. 2014;2014(12):CD005046. https://doi.org/10.1002/14651858.CD005046.pub3.
33. Cheng JW, Li Y, Xing WQ, Lv HW, Wang HR. Laparoscopic Heller myotomy is not superior to pneumatic dilation in the management of primary achalasia: conclusions of a systematic review and meta-analysis of randomized controlled trials. Medicine (Baltimore). 2017;96(7):e5525. https://doi.org/10.1097/MD.0000000000005525.
34. Ofosu A, Mohan BP, Ichkhanian Y, et al. Peroral endoscopic myotomy (POEM) vs pneumatic dilation (PD) in treatment of achalasia: a meta-analysis of studies with ≥ 12-month follow-up. Endosc Int Open. 2021;9(7):E1097–107. https://doi.org/10.1055/a-1483-9406.
35. de Heer J, Desai M, Boeckxstaens G, et al. Pneumatic balloon dilatation versus laparoscopic Heller myotomy for achalasia: a failed attempt at meta-analysis. Surg Endosc. 2021;35(2):602–11. https://doi.org/10.1007/s00464-020-07421-x.
36. Lois AW, Oelschlager BK, Wright AS, Templeton AW, Flum DR, Farjah F. Use and safety of per-oral endoscopic myotomy for achalasia in the US. JAMA Surg. 2022;157(6):490–7. https://doi.org/10.1001/jamasurg.2022.0807.

37. Miller HJ, Neupane R, Fayezizadeh M, Majumder A, Marks JM. POEM is a cost-effective procedure: cost-utility analysis of endoscopic and surgical treatment options in the management of achalasia. Surg Endosc. 2017;31(4):1636–42. https://doi.org/10.1007/s00464-016-5151-z.
38. Ehlers AP, Oelschlager BK, Pellegrini CA, et al. Achalasia treatment, outcomes, utilization, and costs: a population-based study from the United States. J Am Coll Surg. 2017;225(3):380–6. https://doi.org/10.1016/j.jamcollsurg.2017.05.014.
39. Moonen A, Busch O, Costantini M, et al. Economic evaluation of the randomized European achalasia trial comparing pneumodilation with laparoscopic Heller myotomy. Neurogastroenterol Motil. 2017;29(11) https://doi.org/10.1111/nmo.13115.

POEM

Anthony J. Kang, Kevin P. Shah, Mark A. Solinski, and Abdul A. Aadam

Abstract Achalasia is an esophageal motility disorder characterized by impaired relaxation of the lower esophageal sphincter. Per-oral endoscopic myotomy (POEM) has arisen as an effective minimally invasive treatment option for patients with achalasia. In this chapter, each step of per-oral endoscopic myotomy with intraprocedural images is described.

Keywords Per-oral endoscopic myotomy · Achalasia · Third-space endoscopy

Introduction

Per-oral endoscopic myotomy (POEM) is a minimally invasive treatment that has gained widespread use since first performed in 2008. POEM is now a standard treatment option for patients with Type I, II, and III achalasia. POEM offers multiple strengths when compared to other traditional treatment options for achalasia, including laparoscopic Heller myotomy (LHM) and pneumatic dilation (PD). First, it offers a minimally invasive approach to myotomy with quick recovery time. Second, the rate of blown-out myotomy, a pseudodiverticulum that forms around the myotomy site, is lower in POEM when compared to LHM. Lastly, data suggests that the clinical efficacy of POEM is non-inferior to Heller myotomy, and the long-term efficacy of POEM may be greater than pneumatic dilation [1–6].

A. J. Kang · K. P. Shah · M. A. Solinski · A. A. Aadam (✉)
Division of Gastroenterology & Hepatology, Northwestern Feinberg School of Medicine, Chicago, IL, USA
e-mail: abdul.aadam@northwestern.edu

F. Schlottmann, M. A. Masrur (eds.), *Endoscopic, Laparoscopic and Robotic Techniques for Foregut Disorders*, https://doi.org/10.1007/978-3-032-00811-4_24

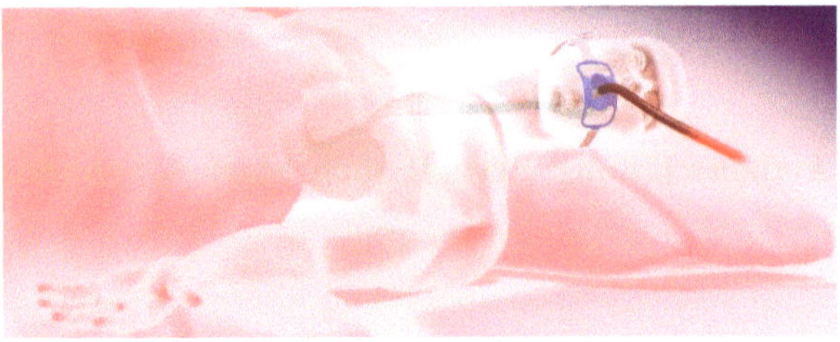

Fig. 1 Patient positioning for POEM procedure

In this chapter, each step of per-oral endoscopic myotomy with intraprocedural endoscopic images is described.

Procedure Description

Pre-procedure Preparation

The patient is placed in left lateral position for this procedure (Fig. 1). General anesthesia should be given with endotracheal intubation. Intravenous antibiotics are administered during the procedure for infectious prophylaxis. A standard gastroscope is utilized with a distal attachment cap.

Procedural Technique

Mucosal Incision and Exposure of the Submucosal Space

The endoscope is inserted through the mouth into the mid-distal esophagus positioned 6–10 cm proximal to the esophagogastric junction (EGJ) (Fig. 2).

The first step involves creating a mucosal incision to allow for access into the submucosal space, which the endoscope will be advanced through. Both an anterior and posterior approach to myotomy have been described for POEM. An anterior approach requires making an incision at the 1 or 2 o'clock position, allowing theoretically for lower risk of post-POEM reflux due to preservation of the gastric cardia sling fibers (Fig. 3).

A posterior approach requires making an incision at the 5 or 6 o'clock position, allowing for a perpendicular axis of the knife to the circular muscle fibers of the

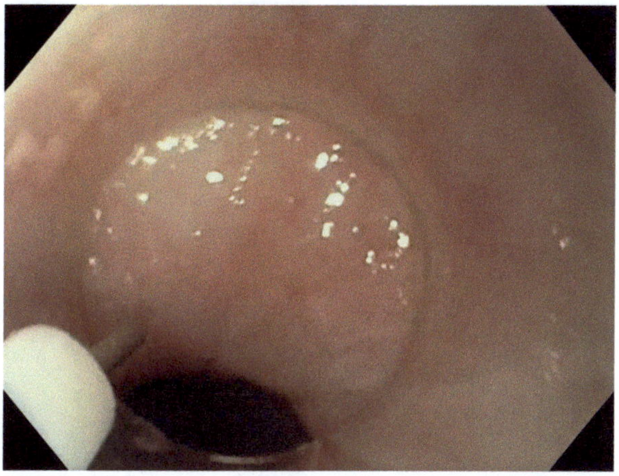

Fig. 2 Positioning 6–10 cm proximal to the gastroesophageal junction (EGJ) for mucosal incision

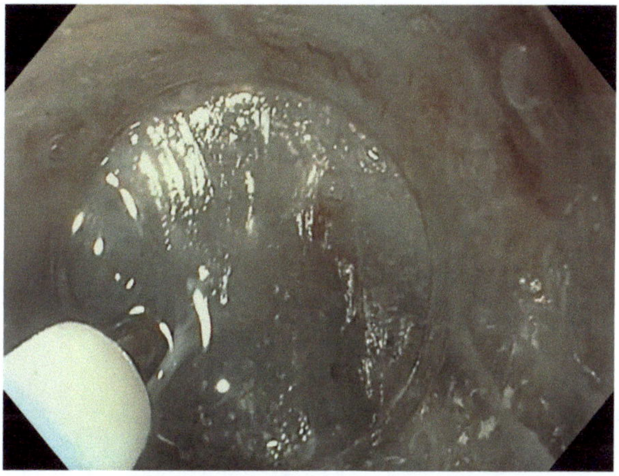

Fig. 3 Anterior approach to creating submucosal space for myotomy

esophagus, thus facilitating a more efficient myotomy (Fig. 4). Literature has demonstrated that both methods have similar clinical success rates; thus, either method may be utilized based on operator preference.

Once the area of mucosal incision has been identified, a solution of methylene blue and saline is injected into the submucosal layer to lift the mucosa (Fig. 5).

A 1.5–2 cm longitudinal incision is made in the mucosa using a ESD knife to expose the submucosal space (Fig. 6).

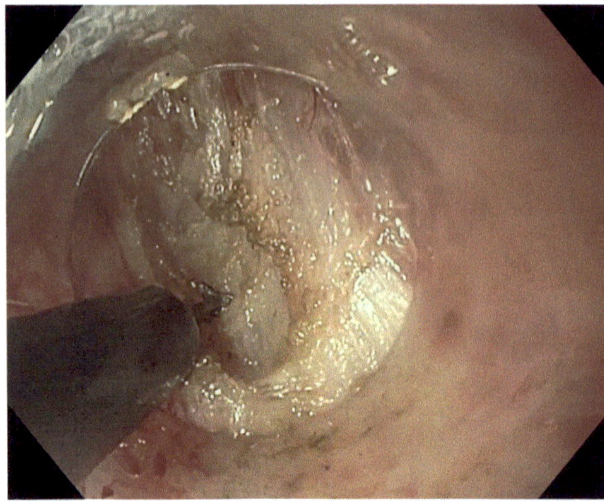

Fig. 4 Posterior approach to creating submucosal space for myotomy

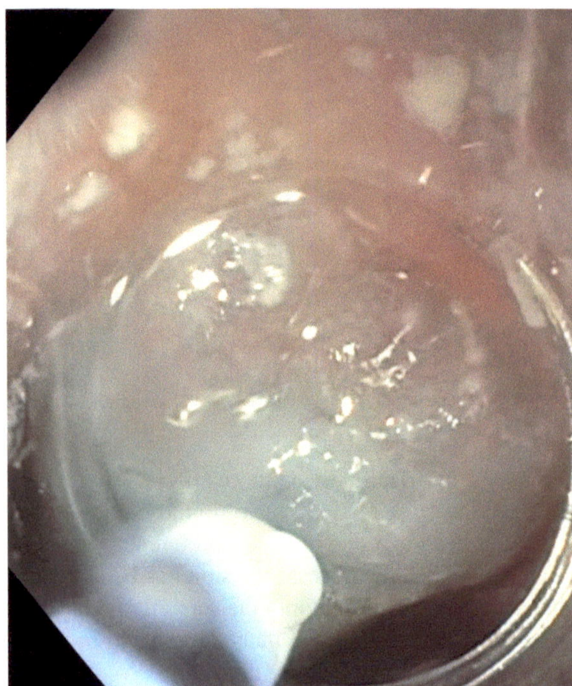

Fig. 5 Injection of methylene blue and saline into submucosal layer to lift the mucosa

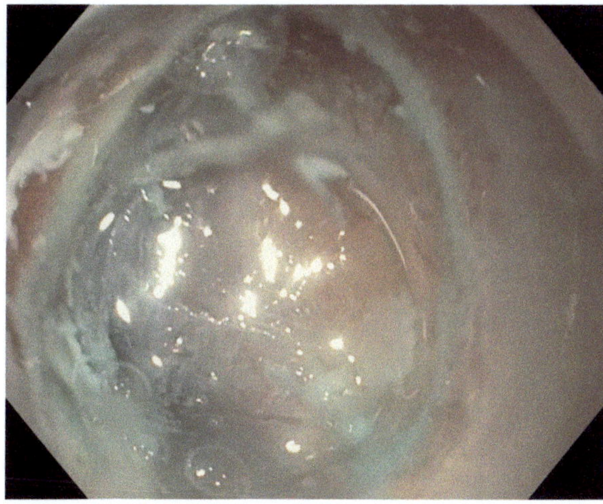

Fig. 6 Longitudinal incision into mucosa using a ESD knife to expose submucosal space

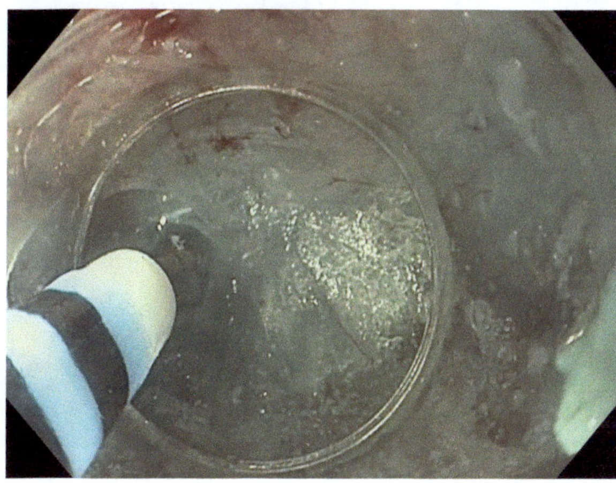

Fig. 7 Inserting endoscope through the created mucosal incision into the submucosal space

Creation of the Submucosal Tunnel

The endoscope with a clear cap is inserted through the mucosal incision into the submucosal space (Fig. 7).

Utilizing electrocautery or a dissection knife, submucosal fibers are dissected to create a submucosal tunnel (Fig. 8).

The tunnel is extended from the point of mucosal incision to 2–3 cm into the gastric cardia (Fig. 9).

An important step in this process is proper identification of the extent of the submucosal tunnel and myotomy. One approach is the double-scope method, where a second ultra-thin endoscope is advanced into the stomach in a retroflexed position, allowing for identification of the gastric cardia This may be especially beneficial in those with abnormal esophageal anatomy where identifying landmarks may be more difficult.

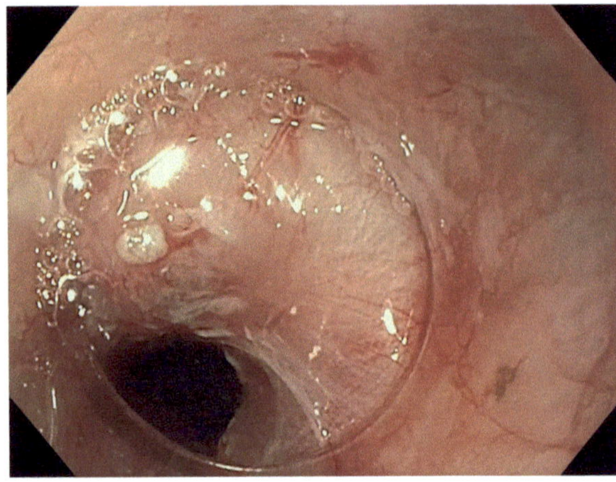

Fig. 8 Dissecting submucosal fibers to create submucosal tunnel

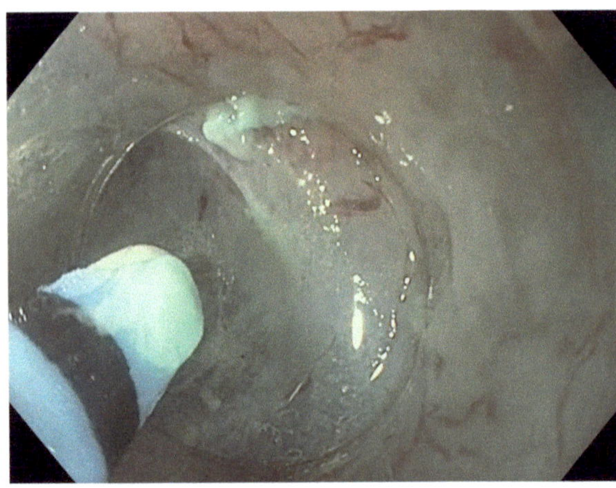

Fig. 9 Extending the tunnel from the point of mucosal incision to 2–3 cm into the gastric cardia

Myotomy

Within the submucosal tunnel, begin cutting the inner circular muscle layer using a Triangular Tip (TT) knife, while ensuring preservation of the outer longitudinal muscle layer (Fig. 10).

Myotomy length in POEM was derived from laparoscopic Heller myotomy length. Thus, a traditional, standard myotomy for Type I and II achalasia typically measures 6–8 cm in length within the esophagus and 2–3 cm in the gastric cardia. However, recent literature suggests that a shorter esophageal myotomy may be non-inferior to traditional myotomy lengths for Type I and II achalasia. Continuation of the esophageal myotomy into the gastric cardia ensures an adequate myotomy through the EGJ. Extension beyond 2–3 cm is associated with increased risk of post-POEM reflux and has not shown improved EGJ distensibility.

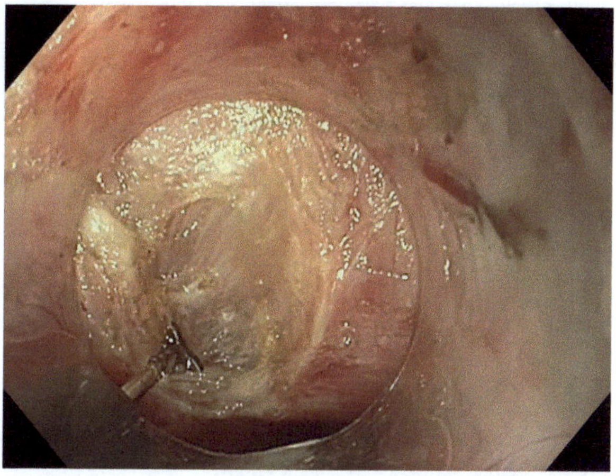

Fig. 10 Cutting the inner circular muscle layer using a Triangular Tip knife

For Type III achalasia, there is special consideration given it is defined by premature/spastic esophageal contractions. The length of the myotomy should be the length of spasticity as measured on pre-interventional manometry.

Assessing Myotomy Adequacy

It is common for operators to utilize a functional lumen imaging probe (FLIP) intraprocedurally as an adjuvant tool during POEM to assess the adequacy of the myotomy. FLIP is a catheter-based system that utilizes impedance planimetry to measure the real-time distensibility index (DI) of the EGJ. Once the myotomy is complete, the endoscope is removed and an EndoFLIP catheter is inserted into the esophagus. Patients with achalasia tend to have a low baseline DI (<2). If intraprocedural DI <2.8, the myotomy is considered inadequate. In this case, the endoscope should be re-inserted and a longitudinal extension of the myotomy is required until DI improves to ≥2.8, which is considered a complete myotomy and associated with higher efficacy of POEM (Fig. 11).

Closure of the Mucosal Incision

Once the myotomy is complete, the mucosal incision is closed using endoscopic clips (Fig. 12). Cautery is used for hemostasis as needed.

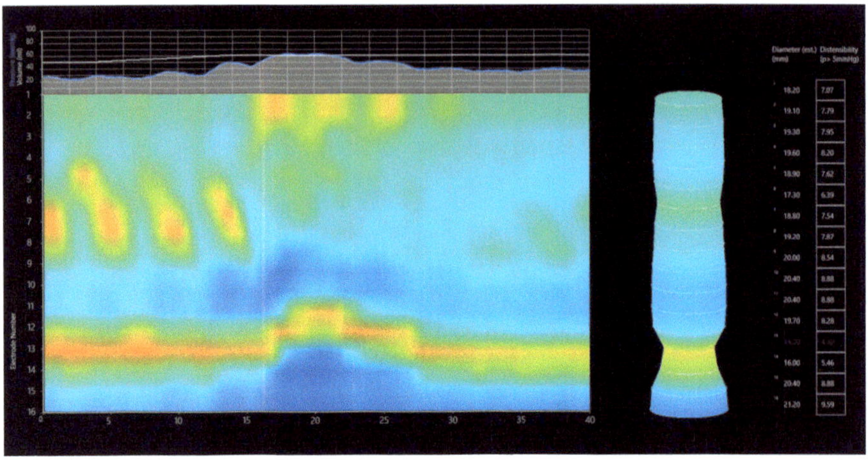

Fig. 11 Intraprocedural FLIP determines myotomy adequacy

Fig. 12 Mucosal incision is closed using endoscopic clips

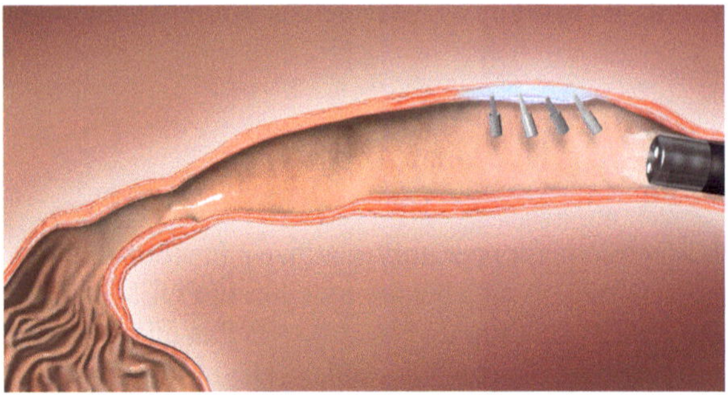

Conclusions

Per-oral endoscopic myotomy is a safe and effective treatment option for achalasia when compared to other standard options, including pneumatic dilation and Heller myotomy. Its utility as a minimally invasive treatment option with quick recovery makes it an appealing choice for many patients. Intraprocedural use of EndoFLIP can help determine myotomy adequacy during POEM. Future studies will examine the efficacy of short-length myotomy compared to standard-length myotomy for Type I and II achalasia.

Conflict of Interest Kevin P. Shah, Mark A. Solinski, Anthony J. Kang, and Abdul A. Aadam declare they have no conflicts of interest.

References

1. Olson D, Liu KC, Aadam AA. Peroral endoscopy Myotomy (POEM) for esophageal motility disorders. Curr Gastroenterol Rep. 2022;24(9):105–14.
2. Ponds FA, Fockens P, Lei A, et al. Effect of Peroral endoscopic Myotomy vs pneumatic dilation on symptom severity and treatment outcomes among treatment-naive patients with achalasia: a randomized clinical trial. JAMA. 2019;322(2):134–44.
3. Rengarajan A, Aadam AA. Peroral endoscopic myotomy and its use in non-achalasia disorders. Dis Esophagus. 2024 Jul 3;37(7):doae014.
4. Rodriguez de Santiago E, Mohammed N, Manolakis A, et al. Anterior versus posterior myotomy during poem for the treatment of achalasia: systematic review and meta-analysis of randomized clinical trials. J Gastrointestin Liver Dis. 2019;24(1):107–15.
5. Rohof WO, Salvador R, Annese V, et al. Outcomes of treatment for achalasia depend on manometric subtype. Gastroenterology. 2013;144(4):718–25.
6. Werner YB, Hakanson B, Martinek J, et al. Endoscopic or surgical Myotomy in patients with idiopathic achalasia. N Engl J Med. 2019;381(23):2219–29.

Laparoscopic Heller Myotomy

Francisco Schlottmann, Sofia Bertona, Mario A. Masrur, and Rudolf Buxhoeveden

Abstract Achalasia is a primary esophageal motility disorder with two main characteristics: lack of esophageal peristalsis and partial/absent relaxation of the lower esophageal sphincter in response to swallowing. The laparoscopic Heller myotomy is associated with excellent outcomes and symptomatic relief in the majority of patients. A partial fundoplication is always added to prevent postoperative gastroesophageal reflux. A properly executed operation is critical to obtain successful outcomes.

Keywords Achalasia · Dysphagia · Heller myotomy · Dor fundoplication · Laparoscopy · Endoscopy

Introduction

Achalasia is a primary esophageal motility disorder with two main characteristics: lack of esophageal peristalsis and partial/absent relaxation of the lower esophageal sphincter in response to swallowing. The most common symptoms are dysphagia, regurgitation, heartburn, and chest pain. Weight loss is also common in patients with achalasia. Unfortunately, there is no curative treatment for the disease. Therapies aim to reduce contractility at the lower esophageal sphincter to ultimately allow for

F. Schlottmann (✉)
Department of Surgery, Hospital Alemán of Buenos Aires, Buenos Aires, Argentina

Department of Surgery, University of Illinois at Chicago, Chicago, IL, USA

S. Bertona · R. Buxhoeveden
Department of Surgery, Hospital Alemán of Buenos Aires, Buenos Aires, Argentina
e-mail: sbertona@hospitalaleman.com; rbuxhoeveden@hospitalaleman.com

M. A. Masrur
Department of Surgery, University of Illinois at Chicago, Chicago, IL, USA
e-mail: mmasrur@uic.edu

F. Schlottmann, M. A. Masrur (eds.), *Endoscopic, Laparoscopic and Robotic Techniques for Foregut Disorders*, https://doi.org/10.1007/978-3-032-00811-4_25

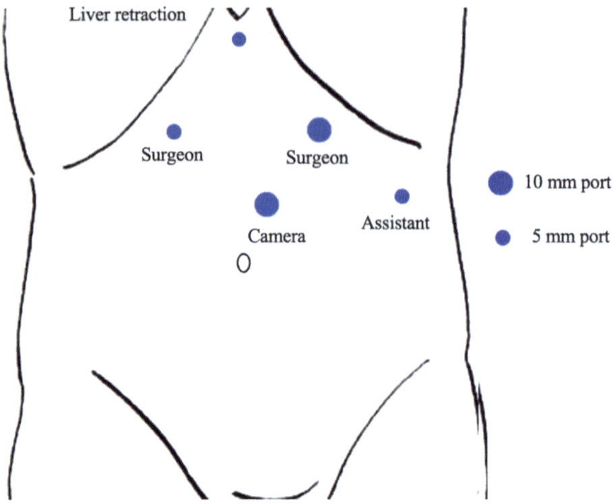

Fig. 1 Ports placement for laparoscopic Heller myotomy

better esophageal emptying. The laparoscopic Heller myotomy (LHM) with a partial fundoplication is considered one of the most effective treatment modalities. A properly executed operation is critical to obtain successful outcomes [1–4].

Procedure Description

Patient Positioning and Trocar Placement

The patient is placed in low lithotomy position with the lower extremities extended on stirrups and with the knees flexed around 20°–30°. The use of pneumatic compression devices for legs is strongly recommended to reduce the risk of deep vein thrombosis. During the entire operation, the surgeon stands between the patient's legs. A total of five laparoscopic ports (two 10 mm and three 5 mm) are commonly used for the operation (Fig. 1).

Division of Short Gastric Vessels

The short gastric vessels are divided using a vessel sealing instrument starting from a point midway along the greater curvature of the stomach towards the fundus. The division of the vessels continues all the way up until de left pillar of the crus. This step of the operation will help obtaining a tension-free fundoplication afterwards (Fig. 2).

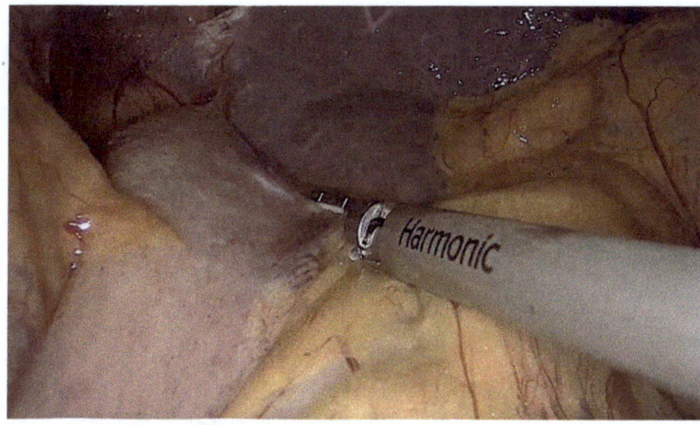

Fig. 2 Division of short gastric vessels

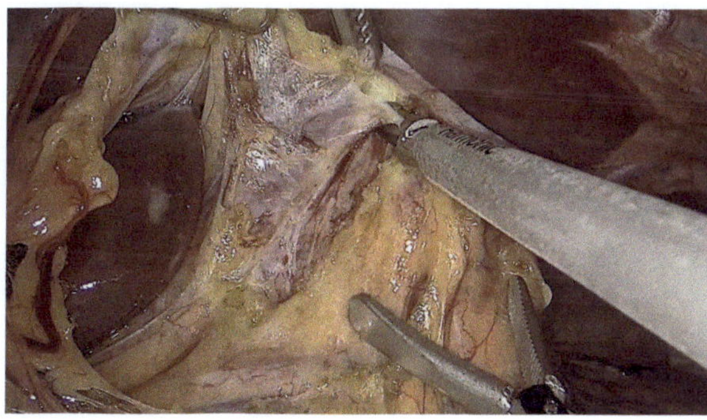

Fig. 3 Division of phrenoesophageal membrane

Division of the Phrenoesophageal Membrane

Once the left pillar is completely dissected, the phrenoesophageal membrane is divided and dissected just above the esophagus (Fig. 3). The anterior vagus is carefully identified and left attached to the esophageal wall to avoid its injury. The left pillar of the crus is separated from the esophagus. Dissection is limited to the anterior and lateral aspects of the esophagus, and no posterior dissection is needed if a Dor fundoplication will be performed.

Division of the Gastrohepatic Ligament

The gastrohepatic ligament is divided with electrocautery or harmonic device starting just above the caudate lobe of the liver. The division continues all the way up until the right pillar of the crus (Fig. 4). The right crus is then dissected all the way down towards the junction with the left crus. The crus is then separated from the esophagus by blunt dissection and the posterior vagus nerve is identified.

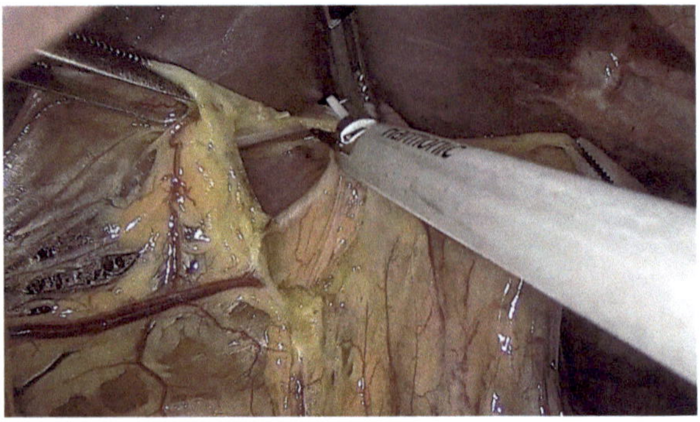

Fig. 4 Division of gastrohepatic ligament

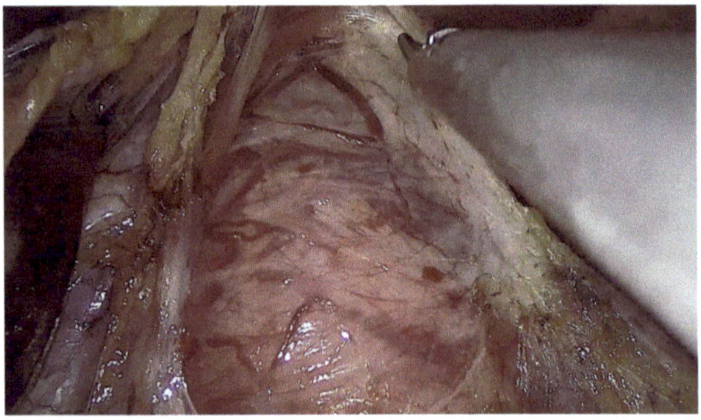

Fig. 5 Anterior mediastinal dissection over a dilated esophagus

Mediastinal Dissection

Once the esophagus is completely detached from the right and left crus, an anterior mediastinal dissection is performed in order to solely expose the anterior aspect of the distal esophagus (Fig. 5). The fat pad over the anterior esophageal and gastric wall is removed in order to expose the gastroesophageal junction.

Esophageal Myotomy

The esophagus is pulled downward and to the left in order to adequately expose the right side of the esophagus. The myotomy is performed at the 11 o' clock position and is started above the gastroesophageal junction with hook electrocautery. Reaching the proper submucosal plane is the most critical step of the operation. In patients with previous therapies (e.g., endoscopic botulinum toxin injection or endoscopic dilation) this can be particularly challenging due to fibrosis and attachments. Once the muscle is divided and the esophageal mucosa is exposed, the use of a Maryland grasper dissector is very useful to guide the

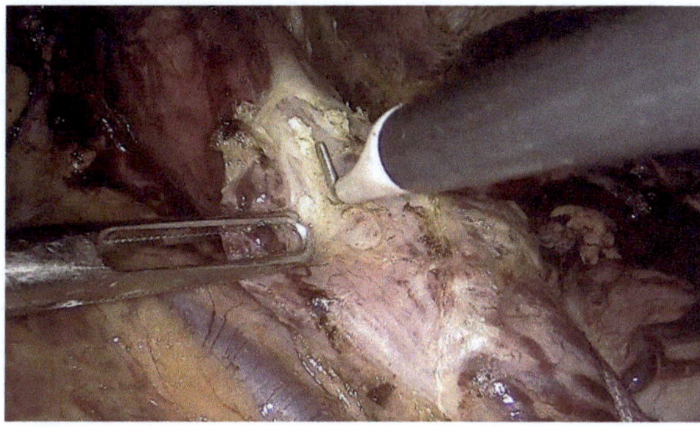

Fig. 6 Starting Heller myotomy with Hook electrocautery

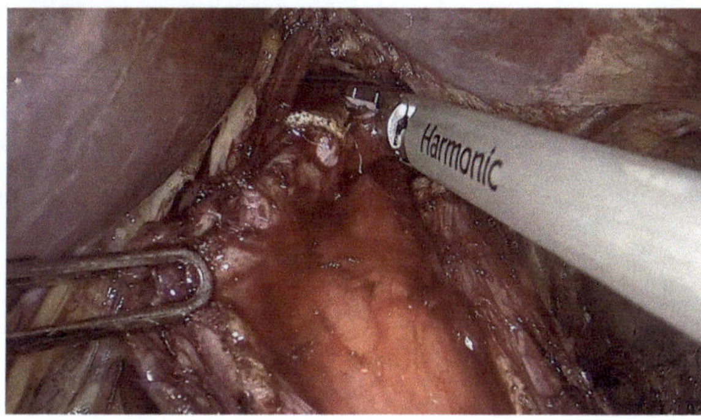

Fig. 7 Proximal extension of Heller myotomy with Harmonic device

myotomy. The myotomy is extended using Harmonic™ Shears device proximally for about 6 cm above the esophagogastric junction and distally for about 2.5 cm onto the gastric wall. The total length of the myotomy is typically about 8–9 cm (Figs. 6, 7, and 8).

If a bleeding is encountered at the muscle fibers divided, compression with gauze is recommended instead of the use of electrocautery. If an esophageal perforation is detected, it should be repaired immediately intraoperatively using a fine absorbable suture.

An upper endoscopy is usually performed to confirm indemnity of the esophageal mucosa and verify the adequate extension of the myotomy (Fig. 9).

Dor Fundoplication

The Dor fundoplication (anterior 180°) has two rows of sutures: one left and one right. The left row includes three stitches: the uppermost stitch incorporates the fundus of the stomach, the esophageal wall, and the left pillar of the crus; the other two incorporate the stomach and the esophageal wall. The gastric fundus is then folded over the exposed mucosa and the greater curvature is placed next to the right

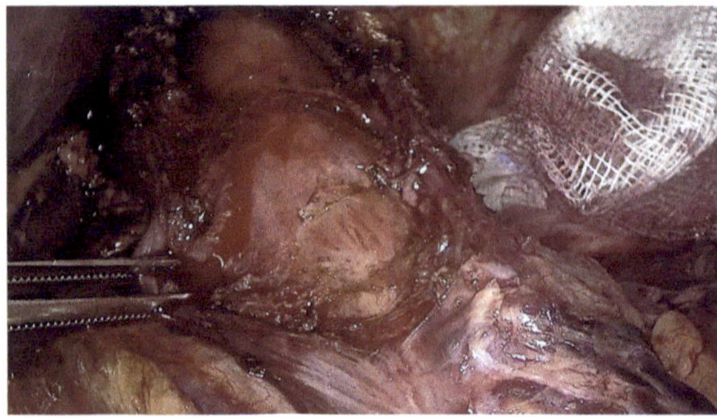

Fig. 8 Distal extension of Heller myotomy into the stomach

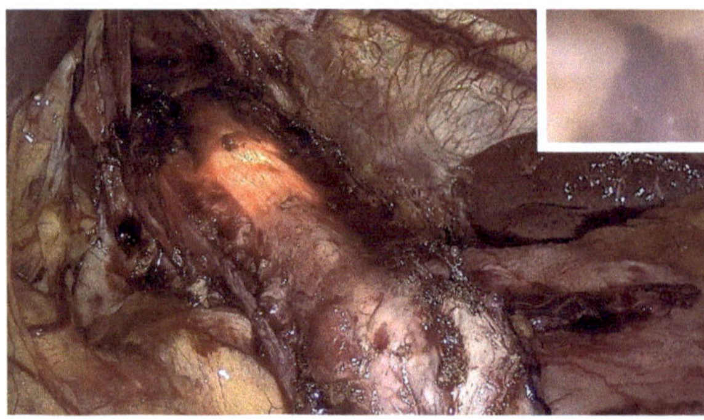

Fig. 9 Intraoperative endoscopy to confirm indemnity of the esophageal mucosa and to evaluate the extension of the myotomy

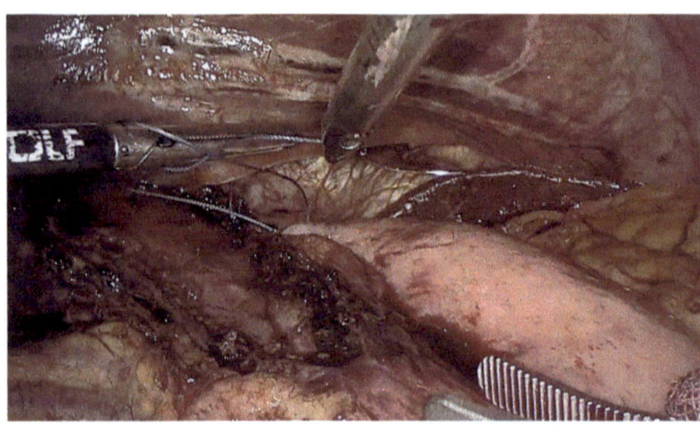

Fig. 10 First (left) row of stitches of Dor fundoplication

pillar of the crus. The second row of stitches comprises three stitches between the fundus and the right pillar of the crus, and commonly two additional stitches between the superior aspect of the fundoplication and the rim of the esophageal hiatus (Figs. 10 and 11).

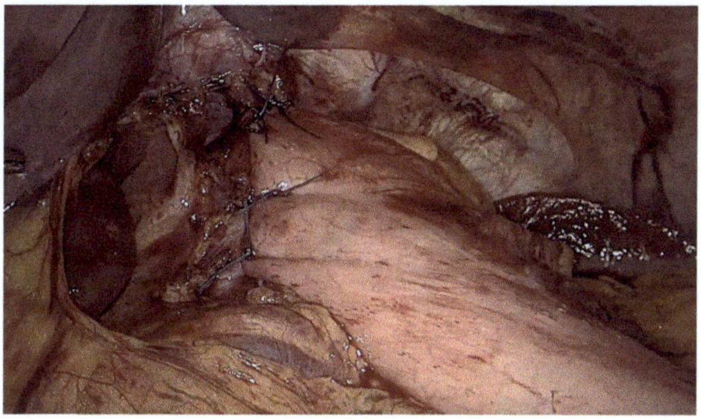

Fig. 11 Second (right) row of stitches of Dor fundoplication

Final Inspection

We remove all trocars under direct vision and check for adequate hemostasis. No abdominal drainages are used, except in cases in which an esophageal perforation was repaired intraoperatively. The fascia of the 10–12 mm ports is closed.

Postoperative Care

Patients can start with clear liquids the day of the operation, and then advance to soft diet as per tolerance. Most patients are discharged within 48 hours of the operation.

Conflicts of Interest The authors have no conflicts of interest.

References

1. Schlottmann F, Patti MG. Esophageal achalasia: current diagnosis and treatment. Expert Rev Gastroenterol Hepatol. 2018;12(7):711–21.
2. Schlottmann F, Neto RML, Herbella FAM, Patti MG. Esophageal achalasia: pathophysiology, clinical presentation, and diagnostic evaluation. Am Surg. 2018;84(4):467–72.
3. Schlottmann F, Herbella FAM, Patti MG. The evolution of the treatment of esophageal achalasia: from the open to the minimally invasive approach. World J Surg. 2022 Jul;46(7):1522–6.
4. Schlottmann F, Nurczyk K, Patti MG. Laparoscopic Heller Myotomy and dor fundoplication: how I do it? J Laparoendosc Adv Surg Tech A. 2020 Jun;30(6):627–9.

Robotic Heller Myotomy

Carlos Galvani

Abstract Achalasia is a relatively uncommon primary motility disorder of the esophagus characterized by failure of the lower esophageal sphincter (LES) to relax and marked absence of esophageal peristalsis. Laparoscopic Heller esophageal myotomy with partial fundoplication has been considered the gold standard in the surgical management of achalasia. Nevertheless, laparoscopic Heller myotomy is a technically challenging operation that has a considerable learning curve. Robotic technology offers numerous advantages over conventional laparoscopy and has gained acceptance amongst esophageal and thoracis surgeons for the treatment of achalasia.

This chapter illustrates our current technique for Robotic Assisted Heller Myotomy and some of the common pearls and pitfalls.

Keywords Achalasia · Esophageal dysmotility · Minimally invasive · Robotic surgery · Heller myotomy

Introduction

Achalasia is a rather uncommon disease process (i.e. incidence 1 in 100,000 individuals), characterized by the absence of the ganglion cells of the myenteric plexus of Auerbach with loss of postganglionic inhibitory neurons. It generally manifests with dysphagia and a variety of foregut symptoms such as regurgitation and chest pain. If untreated, the course of the disease causes a progressive stasis and dilation of the esophagus, with subsequent risk of aspiration, weight loss, and malnutrition. The same consequences could be potentially observed if treatment is suboptimal.

C. Galvani (✉)
Division of General Surgery, Department of Surgery, LSU Health, New Orleans, LA, USA
e-mail: cgalva@lsuhsc.edu

F. Schlottmann, M. A. Masrur (eds.), *Endoscopic, Laparoscopic and Robotic Techniques for Foregut Disorders*, https://doi.org/10.1007/978-3-032-00811-4_26

For that reason, early definitive treatment is essential to prevent potential complications of the disease as well as improve patients' quality of life.

Treatment is always palliative and is aimed to decrease the outflow obstruction at the level of the lower esophageal sphincter (LES). The treatment of the disease has undergone several modifications since 1674, when Willis first reported the a patient with achalasia treated by using dilation with a sponge attached to whalebone, later modified to balloon dilation after Russel's description in 1887 [1]. Subsequently, in 1913, E. Heller performed the first esophagomyotomy using an anterior and posterior esophageal myotomy [1]. Because of the excessive amount of gastroesophageal reflux resulting, this approach was later modified to a single myotomy, which is still today the mainstay of surgical treatment. Subsequently, Pellegrini and Cuscheri in the early 1990s described the minimally invasive approach, showing the obvious benefits of reduced morbidity, shorter postoperative hospital stay, and decreased postoperative pain [2, 3].

The minimally invasive approach offered results at least as good as those from open procedures yielding in addition less postoperative pain, shorter hospital stay, shorter disability, lower cost, and a better cosmetic result than the open approach [4–6] Over the years, because of the high incidence of postoperative reflux and the suboptimal distal myotomy, thoracoscopic Heller myotomy was gradually abandoned and replaced by laparoscopic myotomy. The use of this approach spread rapidly, motivating a change in the treatment algorithm of esophageal achalasia [6].

In the early 2000s, with the introduction of robotic surgery, Melvin and cols. [7] performed the first Robotic assisted Heller myotomy. Several factors such as, the elimination of the surgeon's tremor, the steadiness, the superior control of the tip of the articulated instruments along with 3-D visualization, have contributed to the increasing popularity of this approach. In addition, there is increasing evidence demonstrating lower rate of iatrogenic esophageal perforations [8, 9]. We applied this technology for the treatment of esophageal achalasia with optimal patients outcomes and no esophageal perforations [10, 11].

This chapter illustrates our current technique for Robotic Assisted Heller Myotomy and some of the common pearls and pitfalls.

Procedure Description

Preoperative Management

Achalasia occurs with equal frequency in men and women and is more common in the adult population, but it can also happen in children. For that reason, the preoperative evaluation should be tailored to the specific patient and their preoperative physical status. In addition, patients that undergo previous non-surgical treatment tend to have a longer duration of their disease, which can in fact worsen their physical status. It is essential for the anesthesia team to have a detailed understanding of the surgical procedure in terms of approach, the extent of the operation, and associated complications. It is also recommended for patients to have a clear liquid diet at least 3 days before the surgical procedure to prevent large amount of undigested food in the esophagus and to decrease the risk of aspiration.

Preoperative cardiac and pulmonary morbidity will determine the extent of preoperative cardiac testing as well as the need for pulmonary function testing, especially in those patients with restrictive lung disease secondary to recurrent aspiration pneumonia.

Perioperative

Anesthetic considerations include precautions to reduce the perioperative risk for aspiration. Patients are advised to ingest only clear liquids 2 or 3 days before surgery, to decrease the risk of aspiration during induction of anesthesia. In older patients with several comorbid conditions, a Foley catheter is recommended if the duration of the case is expected to be 2 h or more and usually removed after the case.

Premedication with a prophylactic anti-aspiration is highly recommended. The patient is placed in the supine position before the induction of general endotracheal anesthesia. To minimize the aspiration risk during the induction of anesthesia, the airway can be secured either after a rapid sequence induction with cricoid pressure; or awake, with the aid of a fiberoptic bronchoscope. Standard intraoperative monitoring will suffice for American Society of Anesthesiologists (ASA) physical status class I and II patients. Adequate attention should be paid to the hemodynamic changes resulting from the combined effects of pneumoperitoneum and placing the patient in a reverse Trendelenburg position.

Patient Position

After satisfactory induction of general endotracheal anesthesia, the patient is placed in the supine position. Pneumatic compression stockings are placed on both legs routinely. The legs and pressure points are cushioned appropriately. Once this is established, the abdomen and lower chest are prepped widely and then draped sterile. An orogastric tube is placed, to decompress the esophagus and stomach. The anesthesia team should be aware of the patient's condition while inserting the orogastric tube and avoid pushing the tube against resistance.

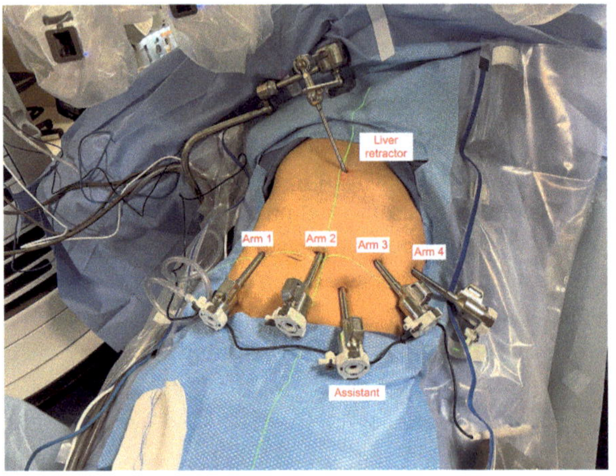

Fig. 1 Port positioning. Four 8-mm trocars (the size of these trocars is specific for the robotic system) and one additional for the assistant if needed. A 0.5 cm incision is made in the subxyphoid area, for the Nathanson liver retractor. One additional 12 mm trocar for the bedside assistant

Abdominal Access and Trocar Positioning

Entry into the abdominal cavity is obtained using an optical trocar technique in the periumbilical area to the left of the midline. Four 8-mm trocars are inserted across the upper abdomen (Camera, and 3 working ports). A 0.5 cm incision is made in the subxyphoid area, and the left lobe of the liver is then retracted anteriorly using the Nathanson liver retractor. An additional 8 mm port is inserted for the bedside assistant in between the camera trocar and the robotic trocar in the left upper quadrant (Fig. 1). The assistant surgeon is positioned on the patient left side. During the case, the assistant oversees instrument exchange, suction, and bringing sutures to the field. At this point, the nursing personnel deploys the robotic surgical cart for docking (Right/Left Upper abdomen). The assistant must prevent collisions between the liver retractor and the robotic arms. Once the arms are docked, the *Da Vinci* (Intuitive Surgical, Sunnyvale, CA) specific instruments are inserted through the three 8 mm working ports. A Force Bipolar is placed in the surgeon's left hand (Arm 1), the robotic 30° down camera in Arm 2, the articulated hook cautery or the Endo Wrist® One Vessel Sealer (Intuitive Surgical, Sunnyvale, CA) in the right hand (Arm 3) and a a Cadiere grasper in Arm 4 (assisting port).

Dissection of the Lower Third of the Esophagus and Division of the Short Gastric Vessels

In patients with no hiatal hernia only anterior and lateral esophageal dissection is performed. If hiatal hernia is present, extensive mediastinal dissection is carried out in order to obtain 2–3 cm of intrabdominal esophagus before starting the esophageal myotomy.

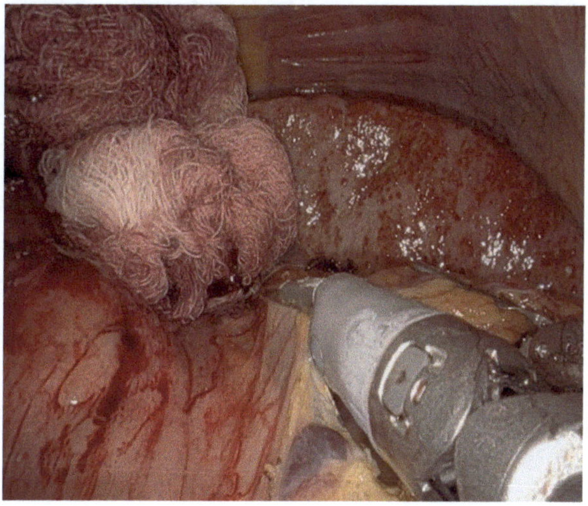

Fig. 2 Division of the short gastric vessels

The operation is started by dividing the peritoneum overlying the left crus of the diaphragm with the Vessel Sealer (Left Crura approach). The phreno-esophageal membrane is transected as well. In order to dissect and separate the esophagus from the left crus a blunt dissection is used to minimize the risk of inadvertent injury or perforation of the esophagus. Once access to the posterior mediastinum is obtained, the uppermost short gastric vessels are then carefully divided. (Fig. 2).

Full mobilization of the fundus is carried out by dividing posterior adhesions to the anterior capsule of the pancreas. The left side of the esophagus is identified by dissecting off the left crus from the esophagus. The dissection is continued in the posterior mediastinum lateral and anterior to expose the lower esophagus, preserving the posterior attachments. Then, attention is centered to the exposure of the right crus. By activating the assisting arm (Arm 4) the surgeon provides traction on the stomach; after this is completed the surgeon using a Cadiere grasper and Vessel Sealer divides the gastrohepatic ligament below the hepatic branch of the vagus nerve and extends the dissection upwards. The peritoneum overlying the anterior surface of the right crus of the diaphragm and the phrenoesophageal membrane is transected. The right crura is recognized and separated from the esophagus by blunt dissection, no posterior dissection is performed as well.

Heller Myotomy

A taper 44 F taper-tip bougie is inserted through the mouth by the anesthesia team. It is of most importance extensive communication between the anesthesiologist and the surgery team to prevent esophageal perforation. The placement of the bougie also helps providing a stable surface for the myotomy. After Bougie insertion, using Arm 4 the surgeon retracts the GE-junction caudally with a Cadiere grasper to

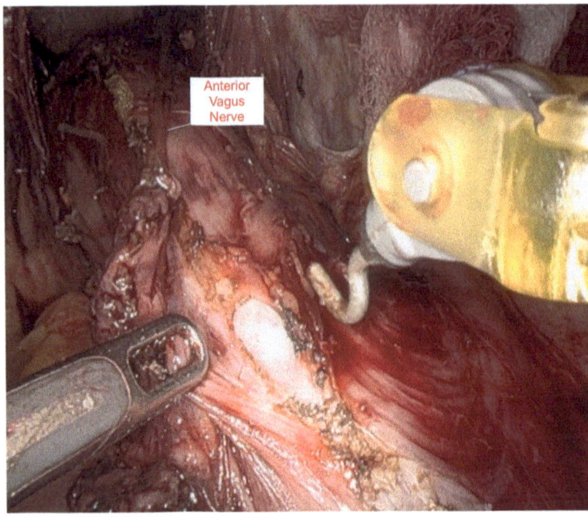

Fig. 3 Beginning of the esophageal myotomy. The myotomy is started out just above the gastroesophageal junction on the 12 o'clock position using the robotic articulated hook electrocautery

increase the length of the intra-abdominal esophagus. For the myotomy. A bipolar Forceps is used in the surgeon's left hand (Arm 1), and the articulated hook cautery in the right hand (Arm 3). It is our routine technique to mobilize the epigastric fat pad along with the anterior vagus nerve from the anterior esophagus in order to perform the myotomy at 12 o'clock (anterior esophagus). This anterior mobilization is carried out as far as possible into the mediastinum to facilitate the proximal extension of the myotomy.

After exposure of the anterior esophagus is complete, tension is created by retracting the esophagus caudally with the Cadiere forceps over the bougie. The myotomy is started out at GE-junction level at the 12 o'clock position using the articulated hook electrocautery (Fig. 3). Methodically marking of the area of the myotomy is performed by scoring the esophagus with the back of the hook electrocautery for about 6–7 cm above the GEJ and at least 3 cm below the GEJ. The submucosal plane is reached in one point by dividing the longitudinal and circular muscle layer. This is followed by extending the myotomy a minimum of 6–8 cm proximally and for at least 3 cm distally into the stomach (Fig. 4).

During the proximal extension of the myotomy the instrument in Arm 1 provides counter-traction of the longitudinal fibers, while the L-hook scores the circular fibers with short burst of energy, hooks and lifts the muscle fibers away from the submucosa with constant gentle upward tension. This maneuver minimizes the use of electrocautery which is key to prevent thermal injuries. Similarly, the myotomy on the gastric side is carried down in a "hockey stick" configuration to transect the sling fibers of the stomach wall. This is the most challenging side of the myotomy. The changing in direction of the muscular fibers, from circular of the esophagus to oblique at the stomach, makes it difficult to develop the necessary submucosal plane to divide the muscular fibers and bleeding is likely. After completion of the myotomy a bulging of the mucosal layer could be observed.

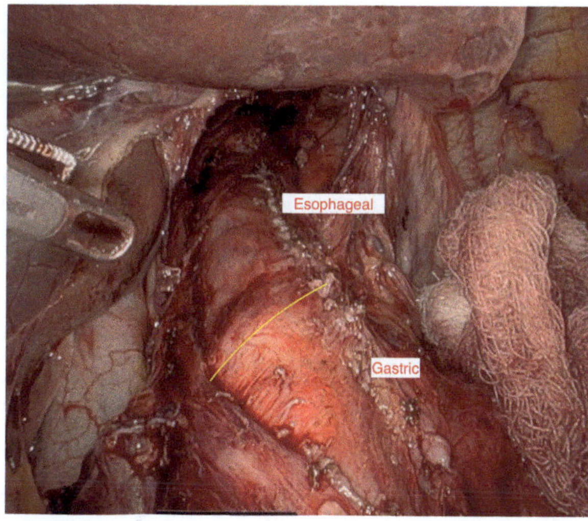

Fig. 4 Completed Heller myotomy, extending a minimum of 6 cm proximally and for about 2 cm distally into the stomach

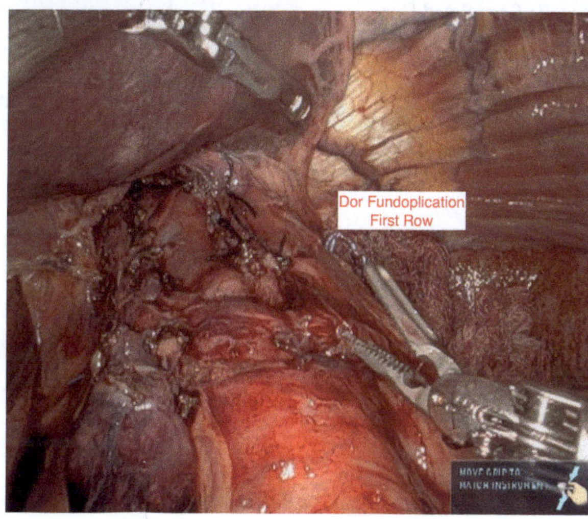

Fig. 5 Dor fundoplication. First row of sutures composed of three stitches. The first stitch includes the gastric fundus, the left crura and the left side of the myotomy

Creation of the Partial Fundoplication (DOR)

In our practice the preferred antireflux procedure is the Dor fundoplication, which is an anterior 180° fundoplication. This type of fundoplication is chosen because it covers the exposed mucosa and is an effective antireflux repair. The Dor fundoplication is composed of two rows of sutures. The first row of suture includes the gastric fundus and left side of the myotomy. The first stitch is a triangular stitch, placed between the fundus, the left pillar and left edge of the myotomy. Two additional stitches incorporate the gastric wall and the left side of the myotomy (Fig. 5). Subsequently, by activating the grasper in Arm 3 the surgeon folds the stomach over

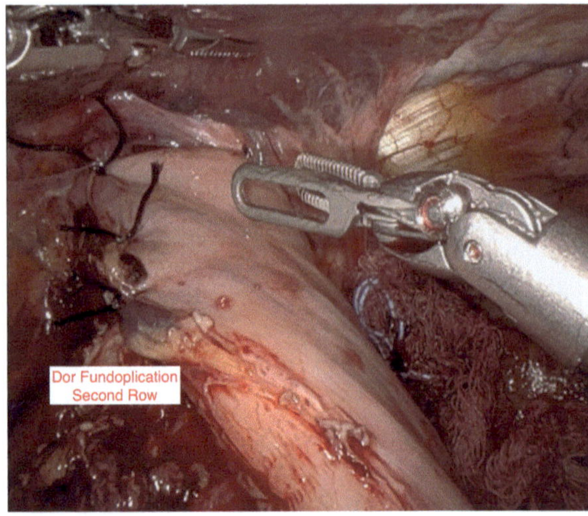

Fig. 6 The second row of sutures are created by placing stitches between the stomach and the right edge of the myotomy

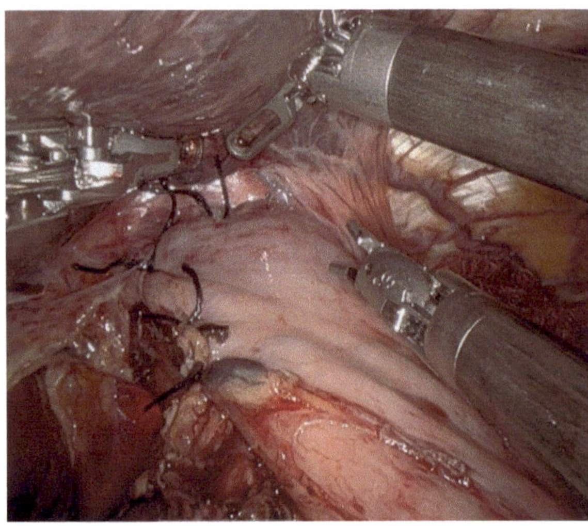

Fig. 7 Completed Dor (180° anterior) fundoplication Two additional stitches are also placed from the fundus to the rim of the hiatus

the exposed mucosa, and the second row of sutures is started. The first stitch is placed between the stomach, the right edge of the myotomy, and the right pillar. The second and the third stitches are placed between the greater curvature of the stomach and the right side of the esophageal muscle. (Fig. 6).

It is vital to avoid including the right pillar in the second and third stitches of the fundoplication since this could represent a reason for dysphagia. Two additional stitches are placed between the gastric fundus and the rim of the hiatus completing in this way the fundoplication. The purpose of these last stitches is to further decrease the tension of the fundoplication and to prevent the lateral rotation of the wrap (Fig. 7).

Fig. 8 Completed Toupet (posterior partial) fundoplication

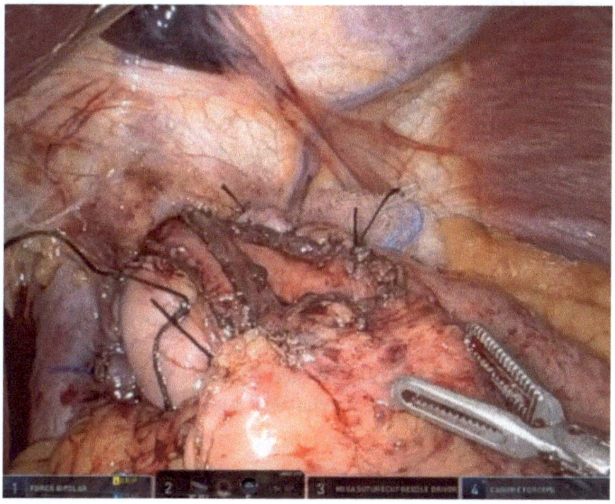

Nevertheless, in patients with hiatal hernia a Toupet fundoplication (posterior partial fundoplication) is preferred. A posterior fundoplication is warranted due to the more extensive mediastinal dissection required to obtain 2–3 cm of intraabdominal esophagus and the need for posterior crural repair (Fig. 8).

Conclusions

Robotic surgery has continuously demonstrated its utility by overcoming some of the pitfalls of laparoscopy. Several factors may play a role in decreasing the morbidity of the procedure. First, the elimination of the surgeon's tremor, the steadiness, and the superior control of the tip of the articulated instruments. In addition, the 3-D vision allows visualizing and dividing each individual muscular fiber, assuring an adequate and safe myotomy.

References

1. Brewer LA 3rd. History of surgery of the esophagus. Am J Surg. 1980;139(6):730–43.
2. Pellegrini C, Wetter LA, Patti M. Thoracoscopic esophagomyotomy. Initial experience with a new approach for the treatment of achalasia. Ann Surg. 1992;216:291–6; discussion 296–9.
3. Shimi S, Nathanson LK, Cuschieri A. Laparoscopic cardiomyotomy for achalasia. J R Coll Surg Edinb. 1991;36(3):152–4.
4. Csendes A, et al. Comparison of forceful dilatation and esophagomyotomy in patients with achalasia of the esophagus. Hepato-Gastroenterology. 1991;38(6):502–5.
5. Patti MG, et al. Minimally invasive surgery for achalasia: an 8-year experience with 168 patients. Ann Surg. 1999;230(4):587–93; discussion 593–4.

6. Patti MG, et al. Impact of minimally invasive surgery on the treatment of esophageal achalasia: a decade of change. J Am Coll Surg. 2003;196(5):698–703; discussion 703–5.
7. Melvin WS, Needleman BJ, Krause KR, Wolf RK, Michler RE, Ellison EC. Computer-assisted robotic heller myotomy: initial case report. J Laparoendosc Adv Surg Tech A. 2001;11:251–3.
8. Milone M, Manigrasso M, Vertaldi S, Velotti N, Aprea G, Maione F, Gennarelli N, De Simone G, De Conno B, Pesce M, Sarnelli G, De Palma GD. Robotic versus laparoscopic approach to treat symptomatic achalasia: systematic review with meta-analysis. Dis Esophagus. 2019;32(10):1–8.
9. Ataya K, Bsat A, Aljaafreh A, Bourji H, Al Ayoubi AR, Hassan N. Robot-assisted Heller Myotomy versus laparoscopic Heller Myotomy: A systematic review and meta-analysis. Cureus. 2023 Nov 8;15(11):e48495.
10. Galvani C, et al. Laparoscopic Heller myotomy for achalasia facilitated by robotic assistance. Surg Endosc. 2006;20(7):1105–12.
11. Horgan S, et al. Robotic-assisted Heller myotomy versus laparoscopic Heller myotomy for the treatment of esophageal achalasia: multicenter study. J Gastrointest Surg. 2005;9(8):1020–9; discussion 1029–30.

Esophageal Cancer

Endoscopic Submucosal Dissection (ESD) for Esophageal Cancer

Kevin P. Shah, Mark A. Solinski, Tony J. Kang, and Abdul A. Aadam

Abstract Esophageal cancer continues to have a high prevalence and incidence worldwide. Endoscopic submucosal dissection (ESD) is an effective treatment modality for superficial esophageal cancers and offers an advantage over traditional endoscopic mucosal resection (EMR) in determining histopathologic assessment. In this chapter, we describe each step of minimally invasive ESD for esophageal neoplasms with intraoperative endoscopic images.

Keywords Endoscopic submucosal dissection (ESD) · Superficial esophageal cancer · Gastrointestinal neoplasms · Endoscopic mucosal resection (EMR)

Introduction

Esophageal cancer continues to have a high prevalence and incidence worldwide. Endoscopic submucosal dissection (ESD) is an effective treatment modality for superficial esophageal cancers, including both squamous cell carcinoma (SCC) and esophageal adenocarcinoma (EAC) in select patients. In this chapter, we describe each step of minimally invasive ESD for esophageal neoplasms with intraoperative endoscopic images.

ESD confers a strong advantage over traditional endoscopic mucosal resection (EMR) for multiple reasons. First, it allows for en-bloc resection of lesions for more accurate histopathologic evaluation of margins. Second, it allows for lesions larger in size in the gastrointestinal tract (>2 cm) to be successfully resected with low rates of recurrence. Third, it offers a minimally invasive alternative that is potentially curative and preserves quality of life compared to surgical intervention.

K. P. Shah · M. A. Solinski · T. J. Kang · A. A. Aadam (✉)
Division of Gastroenterology & Hepatology, Northwestern Feinberg School of Medicine, Chicago, IL, USA
e-mail: abdul.aadam@northwestern.edu

F. Schlottmann, M. A. Masrur (eds.), *Endoscopic, Laparoscopic and Robotic Techniques for Foregut Disorders*, https://doi.org/10.1007/978-3-032-00811-4_27

Appropriate patient selection is crucial for esophageal ESD. Those with low risk of lymph node metastasis are the most ideal candidates to undergo therapy. For patients with esophageal SCC, M1 (intraepithelial) and M2 (invasion into lamina propria) tumors portend the lowest risk of lymph node involvement. Risk increases, but is still acceptable for tumors that are M3 (invasion into the muscularis mucosa) and SM1 (invasion into the superficial layer of submucosa). Lesions with depth of invasion >200 μm or lymphovascular invasion have higher rates of lymph node metastasis and should not undergo ESD.

Patients with Barrett's esophagus (BE)-associated neoplasia traditionally undergo EMR, but the role of ESD in EAC is steadily increasing as it provides a more accurate histopathologic diagnosis, often upstaging pre-ESD histology to invasive cancer. Data suggests that ESD may be particularly useful for patients with inconclusive EMR histopathology, large visible lesions in the distal esophagus or gastro-esophageal junction, or prior endoscopic ablative therapy in the esophagus [1–6].

Procedure Description

Procedure Preparation and Patient Positioning

An endoscope with water-jet capability should be used with insufflation using carbon dioxide which is essential compared to air insufflation. The patient is placed in left lateral decubitus position on the endoscopy table for this procedure. Monitored anesthesia care or general anesthesia can be used for ESD in the esophagus.

Procedure Technique

Identification and Classification of the Lesion

The endoscope is inserted through the patient's mouth and passed into the esophagus with a distal attachment cap. The esophageal lesion is examined using high-definition white light endoscopy and near-focus endoscopy to assess the size and morphology (Fig. 1). The Paris classification system is used to categorize lesions based on morphology, which predicts likelihood of submucosal invasion. The use of digital chromoendoscopy (narrow band imaging) or dye-based chromoendoscopy (iodine for esophageal SCC or acetic acid for BE-associated neoplasia) enhances the ability of the endoscopist to correctly classify the lesion.

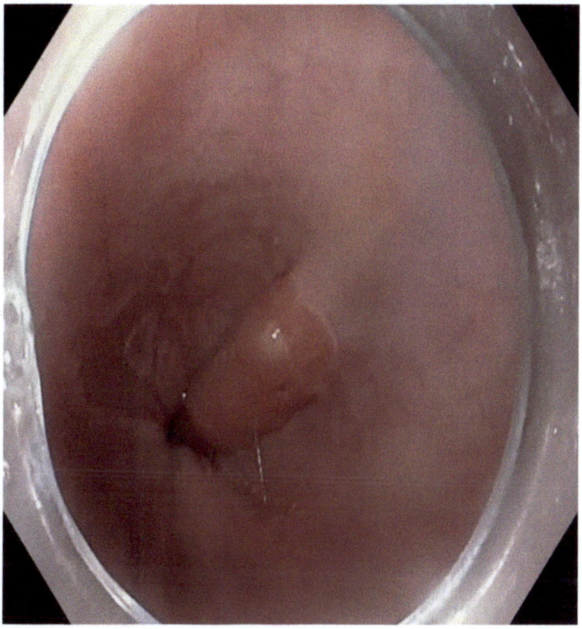

Fig. 1 Examination of esophageal lesion using HD-WLE and near-focus endoscopy to assess size and morphology

Marking the Lesion

After the margins of the lesion are identified, marking dots are made using a dual knife (soft coagulation 50 W) or Forced coagulation (20 W) along the perimeter approximately 5 mm away from the border (Fig. 2). The marking dots serve as a guide for resection.

Submucosal Injection

Submucosal injection is a critical step to ensure safe dissection and reduce the risk of perforation. It allows for increased separation of visible lesions from the muscularis propria layer by expanding the submucosal layer. The first injection is made with normal saline outside the margin where dissection will begin. For circumferential dissections in the esophagus, injection begins in the periphery of the lesion rather than the center (Fig. 3). Injections are continued into the submucosa as needed prior to dissection of tissue. After initial normal saline injection and confirmation of entry into the submucosa, some endoscopists prefer dyes (indigo carmine, methylene blue, etc.) and vasoconstrictors to allow for better delineation of layers and to reduce intraprocedural bleeding, respectively (Fig. 4).

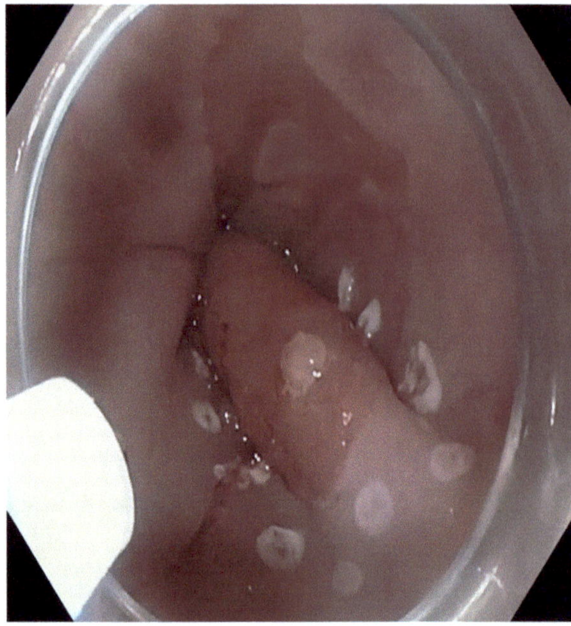

Fig. 2 Marking dots made 5 mm away from the border of the lesion as a guide for resection

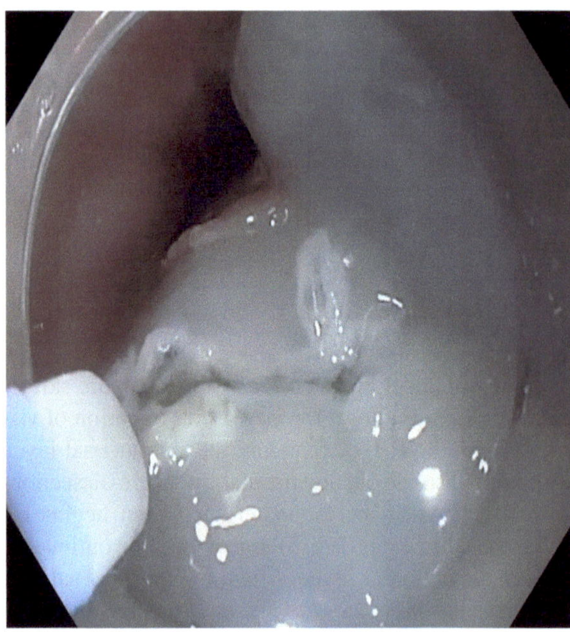

Fig. 3 Submucosal injection to separate a lesion from the muscularis propia layer

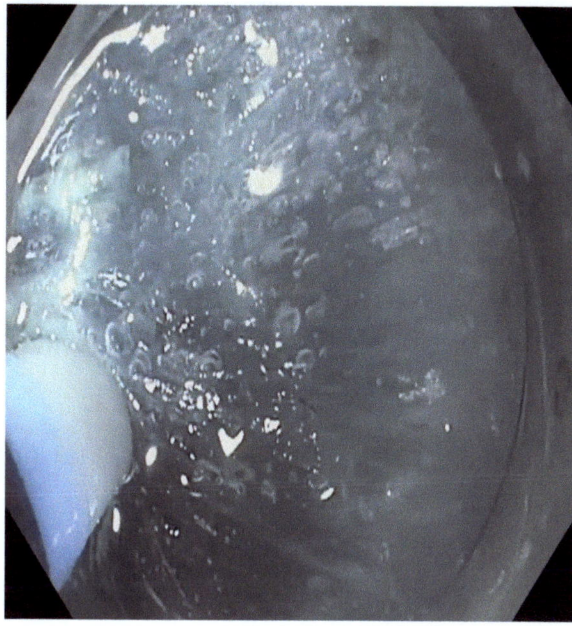

Fig. 4 Submucosal injection with dye to allow for better delineation of layers

Mucosal Incision

The C-shaped incision and dissection technique allows for efficient ESD for esophageal lesions. After the lesion is lifted with submucosal injection, a C-shaped mucosal incision is made circumferentially on the anal and oral side of the lesion using the ESD knife (pulse cut slow 30 W) or Endocut I mode (effect 2, duration 3, interval 2) to access the submucosa (Fig. 5).

A small uncut portion of mucosa is typically left intact by the endoscopist on the non-gravity dependendent lateral aspect to facilitate ease of lateral dissection which is the final step of the procedure. When making the mucosal incision, caution must be taken to account for gravity and maintain the lesion away from pooling of fluid (Fig. 6).

Submucosal Dissection

Once the circumferential mucosal incision is complete, submucosal dissection begins with the use of an ESD knife typically using EndoCut current or PresiceSect settings. The ESD knife is inserted into the submucosal layer parallel to the esophageal wall (Fig. 7). Remaining parallel to the muscularis propria within the submucosa allows for safer dissection and minimizes the risk of perforation.

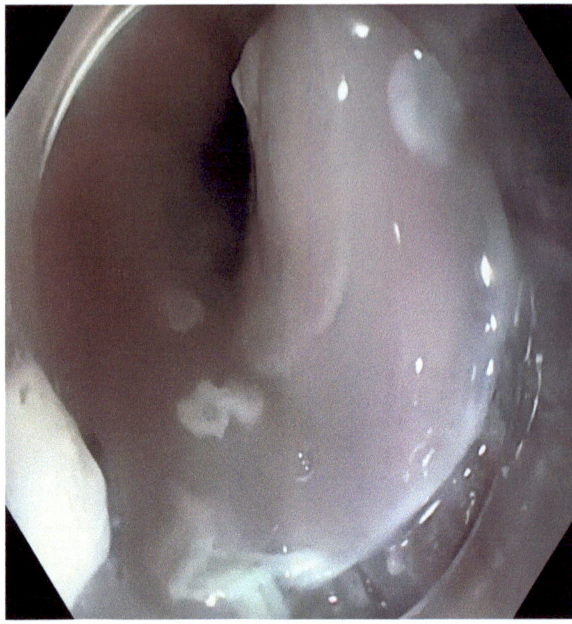

Fig. 5 C-shaped incision and dissection to access the submucosa

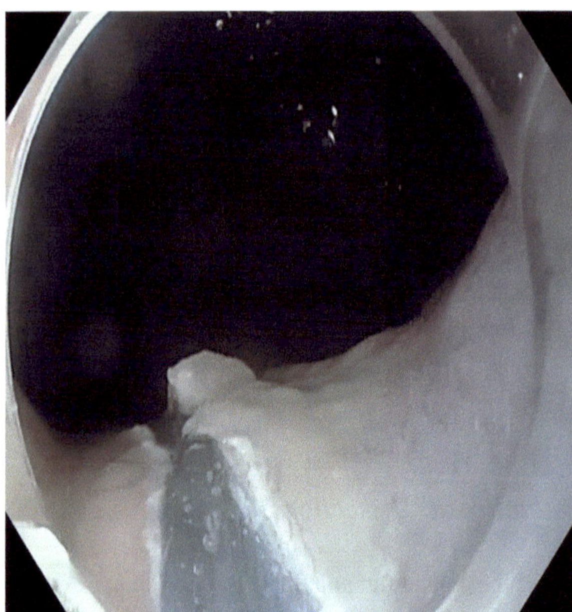

Fig. 6 Maintenance of lesion away from pooling of fluid when making mucosal incision

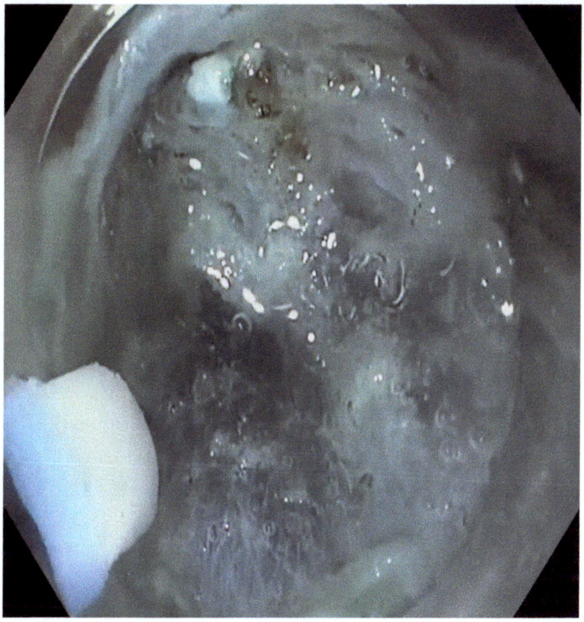

Fig. 7 Insertion of ESD knife into submucosal layer parallel to muscularis propria

Clip-line traction is a commonly utilized method of applying counter traction during submucosal dissection in the esophagus. An endoclip with attached line is deployed on the proximal side of the lesion. The line is pulled through the mouth and used to provide traction during the remainder of the submucosal dissection with the IT knife nano. Visible vessels are treated with the use of a waterjet and coagulation settings with the ESD knife as needed during dissection. If bleeding is obscuring visualization or if large vessels are encountered, a coagulation grasper can be used for hemostasis.

En-Bloc Resection and Defect Management

After submucosal dissection is completed, the lesion is resected en-bloc (Fig. 8). The base of the mucosal defect is examined endoscopically and injected with topical steroid such as triamcinolone to reduce the risk of post-ESD stricturing of the esophagus.

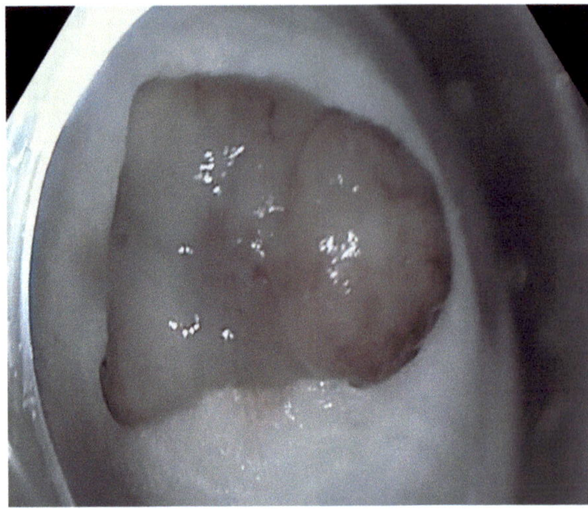

Fig. 8 Resection of lesion en-bloc after submucosal dissection is complete

Conclusions

Endoscopic submucosal dissection allows for safe and effective en-bloc resection of superficial esophageal cancers for more accurate histopathologic diagnosis. It can be used for both esophageal squamous cell carcinoma and esophageal adenocarcinoma in select patients. ESD provides advantages over traditional EMR and surgical approaches to management of lesions in the esophagus without compromising the quality of life of patients.

Conflict of Interest Kevin P. Shah, Mark A. Solinski, Tony J. Kang, and Abdul A. Aadam declare they have no conflicts of interest.

References

1. Draganov PV, Aihara H, Karasik MS, et al. Endoscopic submucosal dissection in North America: a large prospective multicenter study. Gastroenterology. 2021;160(7):2317–27.
2. Aadam AA, Abe S. Endoscopic submucosal dissection for superficial esophageal cancer. Dis Esophagus. 2018;31(7). https://doi.org/10.1093/dote/doy021.
3. Yang D, King W, Aihara H, et al. Effect of endoscopic submucosal dissection on histologic diagnosis in Barrett's esophagus visible neoplasia. Gastrointest Endosc. 2022;95(4):626–33.
4. Saito Y, Abe S, Inoue H, et al. How to perform a high-quality endoscopic submucosal dissection. Gastroenterology. 2021;161(2):405–10.
5. Libânio D, Pimentel-Nunes P, Bastiaansen B, et al. Endoscopic submucosal dissection techniques and technology: European Society of Gastrointestinal Endoscopy (ESGE) technical review. Endoscopy. 2023;55(4):361–89.
6. Ono S, Fujishiro M, Koike K. Endoscopic submucosal dissection for squamous cell carcinoma of esophagus: tips and tricks of experts. Video J Encycl GI Endosc. 2013;1(1):43–5.

Endoscopic Stenting

Saqib Walayat and Zohair Ahmed

Abstract Esophageal cancer is a serious and globally prevalent malignancy associated with high morbidity and mortality rates. The palliative management of dysphagia, a common and debilitating symptom in advanced esophageal cancer, often includes endoscopic stenting. This chapter explores the role of esophageal stenting as a therapeutic intervention, primarily for symptom relief in patients with unresectable tumors or poor prognosis. The efficacy of stents in reducing dysphagia, techniques for their placement, and the selection criteria for patients are discussed, with a focus on optimizing outcomes and minimizing complications. Complications range from mild symptoms, such as pain and reflux, to severe adverse events like stent migration and perforation. Patient selection requires a multidisciplinary approach. Esophageal stenting is not curative, it remains a critical component of palliative care, enhancing the quality of life for esophageal cancer patients.

Keywords Esophageal cancer · Malignant dysphagia · Endoscopic stenting · Esophageal fistula · Stent migration

Introduction

Esophageal cancer is the 8th most common cancer worldwide, known for its significant morbidity, high mortality rate, and poor prognosis. In 2020 alone, there were an estimated 600,000 new cases and 500,000 deaths worldwide, making esophageal cancer the 6th leading cause of cancer-related mortality. Recent trends indicate a

S. Walayat
Carle Health Methodist Hospital, Peoria, IL, USA

Z. Ahmed (✉)
Department of Gastroenterology, University of Illinois, Chicago, IL, USA
e-mail: zahmed23@uic.edu

F. Schlottmann, M. A. Masrur (eds.), *Endoscopic, Laparoscopic and Robotic Techniques for Foregut Disorders*, https://doi.org/10.1007/978-3-032-00811-4_28

rise in adenocarcinoma cases, attributed to increasing obesity rates and lifestyle changes.

One of the most prevalent symptoms of esophageal cancer is dysphagia, which typically begins with difficulty swallowing solids and may progress to liquids as the disease advances. Due to the distensible nature of the esophagus, dysphagia often presents late, by which point approximately 50% of the esophageal lumen may be compromised. This delayed symptomatology contributes to late diagnosis and poor prognosis. The treatment of esophageal cancer usually involves a multimodal approach, including surgery, chemotherapy, and radiation, depending on the stage, tumor location, lesion size, and the presence or absence of metastasis. Unfortunately, more than 50% of esophageal cancer cases are deemed unresectable at the time of diagnosis due to metastasis or patient ineligibility for surgery, and the 5-year survival rate remains below 20%. In such cases, treatment focuses on palliation—primarily aimed at relieving symptoms and improving oral intake. Endoscopic esophageal stenting is one of these treatment modalities aimed at symptom relief and improvement in oral intake.

Esophageal stenting was first introduced in 1845 using an ivory tube to manage malignant dysphagia. Since then, esophageal stent technology has evolved significantly, with a wide array of stents available today [1–5].

Procedure Description

Patient Selection for Esophageal Stent Placement

Effective patient selection is crucial for optimizing outcomes in esophageal stent placement for malignant dysphagia. The decision-making process typically involves a multidisciplinary team that includes gastroenterologists, oncologists, radiologists, and palliative care specialists. Key factors influencing patient selection encompass clinical presentation, tumor characteristics, and overall prognosis.

Clinical Presentation

1. Severity of Dysphagia: The primary indication for esophageal stenting is the management of malignant dysphagia, which often progresses from difficulty swallowing solids to an inability to ingest liquids as the disease advances. Patients presenting with moderate to severe dysphagia, where oral intake is significantly compromised, are prime candidates for stent placement. A dysphagia score is often utilized to quantify symptom severity, with scores of 3 or higher indicating a more urgent need for intervention.
2. Nutritional Status: Malnutrition and weight loss are common in patients with advanced esophageal cancer due to dysphagia. Those experiencing substantial

weight loss (greater than 10% of body weight) or dehydration due to inability to consume adequate nutrition are strong candidates for stenting. In such cases, esophageal stenting can facilitate improved oral intake, nutritional replenishment, and overall quality of life.

3. Patient Symptoms: Beyond dysphagia, other symptoms such as pain and discomfort during swallowing may warrant stent placement. Patients who experience substantial pain, even with liquid intake, may benefit from stenting to alleviate these symptoms.

Tumor Characteristics

1. Tumor Location and Type: The location of the tumor significantly influences patient selection for stenting. Distal esophageal tumors are generally more amenable to stenting due to easier access and reduced risk of complications compared to proximal tumors. Stenting is less effective and often avoided in proximal esophageal lesions due to the higher risk of tracheoesophageal fistula and significant discomfort.
2. Extent of Disease: Patients with localized, unresectable tumors that significantly obstruct the esophagus are better candidates for stenting. In contrast, those with extensive metastatic disease or rapid tumor progression may not derive sufficient benefit from stenting. A thorough evaluation of disease staging and extent via imaging studies such as CT scans or endoscopic ultrasound (EUS) is essential to guide decision-making.
3. Growth Patterns: Tumor characteristics, including growth patterns, are important considerations. Tumors that demonstrate slow growth may allow for stenting to provide longer-term relief, while aggressive tumors may require more immediate interventions, such as chemotherapy or radiation therapy, before considering stenting.

Prognosis and Treatment Goals

1. Life Expectancy and Performance Status: The overall prognosis and performance status of the patient are critical in determining the appropriateness of stenting. The Eastern Cooperative Oncology Group (ECOG) performance status score is commonly used to evaluate patients, with scores of 0–2 indicating a better functional status and potential for benefiting from surgery. Stenting can be used in these patients if they are not surgical candidates. Patients with a poor prognosis, often defined as a life expectancy of less than 6 months, may benefit from stenting for palliative purposes, prioritizing symptom relief and quality of life.
2. Treatment Goals: The primary goals of stenting in esophageal cancer are symptom palliation and improved quality of life. Patients with advanced disease who prioritize symptomatic relief over curative treatment are appropriate candidates

for stenting. A multidisciplinary discussion often helps clarify the goals of care, as some patients may opt for stenting in conjunction with palliative chemotherapy or radiation to enhance overall management.

Contraindications for Stenting

1. Uncontrolled Infection or Esophageal Perforation: Patients with active esophageal infection, significant esophageal perforation, or uncontrolled coagulopathy are generally not candidates for stent placement due to the increased risk of severe complications, including sepsis or exacerbated perforation.
2. Unrealistic Patient Expectations: Patients with unrealistic expectations regarding the benefits of stenting or those who may not fully understand the palliative nature of the procedure may be unsuitable candidates. Comprehensive preprocedural counseling is essential to align patient expectations with clinical realities.

Patient selection is a critical step for successful esophageal stent placement. It is essential to involve a multidisciplinary team, including oncologists, gastroenterologists, and surgeons, to discuss each case individually. Patients with mild dysphagia and a longer life expectancy may respond better to brachytherapy than stenting, as brachytherapy has shown fewer complications in randomized control trials. Stent placement is generally restricted to those with a poor prognosis or who have expressed a preference for this option. Importantly, stents are not typically recommended as a bridge to surgery or before preoperative chemoradiotherapy, as their use has been linked to higher rates of adverse events and complications.

For patients undergoing chemoradiotherapy, studies suggest that stents are of limited benefit. Chemoradiation exposure can increase the risk of stent migration, bleeding, fistula formation, and cause severe pain. Scoring tools are available to assess tumor length, patient performance status, metastasis, age, and gender, helping to determine if stenting is a viable option.

Stent Selection

Type of Esophageal Stents: Metal vs. Plastic Stents/Covered vs. Uncovered Stents

The choice of stent material and type is influenced by patient prognosis, tumor characteristics, and anatomical considerations. Metal stents have largely replaced plastic stents due to their higher efficacy in symptom palliation, reduced rates of complications, and overall cost-effectiveness. Metal stents exhibit greater radial force, which maintains luminal patency, and their self-expanding property allows them to adapt to varying esophageal diameters. Self-expanding metal stents (SEMS) are commonly made of Nitinol, an alloy of nickel and titanium known for its flexibility, shape memory, and resistance to corrosion. Nitinol's elasticity allows stents to conform to angulated segments of the esophagus, making it especially suitable for lesions in the distal or proximal esophagus, where tight angulations are common. Nitinol stents have been associated with better outcomes, as they minimize trauma to the esophageal wall and reduce the risk of stent migration. Stent options include:

1. ***Fully Covered SEMS***: These stents are lined with a silicone or polyurethane membrane, preventing tumor ingrowth and simplifying stent retrieval if necessary. However, fully covered SEMS are more prone to migration due to the absence of tissue ingrowth, which anchors partially covered stents more securely. Migration is particularly problematic in distal tumors where peristaltic forces may displace the stent.
2. ***Partially Covered SEMS***: These stents feature a covered central portion with uncovered ends to facilitate tissue integration at the edges, which reduces migration. However, tissue ingrowth can make removal challenging. If removal is required a fully covered stent can be placed within these stents and left in place for 10–14 days for temporary necrosis of hyperplastic tissue, enabling easier extraction. No significant difference has been observed in the recurrence rates of dysphagia and other adverse events between fully and partially covered SEMS.
3. ***Uncovered SEMS***: Uncovered SEMS are rarely used for malignant dysphagia due to the high risk of tumor ingrowth, which can lead to recurrent obstruction. While they anchor more securely within the esophagus, they are typically reserved for benign conditions or selected cases where tumor in growth is not a significant concern.
4. ***Anti-Reflux Stents***: In cases of distal esophageal malignancy near the gastroesophageal junction, gastroesophageal reflux can be a persistent concern after stent placement. Anti-reflux stents have a one-way valve designed to prevent acid regurgitation. However, randomized control trials have not shown a significant reduction in reflux symptoms with these stents, limiting their utility in clinical practice.

Stent Diameter and Length Considerations

Choosing the appropriate stent size and diameter is critical for optimizing therapeutic outcomes while minimizing complications. Stent size, including both length and diameter, is selected based on the extent and location of the obstruction, patient anatomy, and goals of treatment. Literature on stent sizing highlights the importance of balancing effective luminal patency with potential risks such as stent migration, pain, and tissue injury.

Diameter Considerations

1. ***Optimal Diameter for Obstruction Management***: Studies suggest that a stent diameter between 18–25 mm is generally effective for maintaining luminal patency in malignant esophageal strictures. Larger-diameter stents (≥25 mm) are sometimes preferred in cases of severe dysphagia to improve the swallowing function. However, the larger the diameter, the higher the radial force exerted on the esophageal wall, which can lead to complications like pain, tissue necrosis, and pressure-induced fistulas, particularly in the proximal esophagus. According to recent European Society of Gastrointestinal Endoscopy (ESGE) guidelines, a diameter of around 20–23 mm is recommended to balance dysphagia relief with lower complication rates.
2. ***Small-Diameter Stents and Migration***: Smaller-diameter stents (<18 mm) are associated with a higher risk of migration, particularly in the distal esophagus where peristaltic motion is more pronounced. In clinical trials, the migration rate has been shown to increase when using diameters under 20 mm, especially with fully covered stents, which are not anchored by tissue ingrowth. Migration is particularly problematic in palliative cases, as it can exacerbate dysphagia or lead to additional procedures for repositioning or replacement.
3. ***Impact of Tumor Location***: Proximal esophageal tumors are challenging for stent sizing due to the sensitivity of the upper esophagus and risk of tracheo-esophageal fistula. Larger diameter stents (>23 mm) placed in proximal esophagus can increase patient discomfort, risk of fistula and globus sensation due to pressure on nearby structures [6]. Therefore, stents with a diameter closer to 18–20 mm are often preferred for proximal tumors to reduce these risks. A smaller diameter also reduces the likelihood of tracheal compression and associated respiratory symptoms, which are more common in the upper third of the esophagus. Globus sensation is usually noted when stent is placed within 8 cm of upper esophageal sphincter and may improve after a few days of stent placement. In general, it is recommended that an esophageal stent be placed at least 2 cm below upper esophageal sphincter.
4. ***Palliative Goals and Stent Diameter***: In patients with poor prognosis or limited life expectancy, symptom relief is prioritized over stent durability. For these patients, a slightly larger diameter (23–25 mm) may be chosen to provide rapid improvement in swallowing function. However, studies show that the risk of adverse events, including bleeding and pain, increases with each incremental increase in stent diameter, particularly when fully covered stents are used. Consequently, stent choice should weigh symptom relief with anticipated side effects, with some studies advocating for a "middle-ground" approach of 20–23 mm for the most consistent palliative outcomes.

Length Considerations

1. ***Ensuring Coverage Beyond Tumor Margins***: An adequate stent length should extend at least 1–2 cm beyond both the proximal and distal margins of the stricture to prevent migration and ensure complete tumor coverage. Studies have shown that stents that are too short, failing to cover these margins, are associated with higher rates of stent displacement and recurrent dysphagia due to tumor overgrowth or undergrowth at the edges.
2. ***Effect of Stent Length on Distal vs. Proximal Tumors***: Distal esophageal tumors near the gastroesophageal junction require careful length consideration, as a stent that is too long may cause gastroesophageal reflux due to disruption of the lower esophageal sphincter (LES). Anti-reflux stents have been developed for these cases, featuring a valve to prevent acid regurgitation, though evidence on their efficacy remains mixed. Conversely, in the proximal esophagus, excessively long stents may extend into the upper esophageal sphincter, causing globus sensation and patient intolerance.
3. ***Customizable Stent Length Option***: With the availability of various stent lengths, from 6 cm to over 15 cm, clinicians have greater flexibility in matching stent length to individual patient anatomy and tumor dimensions. Matching stent length closely to the tumor size reduced complications and enhanced patient comfort. When precise lengths are chosen, there is also a decreased risk of stent migration due to inadequate stricture coverage.
4. ***Stent Length and Tumor Dynamics***: Tumor ingrowth and overgrowth are common causes of recurrent dysphagia post-stenting. Tumors with rapid growth patterns may benefit from slightly longer stents (adding at least 1–2 cm to each side of the tumor) to anticipate progression. However, excessive length can exacerbate migration, especially in patients with short or highly angled esophageal segments.

Special Considerations for Complex Tumors

1. Multifocal Tumors or Long Segmental Stenoses: In patients with multifocal esophageal tumors or long-segment strictures, deploying multiple overlapping stents may sometimes be necessary. However, overlapping stents can increase the risk of complications like stent migration, dysphagia due to a "stepped" esophagus, and stent fractures.

Esophageal Stent Placement Technique

Successful esophageal stent placement requires meticulous technique, encompassing patient preparation, marking of the tumor boundaries, stent deployment, and post-placement assessment.

Pre-placement Preparation

1. Tumor Marking: Accurate marking of the proximal and distal tumor ends is crucial for effective stent placement. Techniques include fluoroscopic guidance with external markers, endoscopic clips, and contrast injection. The use of radio-opaque markers has been found to increase placement accuracy, particularly in tumors with indistinct borders (Fig. 1).
2. Dilation Considerations: Historically, dilation of the stricture was recommended before stent placement, but recent studies have shown that dilation may increase the risk of perforation, particularly in malignant strictures. Current practice generally avoids dilation for most patients, although it may still be considered in cases where the tumor creates a severe stricture that prevents passage of the stent delivery system.

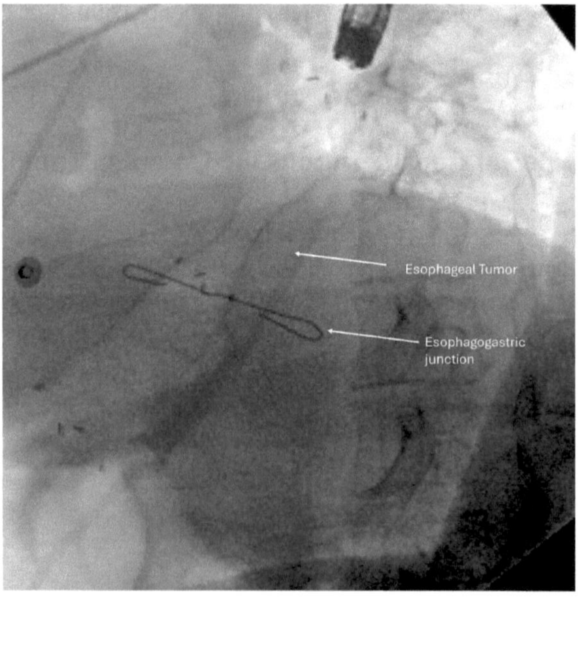

Fig. 1 Fluoroscopic guidance with external marker for stent placement

Stent Deployment

Placement is typically performed under fluoroscopic or combined endoscopic-fluoroscopic guidance to ensure correct positioning. Endoscopic visualization allows real-time confirmation of stent release, reducing the risk of proximal or distal stent misplacement. Once the stent is deployed, it should extend at least 1 cm beyond both the proximal and distal margins of the stricture to minimize migration and ensure complete tumor coverage.

Post-placement Assessment

Post-placement fluoroscopy can confirm stent positioning and identify any immediate complications such as perforation. Dysphagia relief often occurs within 1–2 days of placement, with patients typically progressing from liquid-only diets to a broader range of soft solids. Regular follow-up is recommended to monitor for recurrent dysphagia, pain, or other complications.

Complications of Esophageal Stenting

The complication rate associated with esophageal stent placement is substantial, ranging from 30–35% and varies depending on factors such as tumor location, the presence or absence of fistula, prior history of chemoradiotherapy, tumor vascularity, and stent type. Complications are broadly classified into major and minor categories and include both immediate and delayed effects.

Major Complications

1. Esophageal Hemorrhage: Hemorrhage can occur due to stent irritation, particularly in highly vascularized tumors or if the stent abrades the esophageal wall. Studies suggest that patients with prior radiation therapy are at higher risk for this complication, as tissue friability is increased due to the effects of radiation on local vasculature and tissue integrity.
2. Fistula Formation and Pressure Necrosis: Fistulas can develop between the esophagus and adjacent structures, such as the trachea, bronchus, or even major vessels, like the aorta. This complication is more common in patients with proximal esophageal tumors or those who have undergone extensive radiation therapy. The incidence of tracheoesophageal fistula ranges between 2% and 10%, depending on tumor characteristics and stent type. The high rate of fistula

formation in the proximal esophagus can be attributed to stent-induced pressure necrosis, as the esophagus's natural distensibility may lead to prolonged local pressure. In such cases, multidisciplinary intervention, including the potential need for airway stenting, may be required for symptom management and respiratory stabilization.

3. Esophageal Perforation: Although rare, esophageal perforation occurs in roughly 2% of cases, with a higher incidence in patients who undergo stent placement without preceding dilation. Perforation risk is also elevated in patients with significant prior radiation therapy or friable tumors. Mortality associated with perforation is high due to the potential for mediastinitis and sepsis.

Minor Complications

1. Pain: Pain is one of the most frequently reported side effects, with up to 66% of patients requiring analgesia post-stent placement. This discomfort is often more severe during the first 2 weeks after placement as the esophageal wall adapts to the stent. Pain is particularly pronounced with larger diameter stents, which exert greater radial force. The initial placement and subsequent stent expansion may lead to significant esophageal wall stretch, triggering nociceptive pain that can require opioids for management.
2. Gastroesophageal Reflux Disease (GERD): Reflux occurs in approximately 7% of cases, primarily when the stent is located in the distal esophagus and extends near the gastroesophageal junction. This complication is attributed to the stent's interference with the lower esophageal sphincter's barrier function, leading to acid regurgitation. Anti-reflux stents have been introduced as a potential solution, but recent trials have not demonstrated significant improvement in reflux control compared to conventional stents.
3. Recurrent Dysphagia: Recurrent dysphagia affects about 31% of patients and is commonly due to stent migration, tumor ingrowth, or food impaction within the stent. Tumor overgrowth and ingrowth occur more frequently with uncovered stents, as they allow direct tumor interaction with the stent mesh. Migration is particularly noted in fully covered stents, where the absence of tissue ingrowth allows for potential movement. Food bolus obstruction, another common cause, can often be managed endoscopically.
4. Aspiration Pneumonia: Aspiration pneumonia occurs in approximately 5% of patients, often due to compromised swallowing and increased risk of aspiration after stent placement. Patients with advanced disease, especially those with proximal tumors, are at an elevated risk for this complication. Preventive measures include dietary modifications and head-of-bed elevation.

Conclusions

Endoscopic stenting serves as an effective and essential tool for managing dysphagia and other complications associated with advanced esophageal cancer. While advancements in stent design and placement techniques have improved patient outcomes, complications remain a significant consideration. Patient selection and individualized treatment approaches are key to achieving optimal results, with stenting offering significant relief for those ineligibles for surgery or long-term chemoradiotherapy. Future developments in stent technology and procedural techniques may further enhance the safety and efficacy of this intervention. Overall, esophageal stenting provides critical symptom management in advanced esophageal cancer, improving patients' quality of life and supporting the multidisciplinary palliative care approach.

Conflict of Interest Both authors declare that they have no conflict of interest.

References

1. Liu CQ, Ma YL, Qin Q, Wang PH, Luo Y, Xu PF, Cui Y. Epidemiology of esophageal cancer in 2020 and projections to 2030 and 2040. Thoracic cancer. 2023;14(1):3-11..
2. Layke JC, Lopez PP. Esophageal cancer: a review and update. American family physician. 2006;73(12):2187–94.
3. Vermeulen BD, Siersema PD. Esophageal stenting in clinical practice: an overview. Current treatment options in gastroenterology. 2018;16(2):260–73.
4. Sharma P, Kozarek R, Practice Parameters Committee of the American College of Gastroenterology. Role of esophageal stents in benign and malignant diseases. Official journal of the American College of Gastroenterology| ACG. 2010;105(2):258–73.
5. Spaander MC, Baron TH, Siersema PD, Fuccio L, Schumacher B, Escorsell À, Garcia-Pagán JC, Dumonceau JM, Conio M, De Ceglie A, Skowronek J. Esophageal stenting for benign and malignant disease: European Society of Gastrointestinal Endoscopy (ESGE) Clinical Guideline. Endoscopy. 2016;48(10):939–48.
6. Diamantopoulos A, Roy Choudhury S, Irani FG, Rio Tinto H, Sabharwal T, et al. CIRSE Standards of Practice on Oesophageal and Gastroduodenal Stenting. CardioVascular and Interventional Radiology. 2023;46(5):562–572. https://doi.org/10.1007/s00270-023-03395-0.

Laparoscopic and Thoracoscopic Ivor Lewis Esophagectomy

Manuela Monrabal Lezama, Francisco Schlottmann, and Daniela Molena

Abstract Esophagectomy for esophageal cancer is one of the most challenging operations in thoracic surgery. Minimally invasive Ivor Lewis esophagectomy reduces surgical morbidity while offering comparable oncologic benefits than open surgery. This chapter outlines our surgical approach, providing surgical tips and troubleshooting strategies to improve outcomes and avoid complications.

Keywords Esophageal cancer · Esophagectomy · Minimally invasive · Laparoscopy · Thoracoscopy · Ivor Lewis

Introduction

Minimally invasive esophagectomy (MIE) is a technically demanding procedure requiring expertise in thoracoscopy and laparoscopy. In experienced hands, MIE offers excellent patient outcomes with reduced perioperative morbidity, shorter hospital stay, and fewer pulmonary complications as compared to open surgery.

M. Monrabal Lezama
Department of Surgery, Hospital Aleman of Buenos Aires, Buenos Aires, Argentina

F. Schlottmann
Department of Surgery, Hospital Aleman of Buenos Aires, Buenos Aires, Argentina

Department of Surgery, University of Illinois Chicago, Chicago, IL, USA

D. Molena (✉)
Department of Thoracic Surgery, Memorial Sloan Kettering Cancer Center, New York, NY, USA
e-mail: molenad@mskcc.org

F. Schlottmann, M. A. Masrur (eds.), *Endoscopic, Laparoscopic and Robotic Techniques for Foregut Disorders*, https://doi.org/10.1007/978-3-032-00811-4_29

Oncologic outcomes, including resection completeness, lymphadenectomy, and survival rates, are comparable or even superior to open surgery. Additionally, MIE has shown to significantly improve long-term quality of life [1–5].

Procedure Description

Patient Positioning

The patient is placed in a supine position on a bean bag, with the feet taped securely to a padded footboard. The arms are gently abducted for easy access to the abdomen, which is then prepped and draped thoroughly. Reverse Trendelenburg position is gradually applied during laparoscopy to improve visualization of the upper abdomen.

Abdominal Port Placement

A 5 mm port is inserted under direct vision just below the left costal margin in the midclavicular line. After CO_2 insufflation to 15 mmHg, a 5 mm camera port is placed midline below the falciform ligament, along with a 10 mm port in the right flank and a 5 mm port in the right upper quadrant, allowing smooth access beneath the liver and towards the hiatus. An optional 5 mm port in the left upper quadrant can be added for the assistant. A Nathanson liver retractor is positioned below the xiphoid to lift the left lobe and expose the hiatus (Fig. 1). The primary surgeon stands on the patient's right, using a Harmonic scalpel and an atraumatic grasper, while the assistant, on the left, aids with retraction using graspers in both hands. For mobilization of the stomach's greater curvature, particularly the short gastric vessels and pylorus, the surgeon moves to the left side.

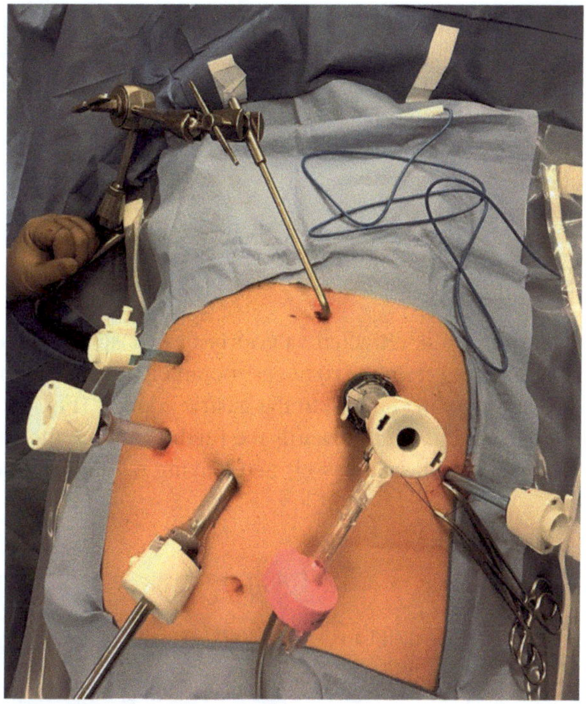

Fig. 1 Abdominal port placement. (From Esophageal Cancer, Diagnosis and Treatment second edition, Springer 2023)

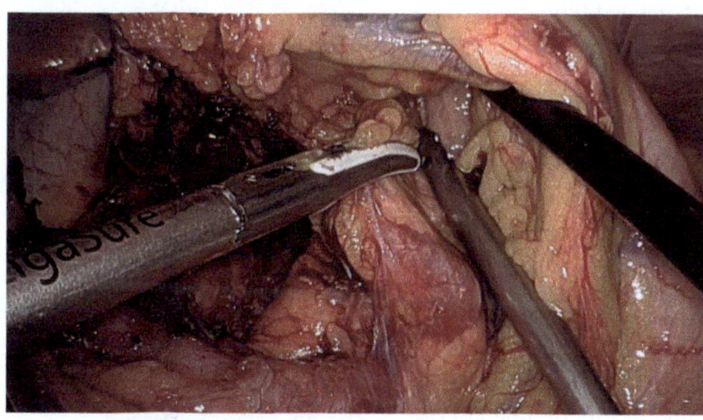

Fig. 2 Superior skeletonization of the hepatic and splenic arteries

Operative Technique

Abdominal Phase

Lymphadenectomy of the Celiac Trunk and Division of the Left Gastric Pedicle

The dissection begins with division of the gastrohepatic ligament, proceeding superiorly until reaching the right crus. The hepatic and splenic arteries are skeletonized superiorly (Fig. 2), and the left gastric vessels are completely dissected at their base before division with vascular stapler, in order to perform a complete dissection of their associated nodes (Fig. 3). Retracting the stomach anteriorly provides access to the celiac artery nodes located between the left gastric artery stump and the diaphragmatic crus. This exposure allows the posterior gastric attachments to be divided, partially mobilizing the tip of the fundus to facilitate later dissection along the greater curve.

Gastric Mobilization

The stomach is retracted anteriorly to expose and divide the gastrocolic ligament, 3–4 cm away from the right gastroepiploic artery, which must be preserved as it will provide vascular supply to the gastric conduit (Fig. 4). Dissection continues along the greater curvature towards the fundus through the gastrosplenic ligament, dividing the short gastric vessels and leaving a long stump on the splenic side to avoid

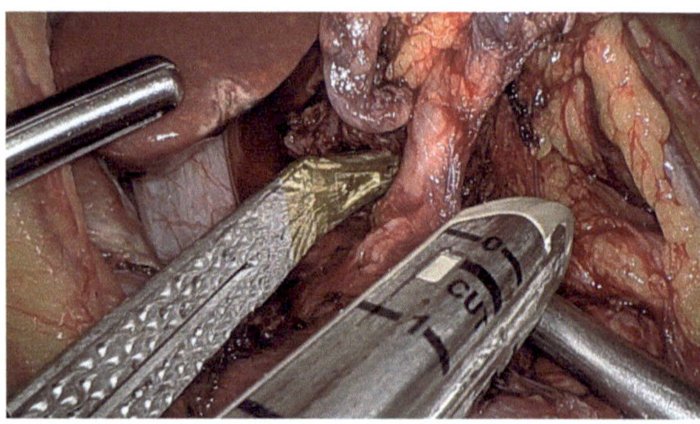

Fig. 3 Complete dissection of the left gastric vessels at their base before division with a vascular stapler, ensuring thorough removal of associated lymph nodes

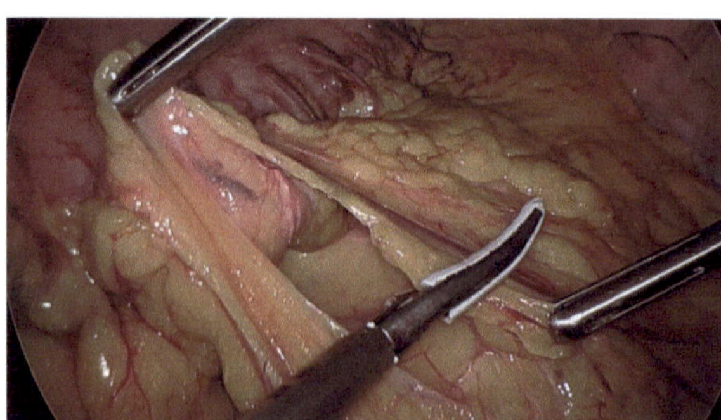

Fig. 4 Retraction of the stomach to expose and divide the gastrocolic ligament 3–4 cm from the right gastroepiploic artery, preserving the artery for vascular supply to the gastric conduit

spleen injury (Fig. 5). The gastrocolic ligament is then divided up to the duodenum, and the right gastroepiploic artery base is dissected to the pancreas's inferior edge (Fig. 6). Complete division of posterior attachments between the pancreas and stomach allows the pylorus to reach the hiatus.

Transhiatal Dissection

The esophagus is circumferentially dissected at the hiatus to facilitate the placement of a Penrose drain, which will act as a handle for retraction (Fig. 7). The dissection

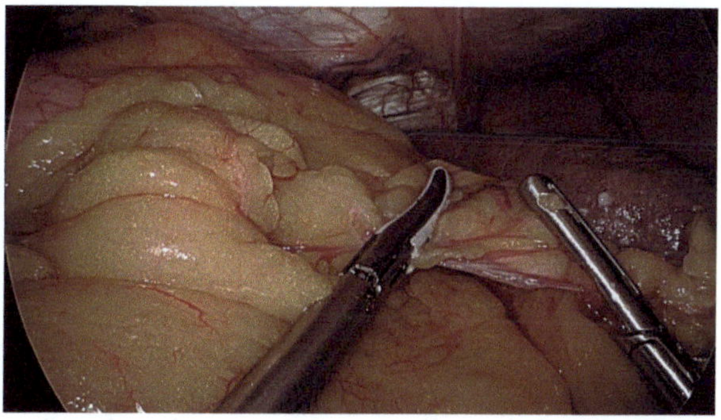

Fig. 5 Dissection along the greater curvature towards the fundus through the gastrosplenic ligament, dividing the short gastric vessels

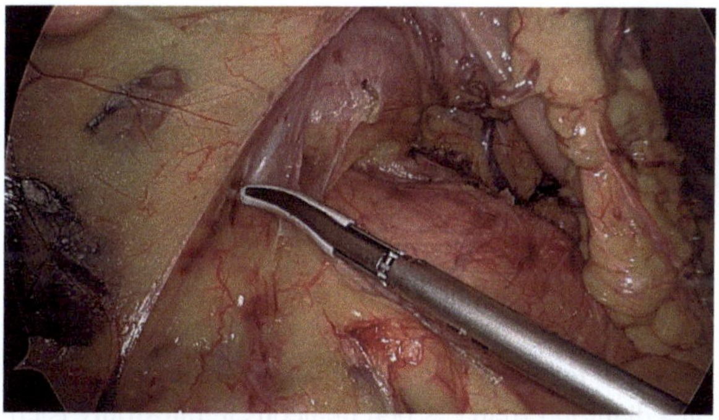

Fig. 6 The gastrocolic ligament is divided up to the duodenum, and the base of the right gastroepiploic artery is dissected to the inferior edge of the pancreas

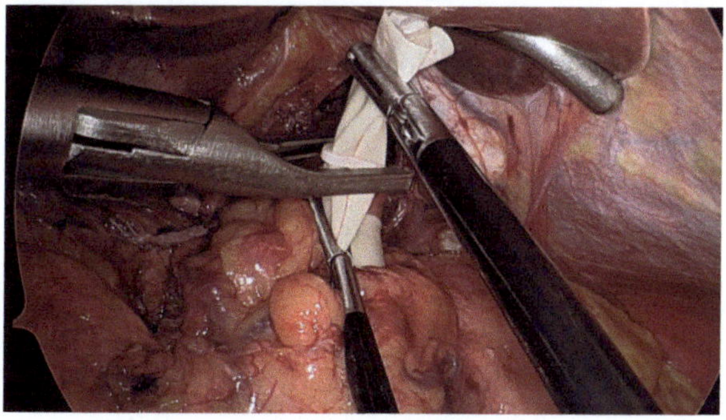

Fig. 7 The esophagus is circumferentially dissected at the hiatus, allowing for the placement of a Penrose drain to serve as a handle for retraction

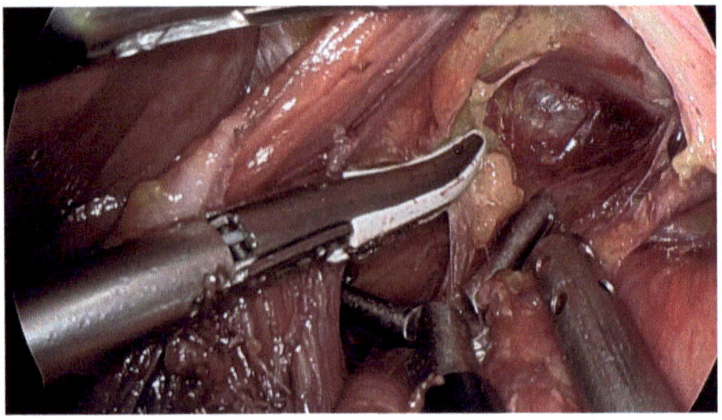

Fig. 8 During transhiatal dissection, the periesophageal and paracardial nodes located between the esophagus and the pericardium are carefully removed

plane extends from pleura to pleura, pericardium to the aorta, to the level of the inferior pulmonary vein. Periesophageal lymph nodes are preserved with the specimen. Additionally, it is crucial to remove the paracardial nodes situated between the esophagus and the pericardium (Fig. 8).

Creation of the Gastric Conduit

A 4- to 5-cm wide gastric conduit is created using surgical staplers, starting about 5 cm proximal to the pylorus on the lesser curvature and extending toward the fundus (Fig. 9). This starting point may vary based on the patient's anatomy and tumor location to ensure a suitable distal margin and conduit placement in the chest or neck. The stomach should be stretched and straightened from fundus to pylorus to prevent staple line spiraling maintaining an adequate distance from the esophagogastric junction (Fig. 10). The final 3–5 cm of the conduit can remain attached for easy retrieval into the chest. If a hiatal hernia is found, it should be closed with stitches to prevent paraconduit herniation.

Creation of Feeding Jejunostomy

A loop of jejunum is anchored to the abdominal wall with absorbable stitches placed on a diamond shape. A percutaneous jejunostomy is created using a Seldinger technique. The 4 anchoring sutures are tied externally within the subcutaneous layer of the abdominal wall. The tube is advanced into the bowel lumen and distal jejunum. An additional stitch is placed distally to the insertion site to avoid torsion of the jejunal loop (Fig. 11).

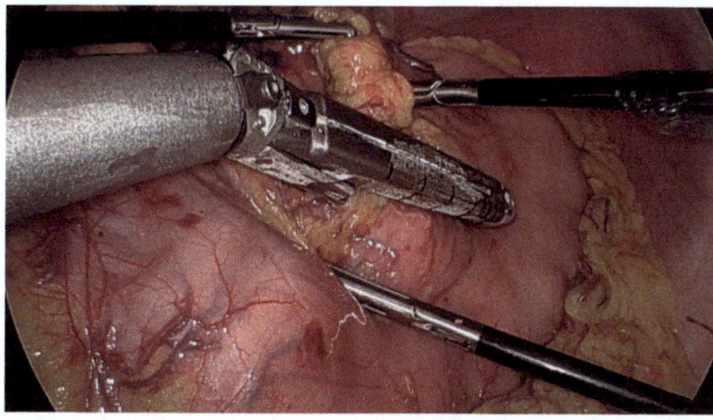

Fig. 9 Creation of A 4- to 5-cm wide gastric conduit is created using surgical staplers

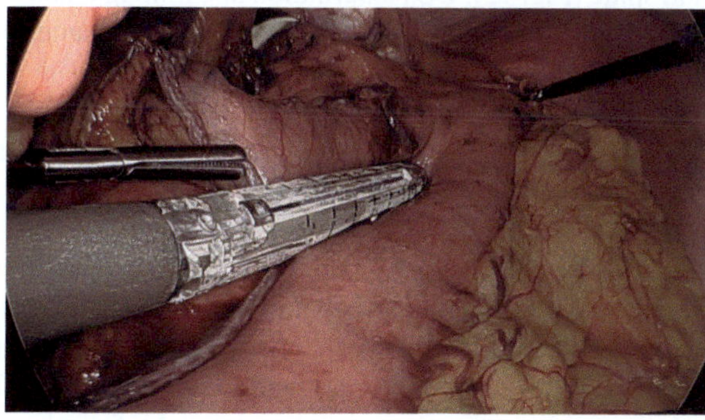

Fig. 10 The stomach is straightened from fundus to pylorus to prevent staple line spiraling, keeping distance from the esophagogastric junction

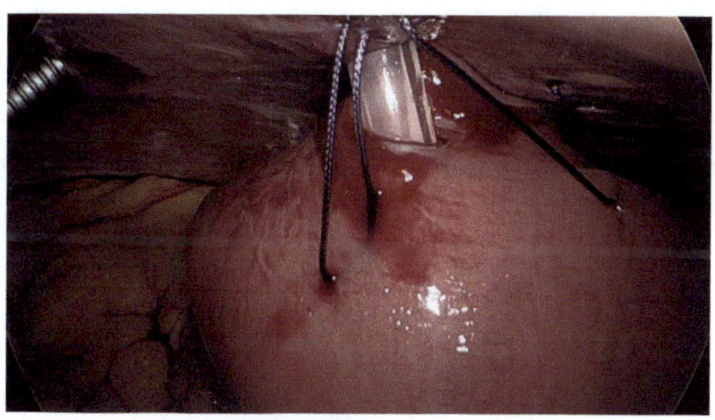

Fig. 11 Creation of percutaneous jejunostomy

Thoracic Phase

Positioning for the Thoracic Phase and Port Placement

The patient is positioned in the left lateral decubitus position, leaning slightly forward on a bean bag with an axillary roll and arm support, and the table flexed. Anesthesia is switched to single lung ventilation. The chest is accessed using a 10 mm optical trocar in the seventh intercostal space, posterior axillary line. Additional ports include a 5 mm camera port in the ninth intercostal space posterior to the first port, a 10 mm port in the fourth or fifth intercostal space in the mid-axillary line, and a 5 mm port in the seventh intercostal space, between the scapula and spine (Fig. 12). CO_2 insufflation at 8 mmHg enhances exposure by flattening the diaphragm and collapsing the lungs towards the anterior mediastinum.

Thoracoscopic Dissection: Opening of the Anterior and Posterior Pleura and Division of the Azygous Vein

The inferior pulmonary ligament is divided up to the level of the inferior pulmonary vein, and the associated lymph nodes are removed (Fig. 13). The mediastinal pleura is dissected anteriorly between the esophagus and lung, up to the azygos vein, which is then divided with a vascular load stapler (Fig. 14). Dissection continues posteriorly between the esophagus and aorta, and inferiorly to the diaphragm, connecting with the transhiatal dissection from the abdominal phase (Fig. 15). The pleura above the azygos vein is preserved and will be used to support the gastric conduit at the end of the procedure.

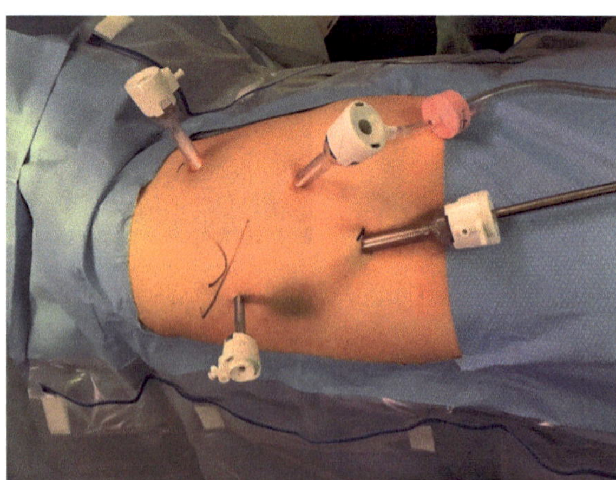

Fig. 12 Thoracic phase port placement. (From Esophageal Cancer, Diagnosis and Treatment second edition, Springer 2023)

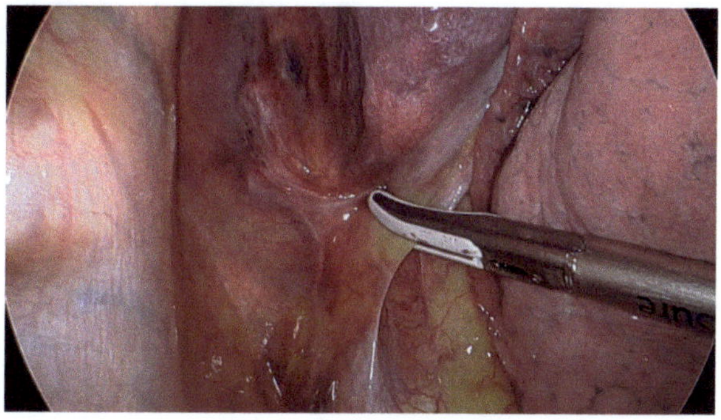

Fig. 13 Division of the inferior pulmonary ligament up to the level of the inferior pulmonary vein, and removal of the associated lymph nodes

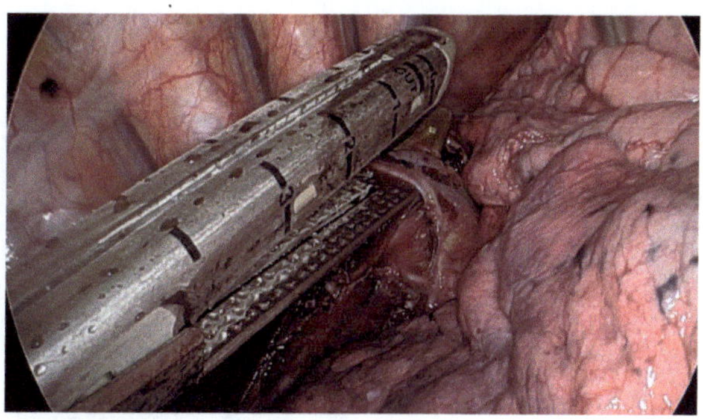

Fig. 14 The azygos vein is divided with a vascular load stapler

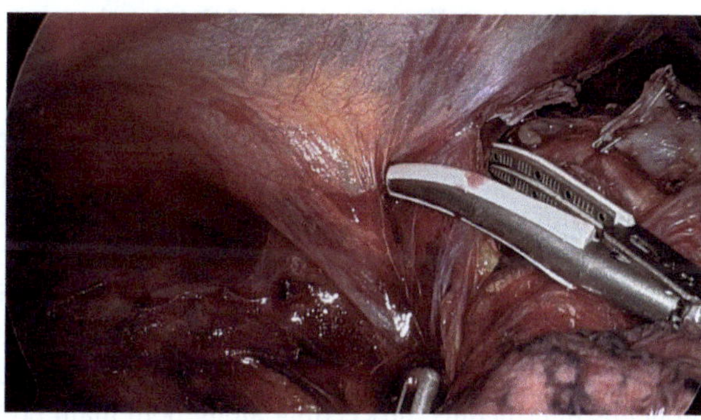

Fig. 15 Dissection continues posteriorly between the esophagus and aorta, and inferiorly to the diaphragm

Circumferential Mobilization of the Esophagus, Identification of Airways, and Division of the Esophagus

As dissection moves inferiorly toward the diaphragm, we will eventually meet the transhiatal dissection. Locate the Penrose drain and use this as a retraction handle (Fig. 16). The esophagus is dissected out of its mediastinal bed towards the azygos vein. Care must be taken near the aorta and left mainstem bronchus (Fig. 17). For gastroesophageal junction tumors, staying close to the esophagus reduces airway risk. It is essential to identify and clip lymphatic branches from the thoracic duct and arterial branches from the aorta to avoid complications.

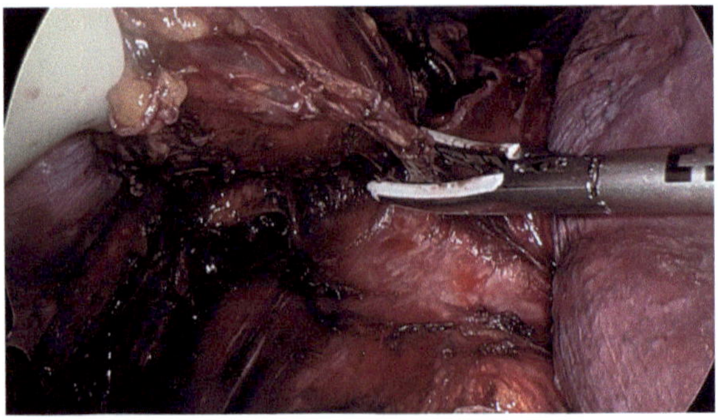

Fig. 16 Dissection proceeds inferiorly to meet the transhiatal dissection, using the Penrose drain for retraction

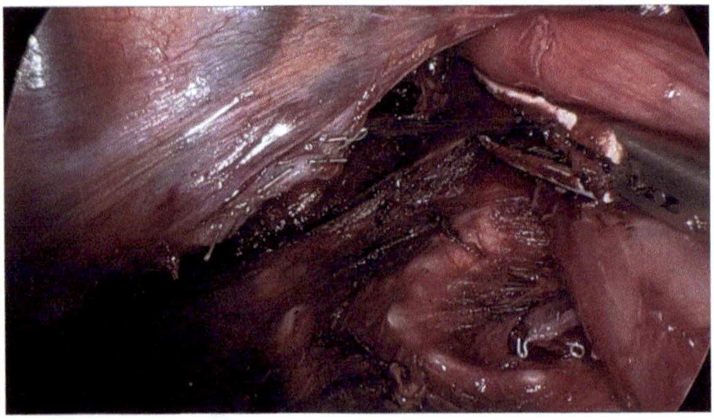

Fig. 17 The esophagus is dissected from its mediastinal bed towards the azygos vein, with careful attention near the aorta and left mainstem bronchus

Gastric Conduit Pullup, Division of the Specimen, Pathological Assessment of Margin, and Mediastinal Lymphadenectomy

The esophagus is sectioned with an adequate proximal margin using a linear stapler (Fig. 18). The gastric conduit is pulled up carefully, ensuring its orientation to avoid twisting, with the staple line facing right (Fig. 19). A linear stapler divides the specimen, preserving the distal margin near the gastroesophageal junction. After enlarging the seventh intercostal space incision, the specimen is removed in a bag and sent for pathologic assessment. While awaiting frozen section results, subcarinal lymph node dissection is performed, starting between the right inferior pulmonary vein and bronchus intermedius, proceeding along both main bronchi to the carina (Fig. 20). Care must be taken to avoid injuring the airway in order to prevent tracheoesophageal fistula.

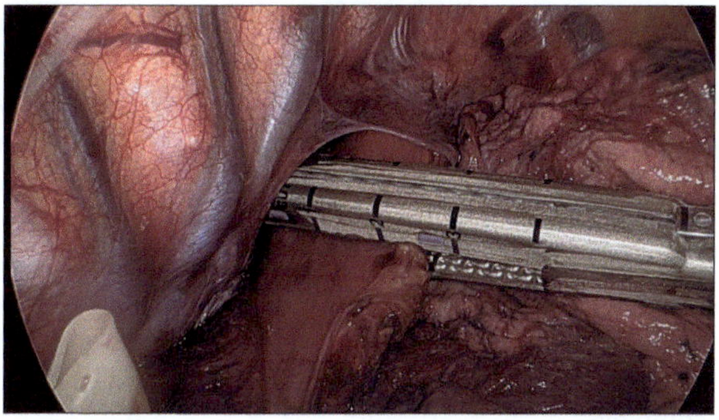

Fig. 18 The esophagus is sectioned with an adequate proximal margin using a linear stapler

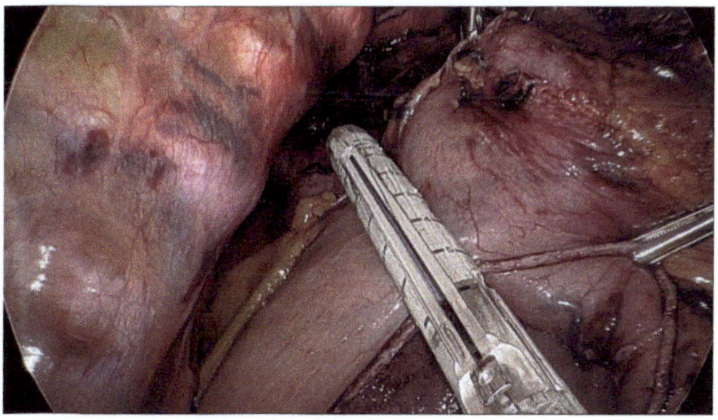

Fig. 19 The gastric conduit is carefully pulled up with the staple line facing right, and a linear stapler divides the specimen

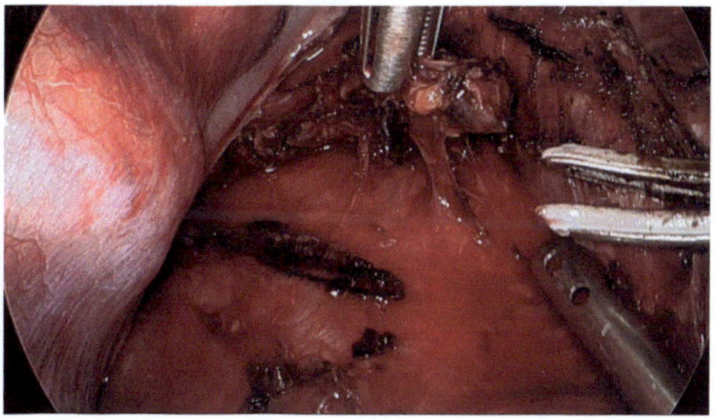

Fig. 20 Subcarinal lymph node dissection is performed between the right inferior pulmonary vein and bronchus intermedius, extending to the carina, while awaiting frozen section results

Passage of the OrVil and Assessment of Conduit Perfusion

The anesthesiologist advances the oral anvil of the OrVil until it reaches the proximal staple line. The esophageal stump is stabilized with graspers, and an opening is made on the posterior right side of the staple line to pass the anvil (Fig. 21). This minimizes ischemic tissue at the anastomotic site. The OrVil is passed through the right corner of the staple line to reduce potential leakage. A pursestring stitch with reabsorbable suture is placed around the anvil to ensure a tight seal around the device (Fig. 22). The conduit is then pulled up, and perfusion is checked with indocyanine green. Areas of poor perfusion should be resected after the anastomosis is complete.

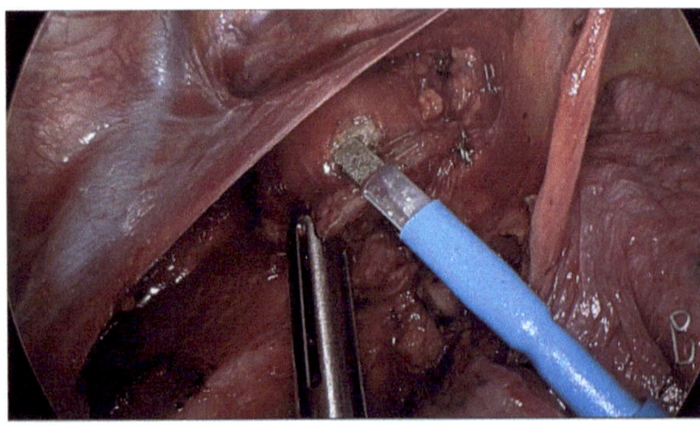

Fig. 21 The anesthesiologist advances the OrVil anvil to the proximal staple line, where an opening is made on the posterior right side to pass the anvil

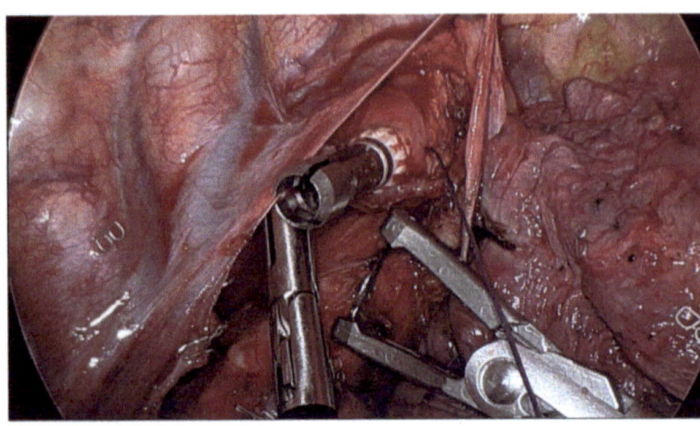

Fig. 22 A pursestring stitch with absorbable suture is placed around the anvil to ensure a tight seal around the device

Esophagogastric Anastomosis

The anastomosis is performed after the pathologist has confirmed negative margins. The conduit's proximal tip is opened with cautery, allowing insertion of the circular stapler (Figs. 23, 24, and 25). The anastomosis is performed where conduit perfusion is good and tension-free, preserving greater curvature vessels to protect the airways (Fig. 26). After firing the circular stapler, two stay sutures are placed: one at the lateral anastomosis for reinforcement and buttressed with omentum, and other medially to relieve tension. A nasogastric tube is inserted, and the conduit is closed with a linear stapler, ensuring separation from the gastric staple line to avoid ischemia (Figs. 27 and 28).

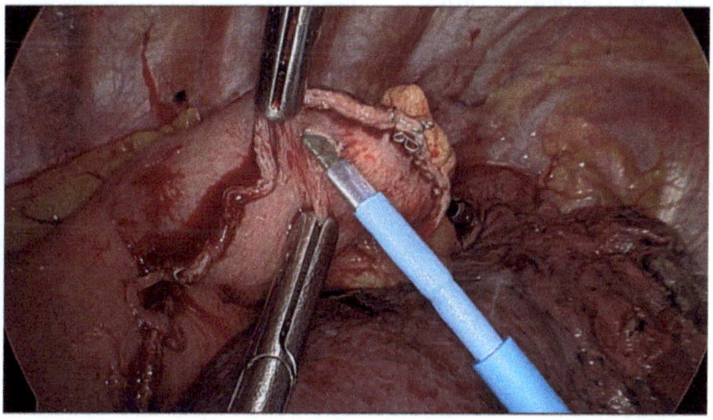

Fig. 23 The conduit's proximal tip is opened using cautery to allow insertion of the circular stapler

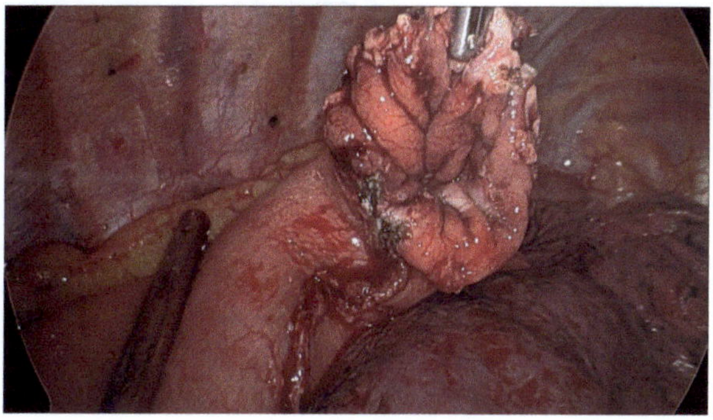

Fig. 24 Conduit's proximal tip opened

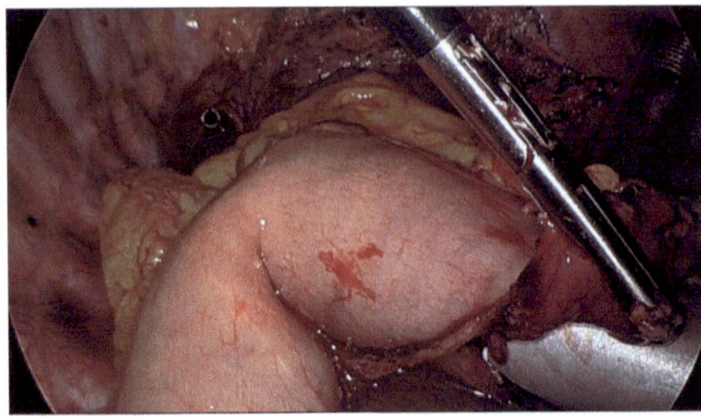

Fig. 25 Insertion of the circular stapler

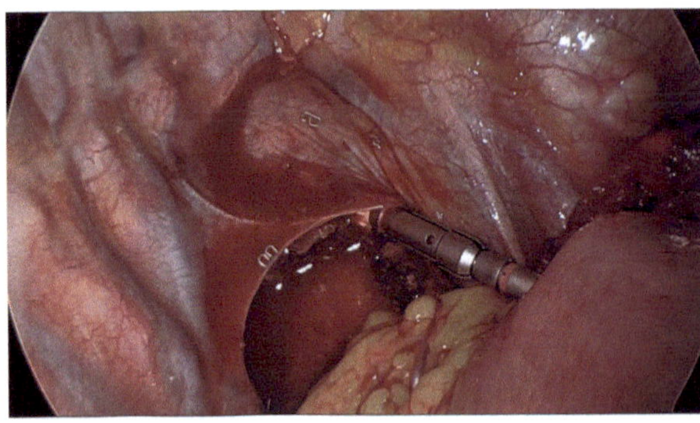

Fig. 26 Esophagogastric anastomosis

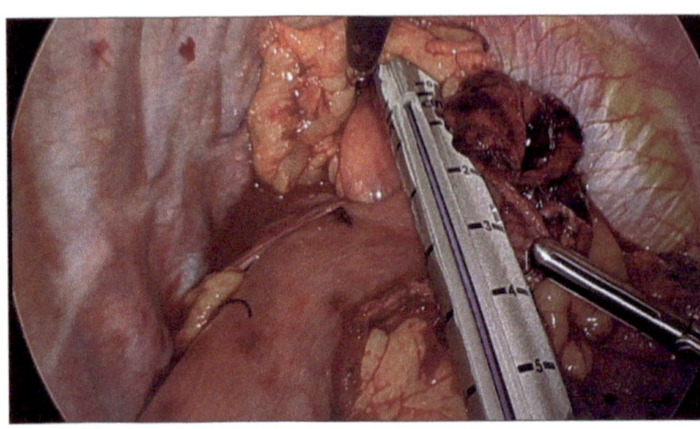

Fig. 27 The conduit is closed with a linear stapler, ensuring separation from the gastric staple line to avoid ischemia

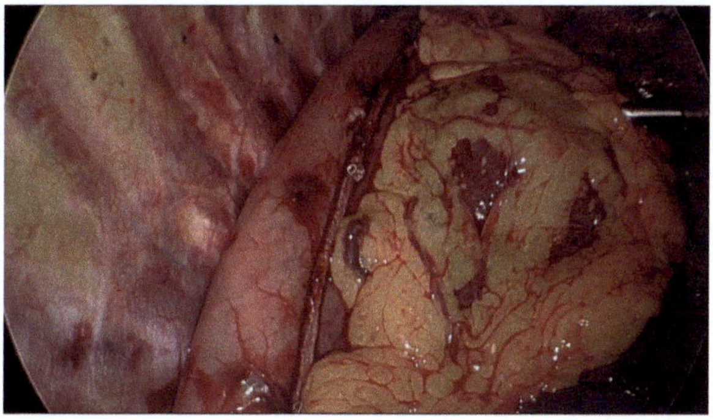

Fig. 28 Gastric conduit

Anastomosis Assessment and Chest Tube Placement

Intraoperative gastroscopy can assess the anastomosis and perform a leak test with insufflation under water. The anesthesiologist advances a nasogastric tube under direct vision into the distal conduit. The conduit may be tacked to the diaphragm with non-absorbable sutures to prevent paraconduit herniation. A straight 28 Fr chest tube is placed and the lung re-expanded. Incisions are closed in the standard fashion.

Conclusions

Minimally invasive Ivor Lewis esophagectomy is a technically demanding operation requiring careful dissection with attention to detail and purposeful care after surgery. Key technical elements should be taken into account throughout the procedure to reduce risks of surgical complications.

Conflict of Interest Manuela Monrabal Lezama, Francisco Schlottmann and Daniela Molena declare that they have no conflicts of interest.

References

1. Luketich JD, Pennathur A, Franchetti Y, Catalano PJ, Swanson S, Sugarbaker DJ, et al. Minimally invasive esophagectomy: results of a prospective phase II multicenter trial-the Eastern Cooperative Oncology Group (E2202) Study. Ann Surg. 2015;261(4):702–7.
2. Mungo B, Lidor AO, Stem M, Molena D. Early experience and lessons learned in a new minimally invasive esophagectomy program. Surg Endosc. 2016;30:1692–8.
3. Litle VR, Buenaventura PO, Luketich JD. Minimally invasive resection for esophageal cancer. Surg Clin North Am. 2002;82(4):711–28.
4. Bras Harriott C, Angeramo CA, Casas MA, Schlottmann F. Open versus hybrid versus totally minimally invasive Ivor Lewis esophagectomy: systematic review and meta-analysis. J Thorac Cardiovasc Surg. 2022;164:e233–54.
5. Bograd AJ, Molena D. Minimally invasive esophagectomy. Curr Prob Surg. 2021;58:100984.

Robotic Ivor Lewis Esophagectomy

Manuela Monrabal Lezama, Francisco Schlottmann, and Daniela Molena

Abstract Robotic thoracic surgery has been increasingly adopted due to its articulating instruments, improved visualization, and better ergonomics. This has helped surgeons transition from open to minimally invasive surgery or increase complexity in minimally invasive procedures. Robotic assisted minimally invasive esophagectomy (RAMIE) faces challenges due to a steep learning curve. However, as more surgeons are trained, the benefits of RAMIE for both patients and surgeons will become clearer. This chapter covers the Robotic Assisted Ivor Lewis esophagectomy technique.

Keywords Robotic · Ivor Lewis · Esophagectomy · Esophageal cancer · Minimally invasive esophagectomy · RAMIE

Introduction

Robotic thoracic surgery has seen increasing adoption, with many surgeons finding the articulating instruments, enhanced visualization, and improved ergonomics highly beneficial. These advancements have facilitated the transition from open to minimally invasive approaches and allowed for increased complexity while maintaining minimal invasiveness. Robotic assisted minimally invasive esophagectomy

M. Monrabal Lezama
Department of Surgery, Hospital Aleman of Buenos Aires, Buenos Aires, Argentina

F. Schlottmann
Department of Surgery, Hospital Aleman of Buenos Aires, Buenos Aires, Argentina

Department of Surgery, University of Illinois Chicago, Chicago, IL, USA

D. Molena (✉)
Department of Thoracic Surgery, Memorial Sloan Kettering Cancer Center, New York, NY, USA
e-mail: molenad@mskcc.org

F. Schlottmann, M. A. Masrur (eds.), *Endoscopic, Laparoscopic and Robotic Techniques for Foregut Disorders*, https://doi.org/10.1007/978-3-032-00811-4_30

(RAMIE), however, is still in its early stages and is challenged by a steep learning curve. However, as more surgeons become proficient with robotics, the benefits of RAMIE for both patients and surgeons are expected to become more evident. RAMIE is largely similar to minimally invasive esophagectomy, as described earlier in this volume. However, the robotic platform introduces a few key differences, which we will be highlighted throughout the procedure [1–7].

Procedure Description

Patient Positioning

The patient is placed in a supine position on the operating table with arms secured and a footboard for support, as we typically use a steep reverse Trendelenburg position during the abdominal phase of the procedure.

Abdominal Port Placement

The abdomen is prepped and draped from the nipple line to the pubis. Veress needle entry is used at Palmer's point. Our trocar setup includes three 8 mm robotic trocars, one 12 mm robotic trocar, an 8 mm AirSeal trocar, and a 5 mm laparoscopic trocar for the liver retractor. CO_2 insufflation is set at 15 mmHg with a flow of 40 L/min. The first 8 mm trocar (Arm 2, 30° camera) is placed blindly 15 cm subxiphoid and paramedian, with the rest placed under direct visualization: an 8 mm trocar (Arm 4), an 8 mm trocar (Arm 3), a 12 mm trocar (Arm 1), and the AirSeal in the right lower quadrant. The liver retractor is placed just below the liver and secured, and the robot is docked using the "Upper abdomen" setting.

Operative Technique

Abdominal Phase

Lymphadenectomy of the Celiac Trunk and Division of the Left Gastric Pedicle

The dissection starts by dividing the gastrohepatic ligament and proceeds upward until reaching the right crus (Figs. 1 and 2). The left gastric vessels are fully dissected at their base and then divided using a vascular stapler, ensuring complete removal of the associated lymph nodes (Figs. 3, 4, and 5). Anterior retraction of the stomach exposes the celiac artery nodes located between the stump of the left

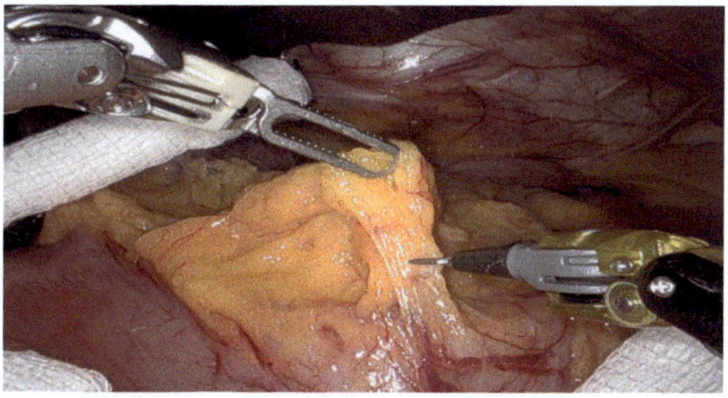

Fig. 1 Division of the gastrohepatic ligament

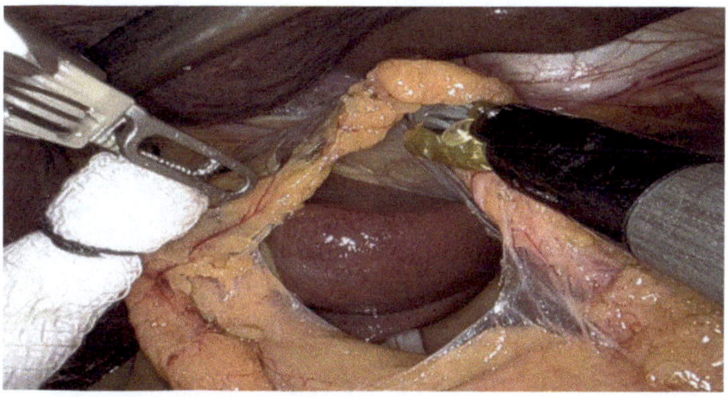

Fig. 2 Further dissection on the lesser curvature

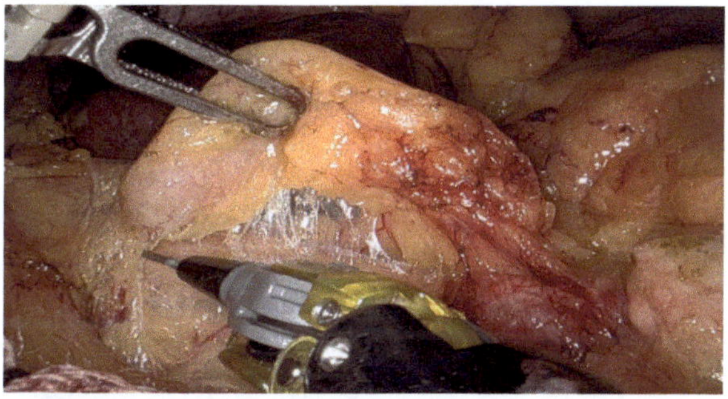

Fig. 3 Lymphadenectomy at the celiac trunk

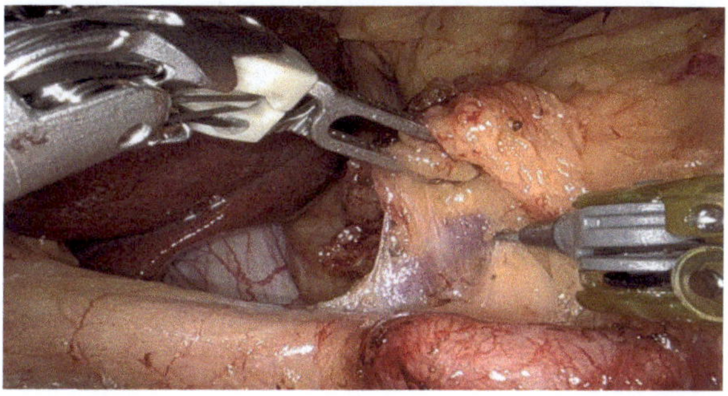

Fig. 4 Dissection of the left gastric vessels ensuring complete removal of the associated lymph nodes

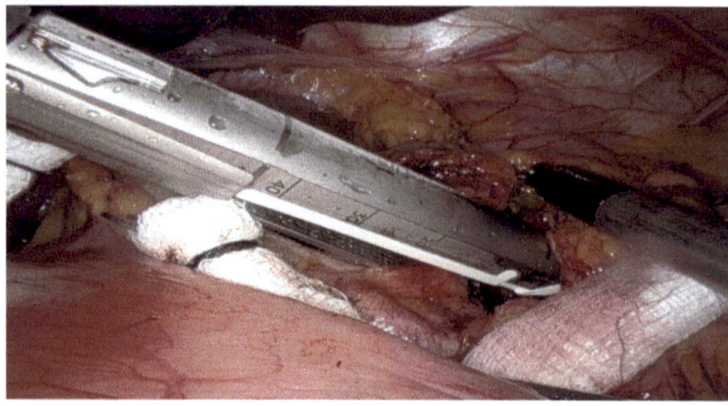

Fig. 5 Division of left gastric vessels using a vascular stapler

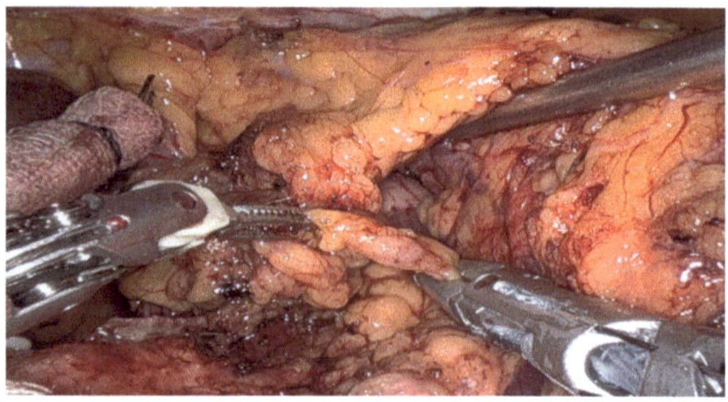

Fig. 6 Anterior retraction of the stomach exposes the celiac artery nodes located between the stump of the left gastric artery and the diaphragmatic crus

gastric artery and the diaphragmatic crus (Fig. 6). This exposure allows division of the posterior gastric attachments, partially mobilizing the fundus tip to facilitate further dissection along the greater curvature.

Gastric Mobilization

The mobilization of the greater curvature begins by elevating the gastrocolic ligament and identifying the right gastroepiploic artery, which must be carefully preserved along its course (Fig. 7). The greater omentum is divided with a vessel sealer, creating a vascularized omental pedicle that will serve as a buttress for the anastomosis and a barrier between the airway and anastomosis (Fig. 8). At the level of the short gastric vessels, dissection continues closer to the stomach, dividing the gastrosplenic ligament and mobilizing the fundus (Fig. 9). The gastrocolic ligament is divided up to the duodenum, and the base of the right gastroepiploic artery is dissected down to the lower edge of the pancreas (Fig. 10). Complete separation of the posterior attachments between the stomach and pancreas enables the pylorus to reach the hiatus.

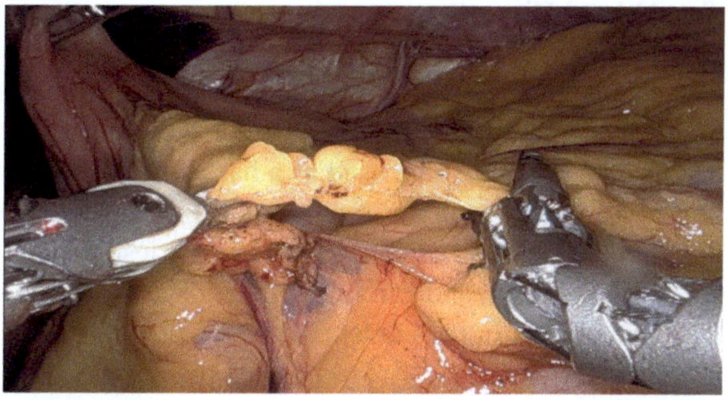

Fig. 7 After identifying the right gastroepiploic artery, the greater omentum is divided with a vessel sealer

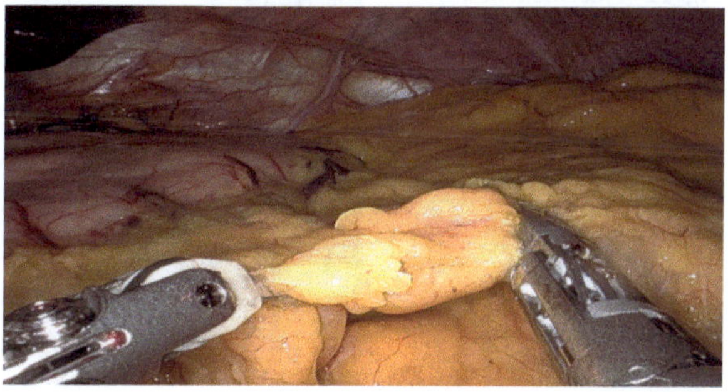

Fig. 8 Creation of a vascularized omental pedicle that will serve as a buttress for the anastomosis and a barrier between the airway and anastomosis

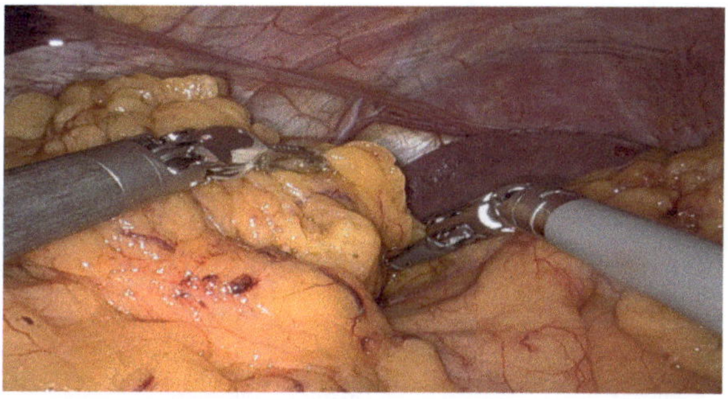

Fig. 9 The short gastric vessels are dissected closer to the gastric side

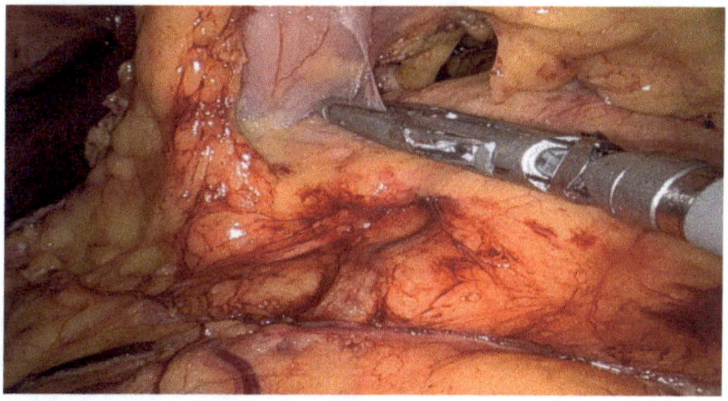

Fig. 10 The base of the right gastroepiploic artery is dissected down to the lower edge of the pancreas. Attachments between the stomach and pancreas are separated in order to let the pylorus reach the hiatus

Transhiatal Dissection

The esophagus is circumferentially mobilized from the hiatus, with the dissection extending upward towards the inferior pulmonary veins. Placing a Penrose drain can be useful as it can be used as a handle for retraction (Fig. 11). A tip-up grasper is used to provide counter-traction throughout the process, minimizing the need to handle the specimen directly (Fig. 12). Periesophageal lymph nodes are preserved with the specimen, and careful removal of the paracardial nodes between the esophagus and pericardium is essential (Fig. 13).

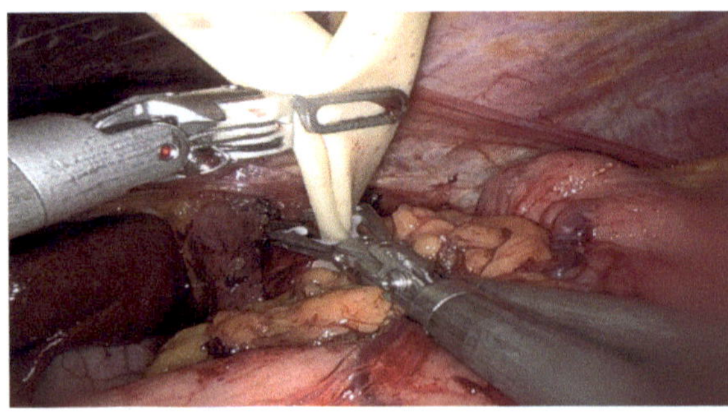

Fig. 11 Placement of a Penrose drain around the esophagus facilitates transhiatal dissection

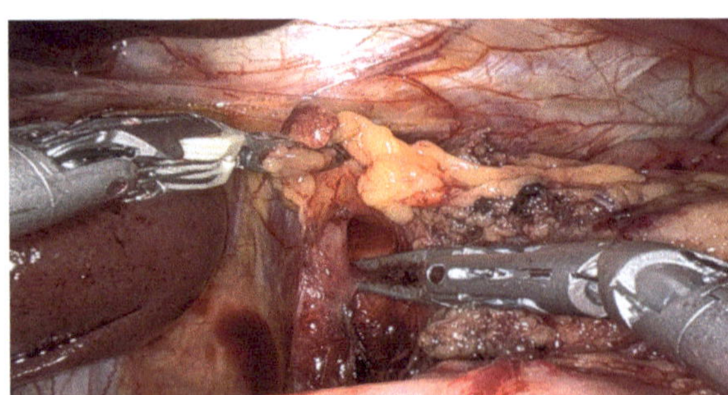

Fig. 12 Transhiatal dissection of the distal esophagus

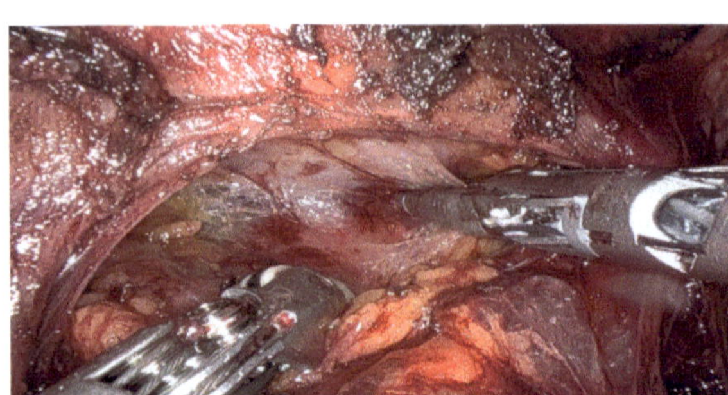

Fig. 13 Careful removal of the paracardial nodes between the esophagus and pericardium

Creation of the Gastric Conduit

A 4- to 5-cm wide gastric conduit is fashioned using surgical staplers, beginning approximately 5 cm proximal to the pylorus along the lesser curvature and extending toward the fundus (Fig. 14). The stomach is straightened from fundus to pylorus to prevent spiraling of the staple line, ensuring sufficient distance from the esophagogastric junction (Fig. 15). The Firefly™ technology integrated into the robotic platform aids in guiding the conduit creation, especially near the proximal stomach. The final 3–5 cm of the conduit remains attached for easy retrieval into the chest.

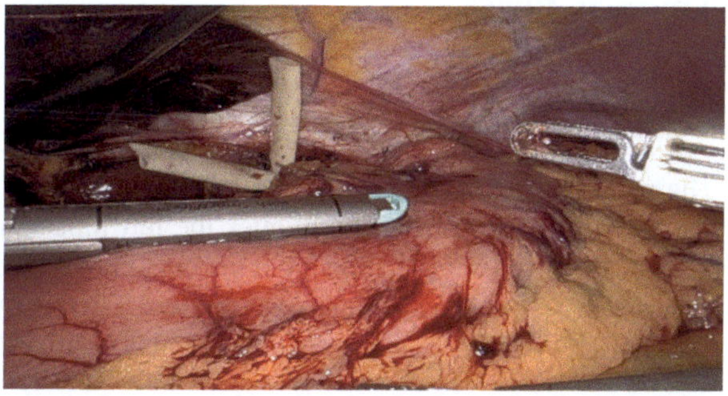

Fig. 14 Creation of gastric conduit with surgical staplers

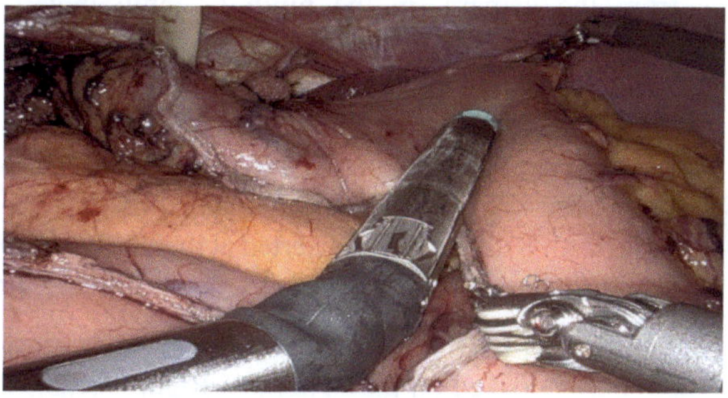

Fig. 15 The stomach is straightened from fundus to pylorus to prevent spiraling of the staple line, ensuring sufficient distance from the esophagogastric junction

Creation of Feeding Jejunostomy

For robotic jejunostomy tube insertion, it is often more efficient to move the camera to Arm 3 and use Arms 2 and 4 for the Cadiere forceps and needle driver, respectively. A loop of jejunum is secured to the abdominal wall with absorbable sutures arranged in a diamond shape. A percutaneous jejunostomy is then created using the Seldinger technique. The four anchoring sutures are tied externally within the subcutaneous layer of the abdominal wall. The tube is advanced into the bowel lumen and distal jejunum, and an additional suture is placed distally to prevent torsion of the jejunal loop (Fig. 16).

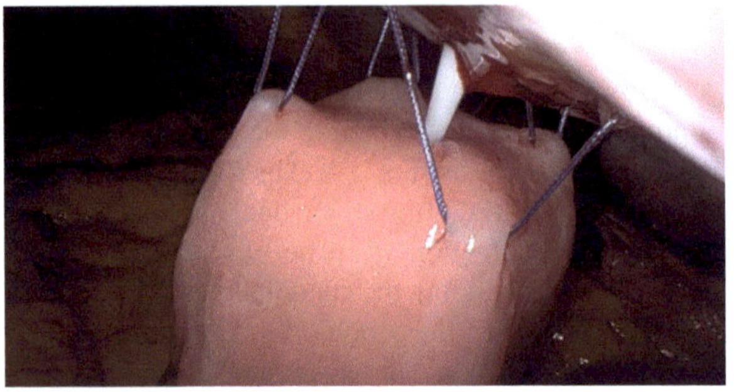

Fig. 16 Creation of feeding jejunostomy

Thoracic Phase

Positioning for the Thoracic Phase and Port Placement

The patient is repositioned into the left lateral decubitus with the bed flexed. The anesthesia team selectively ventilates the left lung via a dual-lumen endotracheal tube. Thoracic trocar placement begins with an 8 mm camera trocar inserted at the fifth intercostal space along the posterior axillary line. A 30° camera is inserted, and insufflation is initiated at 8 mmHg CO_2 and 40 L/min flow.

- Arm 1: An 8 mm trocar is placed posteriorly and inferiorly, two handbreadths from the camera, in the ninth or tenth intercostal space, just above the diaphragm.
- Arm 2: A 12 mm trocar is placed one handbreadth inferior to the camera port and one handbreadth anterior to Arm 1, typically at the seventh intercostal space.
- AirSeal port: This is triangulated between Arm 2 and Arm 3, placed as far anterior as possible without injuring the diaphragm.
- Arm 4: An 8 mm trocar is inserted at the third intercostal space, high in the axilla, staying anterior to the latissimus dorsi and allowing enough space for proper angling of the robot towards the lower chest.

The robot is docked on the "Thoracic Right" preset. The instruments are inserted, and the the surgery continues with the intrathoracic esophageal dissection.

Thoracic Dissection: Opening of the Anterior and Posterior Pleura and Division of the Azygous Vein

The thoracic dissection starts by opening the inferior pulmonary ligament with electrocautery, extending the pleural incision along the esophagus up to the azygos vein (Fig. 17). The azygous vein is mobilized from the underlying esophagus and then transected with a vascular stapler (Fig. 18). Dissection proceeds posteriorly between the esophagus and the aorta, and inferiorly towards the diaphragm, connecting with the transhiatal dissection performed during the abdominal phase (Fig. 19).

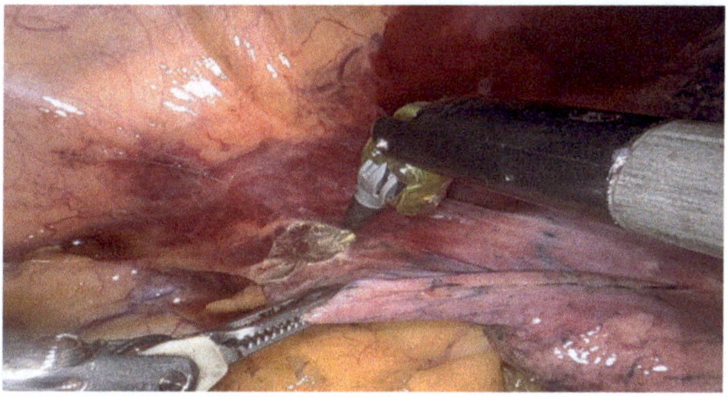

Fig. 17 Thoracic dissection starts by opening the inferior pulmonary ligament, extending the dissection up to the azygos vein

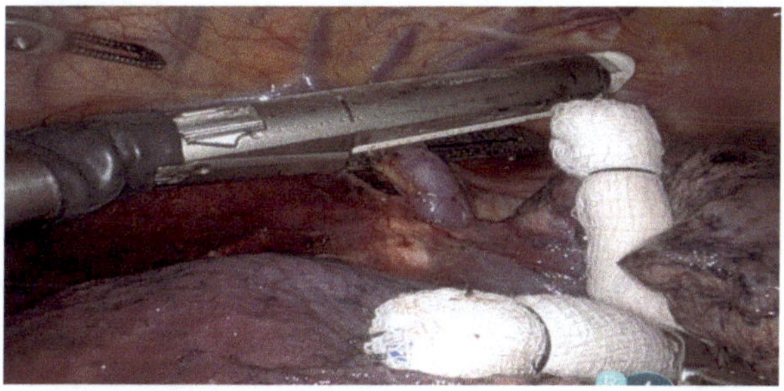

Fig. 18 The azygos vein is mobilized and then transected using a vascular stapler

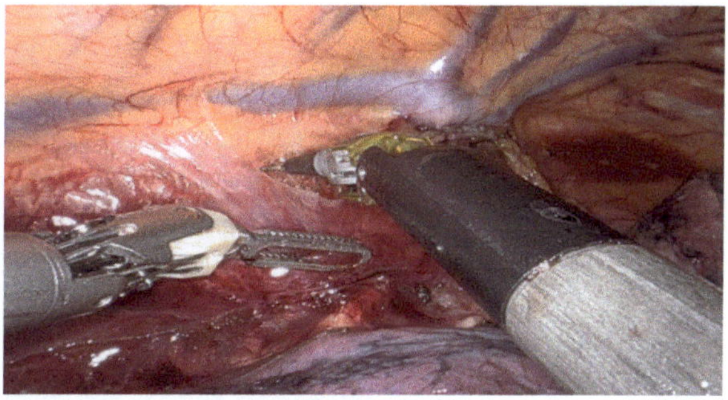

Fig. 19 Dissection proceeds posteriorly and inferiorly, in order to reach the transhiatal dissection

Circumferential Mobilization of the Esophagus, Identification of Airways, and Division of the Esophagus

As dissection progresses toward the diaphragm, we will eventually meet with the transhiatal dissection (Fig. 20). The Penrose drain is used as a retraction handle, allowing us to carefully dissect the esophagus from the posterior mediastinum while avoiding the thoracic duct and ensuring meticulous hemostasis of the bronchial arteries. The vessel sealer is ideal for this task. A crucial step is mobilizing the esophagus from the airway, using minimal energy dissection (Fig. 21). Lymphatic branches from the thoracic duct and arterial branches from the aorta are identified and clipped to prevent complications. The esophagus is then transected with a linear stapler, ensuring an adequate proximal margin (Fig. 22).

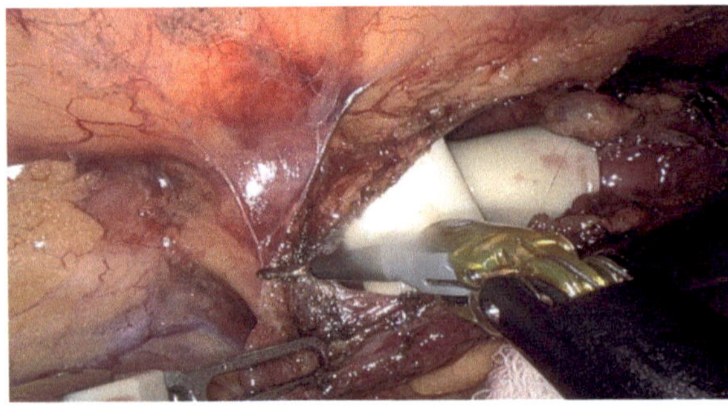

Fig. 20 Once the transhiatal dissection is encountered, the Penrose drain may be useful as a retraction handle, allowing to dissect the esophagus from its attachments

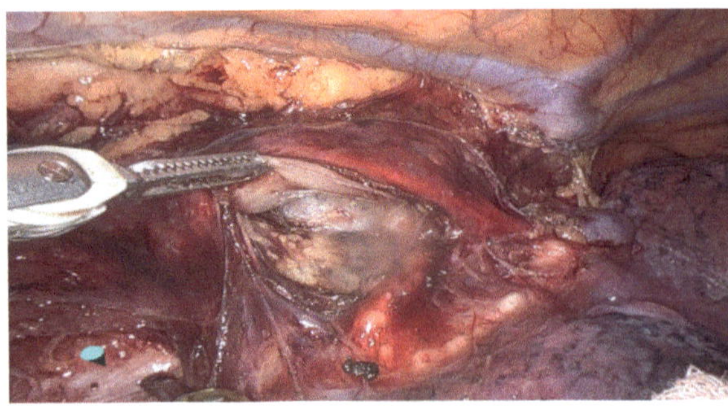

Fig. 21 The esophagus is dissected close to the airway using minimal energy dissection

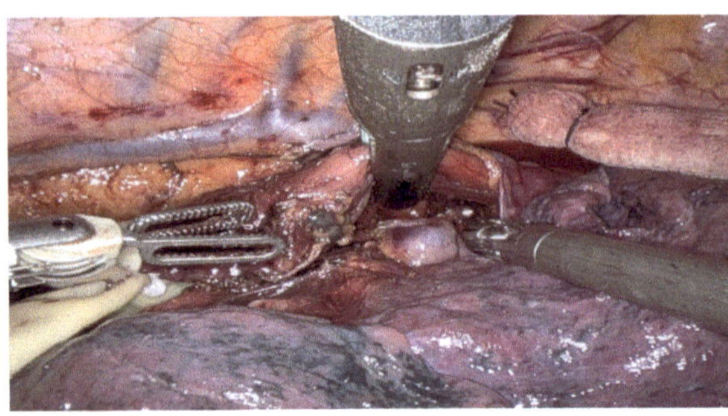

Fig. 22 Transection of the esophagus using a linear stapler, ensuring an adequate proximal margin

Gastric Conduit Pullup, Division of the Specimen, Pathological Assessment of Margin, and Mediastinal Lymphadenectomy

The gastric conduit is carefully pulled up, ensuring proper alignment to avoid any twisting, with the staple line facing right. The specimen is divided using a linear stapler, maintaining the distal margin near the gastroesophageal junction (Fig. 23). The specimen is removed in a bag after enlarging the seventh intercostal space incision, and sent for pathological evaluation. While awaiting the frozen section results, subcarinal lymph node dissection is performed, starting between the right inferior pulmonary vein and bronchus intermedius and extending along the main bronchi to the carina (Fig. 24). Careful attention is given to avoid airway damage and lower the risk of tracheoesophageal fistula.

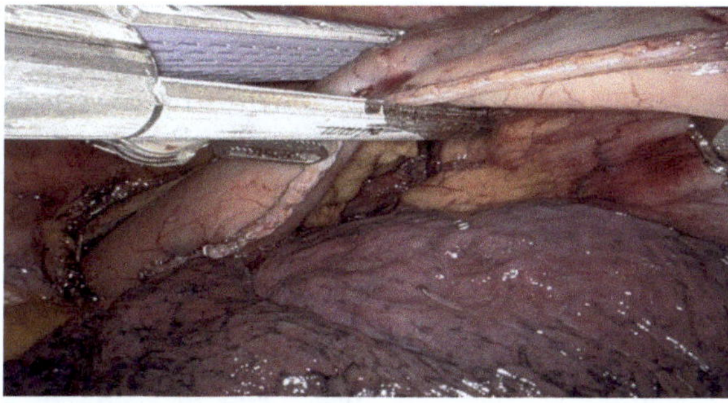

Fig. 23 Division of the specimen using a linear stapler

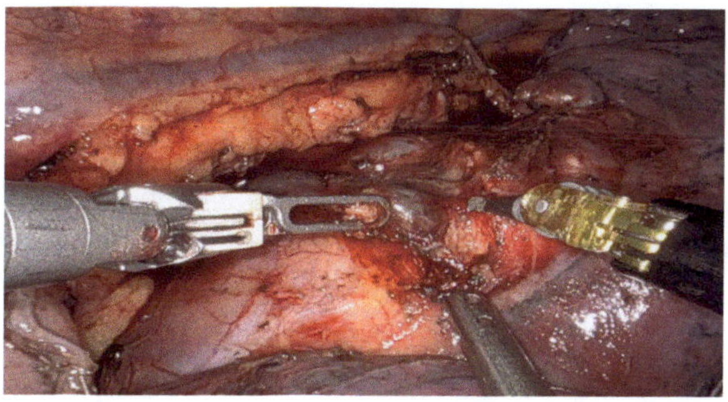

Fig. 24 Subcarinal lymph node dissection is performed while awaiting the frozen section results

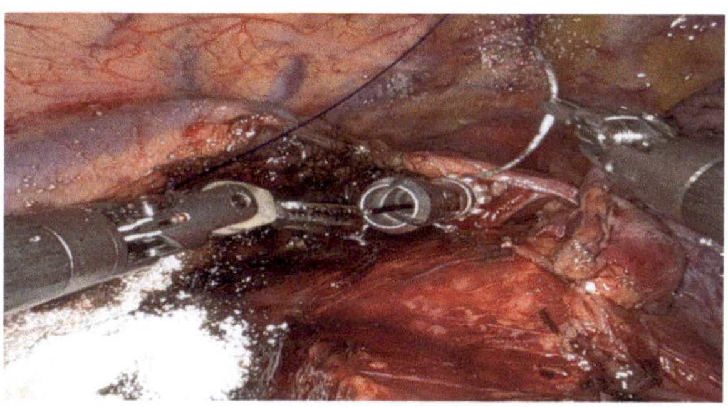

Fig. 25 The OrVil is passed through the right corner of the staple line to minimize the risk of leakage. A purse-string stitch using absorbable suture is placed around the anvil to create a secure seal

Passage of the OrVil and Assessment of Conduit Perfusion

The anesthesiologist advances the OrVil oral anvil until it reaches the proximal staple line. The esophageal stump is secured with graspers, and an opening is created on the posterior right side of the staple line to insert the anvil. The OrVil is passed through the right corner of the staple line to minimize the risk of leakage. A purse-string stitch using absorbable suture is placed around the anvil to create a secure seal (Fig. 25). The conduit is then pulled up, and its perfusion is assessed with indocyanine green (Fig. 26). Any poorly perfused areas should be resected after completing the anastomosis. It's important to avoid excess conduit length, which can cause redundancy and delayed emptying.

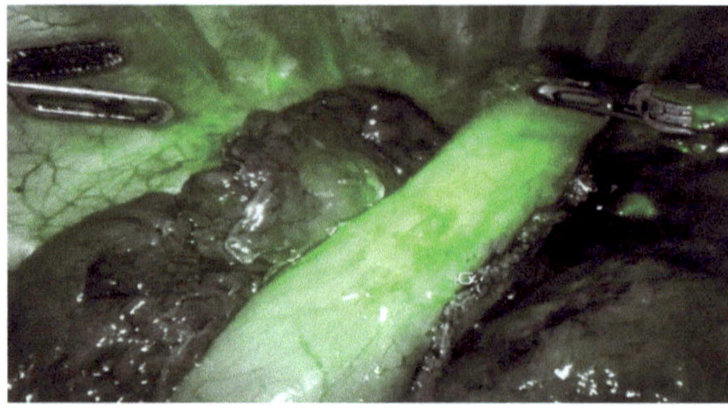

Fig. 26 Assessment of conduit perfusion using indocyanine green

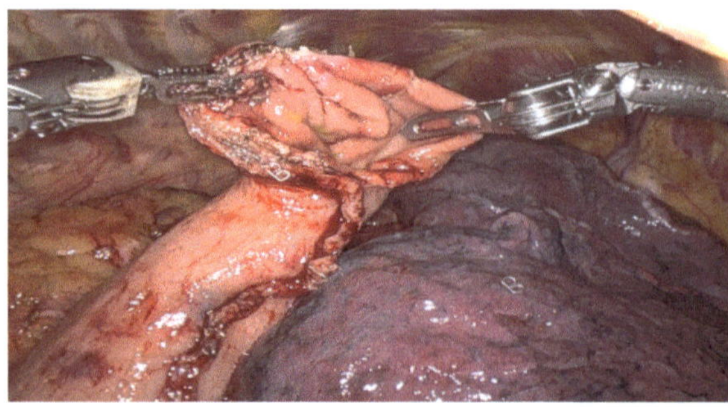

Fig. 27 The conduit's proximal tip is opened using cautery to allow insertion of the circular stapler

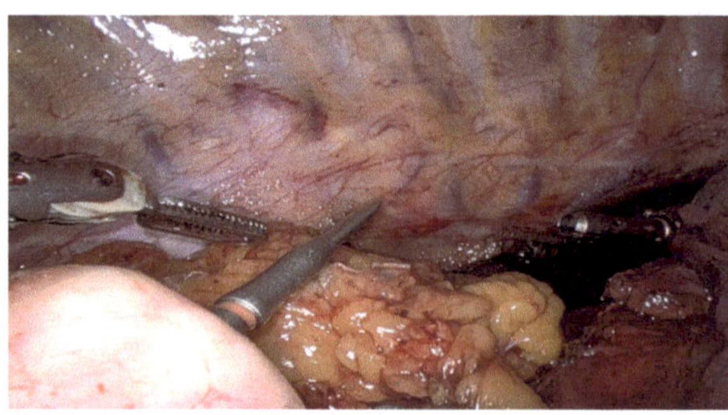

Fig. 28 The circular stapler inside the conduit is aligned with the anvil placed at the esophagus

Esophagogastric Anastomosis

The anastomosis is performed once the pathologist confirms clear margins. The proximal tip of the conduit is opened using cautery to allow insertion of the circular stapler (Fig. 27). The anastomosis is performed in an area of the conduit with good perfusion and minimal tension, preserving the greater curvature vessels to protect the airways (Figs. 28, 29, and 30). After the circular stapler is fired, two stay sutures are placed: one laterally for reinforcement, buttressed with omentum, and the other medially to reduce tension. A nasogastric tube is inserted, and the conduit is closed using a linear stapler, ensuring it is separated from the gastric staple line to prevent ischemia (Fig. 31).

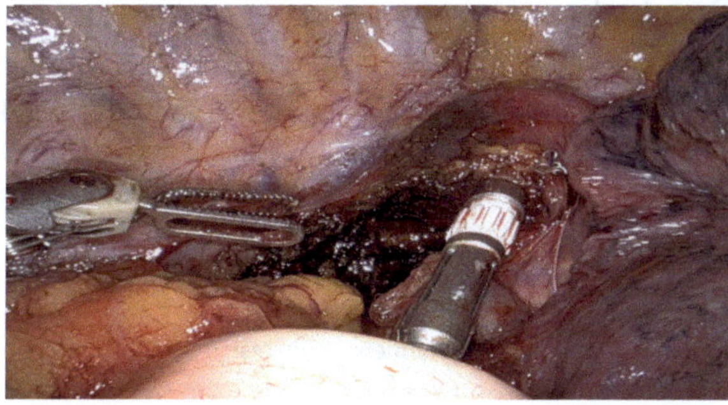

Fig. 29 Esophagogastric anastomosis

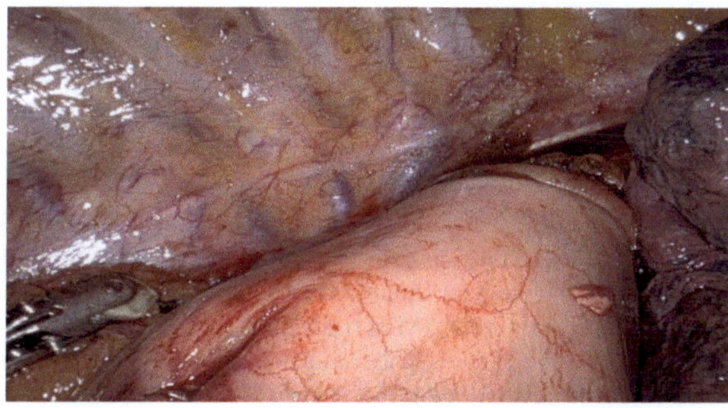

Fig. 30 Esophagogastric anastomosis completed

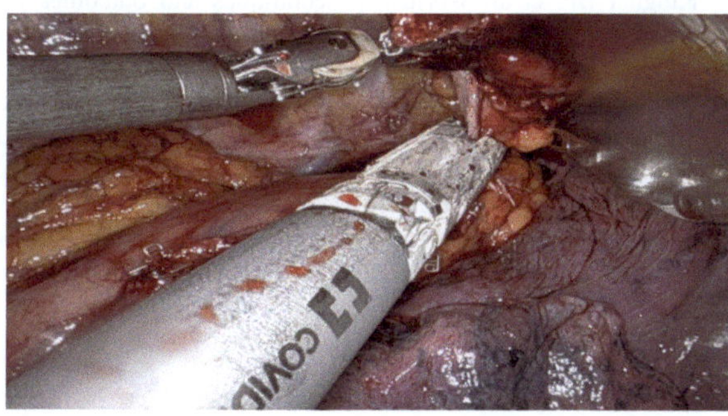

Fig. 31 The conduit is closed with a linear stapler, ensuring separation from the gastric staple line to avoid ischemia

Anastomosis Assessment and Chest Tube Placement

Intraoperative gastroscopy can be used to assess the anastomosis and perform a leak test by insufflating air under water. The anesthesiologist advances a nasogastric tube into the distal conduit under direct visualization. Non-absorbable sutures may be used to tack the conduit to the diaphragm, preventing paraconduit herniation. A straight 28 Fr chest tube is inserted, and the lung is re-expanded. The incisions are then closed in the standard fashion.

Conclusions

Ivor Lewis esophagectomy remains a highly demanding procedure. The use of robotic platform can significantly enhance precision, efficiency, and surgeon ergonomics. These clear benefits for the surgeon might potentially improve surgical and oncological outcomes.

Conflict of Interest Manuela Monrabal Lezama, Francisco Schlottmann and Daniela Molena declare that they have no conflicts of interest.

References

1. Young A, Alvarez Gallesio JM, Sewell DB, Carr R, Molena D. Outcomes of robotic esophagectomy. J Thorac Dis. 2021;13:6163–8.
2. Cerfolio RJ, Bryant AS, Hawn MT. Technical aspects and early results of robotic esophagectomy with chest anastomosis. J Thorac Cardiovasc Surg. 2013;145:90–6.
3. Yang Y, et al. Robot-assisted versus conventional minimally invasive esophagectomy for resectable esophageal squamous cell carcinoma: early results of a multicenter randomized controlled trial: the RAMIE trial. Ann Surg. 2022;275:646–53.
4. van der Sluis PC, et al. Robot-assisted minimally invasive esophagectomy with intrathoracic anastomosis (Ivor Lewis): promising results in 100 consecutive patients (the European experience). J Gastrointest Surg. 2021;25:1–8.
5. Kingma BF, et al. Worldwide techniques and outcomes in robot-assisted minimally invasive esophagectomy (RAMIE): results from the multicenter international registry. Ann Surg. 2022;276:e386–92.
6. Babic B, et al. Robot-assisted minimally invasive esophagectomy (RAMIE) versus hybrid minimally invasive esophagectomy: propensity score matched short-term outcome analysis of a European high-volume center. Surg Endosc. 2022;36:7747–55.
7. Angeramo CA, Bras Harriott C, Casas MA, Schlottmann F. Minimally invasive Ivor Lewis esophagectomy: robot-assisted versus laparoscopic-thoracoscopic technique. Systematic review and meta-analysis. Surgery. 2021;170(6):1692–701.

Laparoscopic McKeown Esophagectomy

Sergio Bustos and Roberto Bustos

Abstract This chapter describes esophagectomy in prone position for dissection of the thoracic esophagus, associated with laparoscopy access and cervicotomy for the abdominal and cervical portions of the esophagus, respectively. This approach offers an improved visualization of all structures of the mid and posterior mediastinum, with the caveat of requiring further understanding of this area from a posterior approach.

Keywords Esophagectomy in prone position · Esophageal cancer · Laparoscopy · Thoracoscopy · Neck approach for gastric conduit anastomosis

Introduction

This technique consists in dissection of the thoracic esophagus via thoracosopic approach in prone position. Patient is then positioned supine for the laparoscopic portion to fashion the gastric conduit which will be later brought to the neck. A left cervicectomy is performed to access the esophageal remnant and the gastric conduit to create the esophago-gastric anastomosis [1–4].

S. Bustos (✉)
Department of Surgery, Servicio de Cirugia Clinica Francesa, Mendoza, Argentina

R. Bustos
Saint Louis University Hospital, St Louis, MO, USA

F. Schlottmann, M. A. Masrur (eds.), *Endoscopic, Laparoscopic and Robotic Techniques for Foregut Disorders*, https://doi.org/10.1007/978-3-032-00811-4_31

Procedure Description

Patient Positioning

Initially, patient is supine and general anesthesia is induced with selective intubation of left bronchus. Sequential compression devices are also used. Patient is then placed prone with a shoulder roll underneath the upper chest with arms extended forward (avoiding hyperextension to prevent brachial plexus injury). Padding is placed also underneath the ankles.

Thoracoscopic Port Placement

The first 10–12 mm trocar for the scope is placed between the spine and internal border of the scapula at the 5th intercostal space If at entry the lung is not sufficiently collapsed, CO_2 can be insufflated at 8 mm Hg. It is preferable to keep the lung collapsed instead of atelectatic to avoid compromising gas exchange. A second 10–12 mm trocar will be placed for the surgeon's right hand (to the right and higher than the first one) and a third 5 mm trocar for the surgeon's left hand (to the left and higher than the first one). This configuration allows identifying clearly the lung and right hilum with intact mediastinal pleura.

Thoracoscopic Dissection of Thoracic Esophagus

The mediastinum is accessed by opening the right mediastinal pleura with hook electrocautery over the arch formed by the Azygos vein. The vein is then dissected bluntly from the esophagus. The vein is dissected and sectioned between hem-o-loks or with vascular stapler. The mediastinal pleura opening continues towards the diaphragm exposing the esophagus and periesophageal fat that contains lymphatic nodes. Dissection continues down to the hiatus. The esophagus is encircled with a Penrose drain to facilitate mobilization (Fig. 1).

The bronchial, suprabronchial and retrotracheal portions of the esophagus are then dissected with their corresponding lymph nodes. It is critical to carefully dissect the esophagus from the posterior aspect of right bronchus, as the bronchial membrane is occupied by the bronchial balloon. If the balloon is overinflated during this dissection, the bronchial membrane which lacks protecting cartilage can be injured. Therefore, before this step, the anesthesiologist should decrease the pressure of the balloon.

Dissection of the esophagus and surrounding nodes continues up to the sternal notch. Hemostasis is checked and pleural drain is placed at the 9th intercostal space

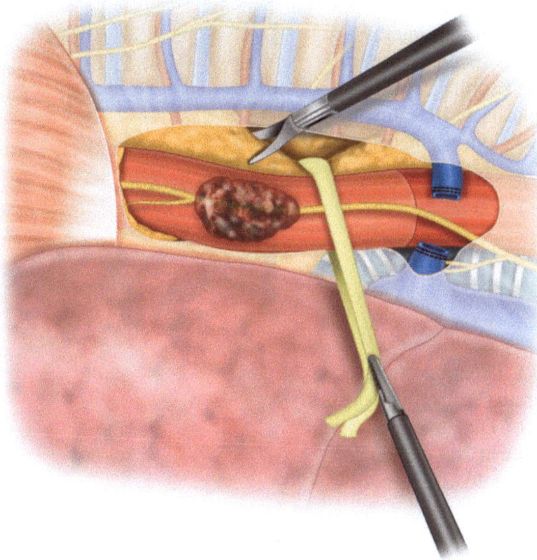

Fig. 1 Mediastinal dissection of the esophagus in prone position

at the posterior axillary line. The thoracostomy tube should be immediately connected to water seal to maintain the lung expanded throughout the rest of the surgery.

Laparoscopic Port Placement

Patient is now placed supine in low lithotomy position with the lower extremities extended on stirrups and with the knees flexed around 20°–30°. The surgeon is positioned between the legs and the first assistant to the left of the patient. Pneumoperitoneum is obtained with a Veress needle at the location of the first 10–12 mm trocar (left transrectal around one fist below the costal margin). After the 30-degree scope is introduced, the second and third trocars are placed in the left flank and right pararectal at the same height as the first trocar. An additional 5 mm trocar can be placed subxiphoid for liver retraction. Trocar for linear stapler is placed in the right flank just before it is needed.

Laparoscopic Gastric Mobilization

The gastrocolic ligament is opened sparing the vascular arcade in the greater curvature (i.e., right gastroepiploic artery) (Fig. 2). Dissection continues cranially towards the spleen taking down the short gastric vessels until the base of the left crus is

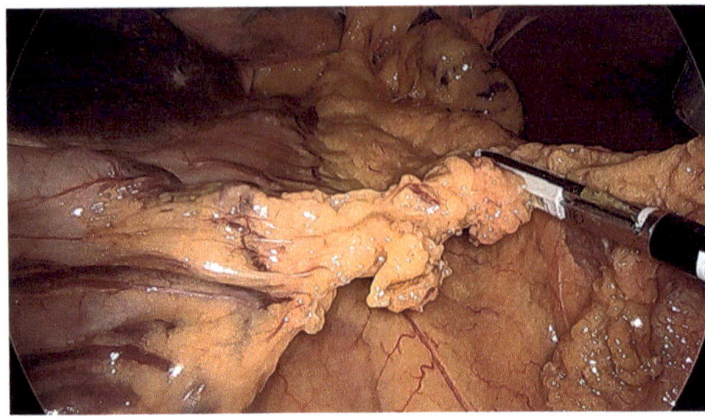

Fig. 2 Dissection of greater curvature of the stomach preserving the right gastroepiploic artery. (From Esophageal Cancer, Diagnosis and Treatment 2nd edition, Springer 2023)

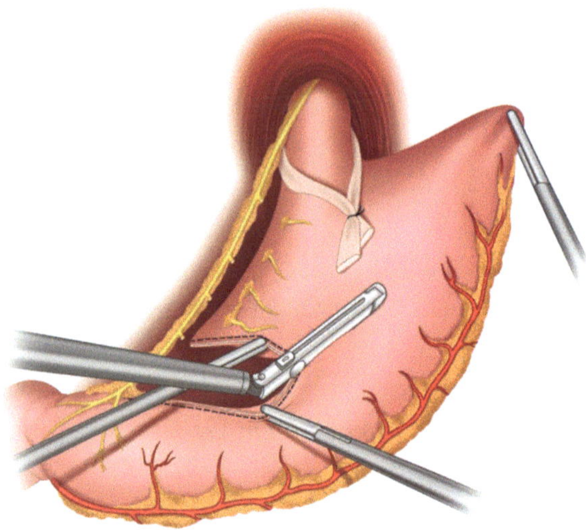

Fig. 3 Creation of gastric conduit. (From Esophageal Cancer, Diagnosis and Treatment 2nd edition, Springer 2023)

reached. Then dissection is continued towards the antrum and duodenum preserving the gastroepiploic arcade. The posterior peritoneum is incised above the first and second portion of the duodenum. The duodenal dissection should allow mobilizing the pylorus towards the midline.

The pars flaccida of the lesser omentum is accessed and dissected laterally, preserving the pyloric artery. The stomach is flipped cranially and above the pancreas until the root of the left gastric artery can be identified. The left gastric artery and coronary vein are sectioned at their base with a vascular stapler.

The phrenoesophageal ligament is taken down with cautery and the distal esophagus is mobilized reaching the dissection performed during the thoracic phase of the operation. A trocar is now placed at the right flank and a linear stapler is introduced. The gastroplasty is carried out above the incisura angularis up to the gastric fundus

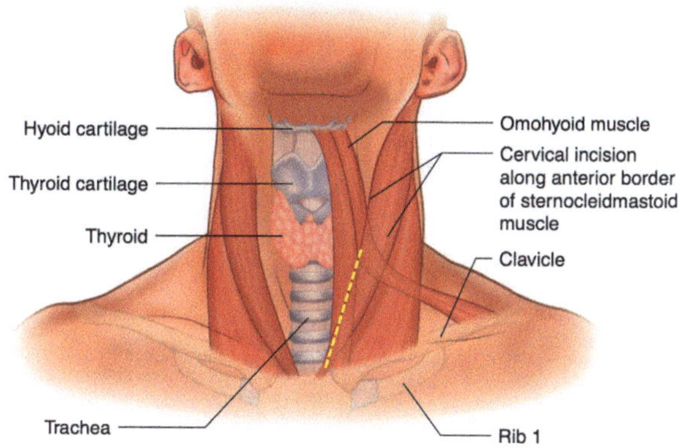

Fig. 4 Cervical incision (yellow dotted line). (From Esophageal Cancer, Diagnosis and Treatment 2nd edition, Springer 2023)

about 4 cm from the cardias (Fig. 3). At this level about 3 cm are left without resecting, allowing traction to bring the stomach transhiatally afterwards.

Cervical Incision and Esophagogastric Anastomosis

A left cervical incision is done following the anterior border of the sternocleidomastoid muscle (Fig. 4). Upon section of the platysma and superficial cervical fascia, the omohyoid muscle is transected to improve exposure. Dissection continues medially until the carotid artery is identified. Middle thyroid vessels are transected between ligatures or clips. Recurrent laryngeal nerve is identified between the trachea and the esophagus in a dihedral angle. The nasogastric tube helps to identify and dissect esophagus while palpated. The esophageal dissection continues behind the trachea and the recurrent nerve. Once the esophagus is freed, it is encircled with a rubber band and retracted. The cervical esophagus is dissected with blunt maneuvers towards the thorax. The simultaneous traction and finger dissection allows reaching the dissection done during thoracoscopy (Figs. 5 and 6).

While in the abdomen the surgeon pushes the stomach through the hiatus avoiding any twisting, the surgeon at the neck pulls the esophagus, dragging the partially transected stomach until the stomach is visualized through the cervicotomy. Once the esophagus and the stomach are exteriorized at the neck, the stomach is transected completely with a linear stapler load.

The gastric fundus is completely transected and closed (started in the laparoscopic portion) and the anterior aspect is approximated to the posterior aspect of the cervical esophagus. The gastric conduit is opened with electrocautery and the esophago-gastric anastomosis is performed with a running suture. Once the

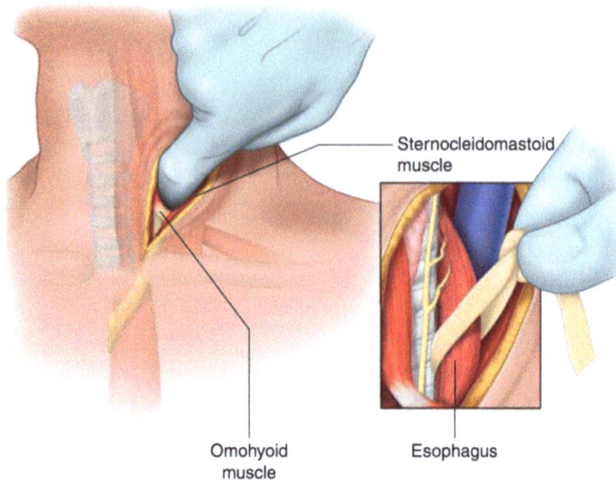

Fig. 5 The tracheoesophageal groove and recurrent nerve are constantly protected with the surgeon's finger, and a Penrose drain is used to encircle the esophagus. (From Esophageal Cancer, Diagnosis and Treatment 2nd edition, Springer 2023)

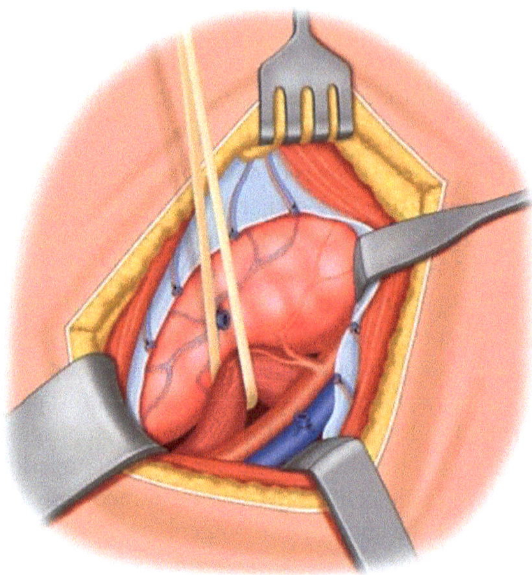

Fig. 6 The middle thyroid vein and inferior thyroid artery divided. (From Esophageal Cancer, Diagnosis and Treatment 2nd edition, Springer 2023)

posterior row of the anastomosis is completed, a nasogastric tube is passed through the anastomosis. Then, the anterior aspect of the anastomosis is closed with a running suture. Before closing the cervical incision in layers, a Jackson-Pratt drain (exteriorized lateral to the upper portion of the incision) is placed next to the anastomosis and in the upper mediastinum.

Conflict of Interest Sergio Bustos Navarrete y Roberto Bustos declare that they have no conflicts of interest.

References

1. El-Serag HB, Graham DY, Satia JA, et al. Obesity is an independent risk factor for GERD symptoms and erosive esophagitis. Am J Gastroenterol. 2005;100(6):1243–50.
2. Jakobsen GS, Smastuen MC, Sandbu R, et al. Association of bariatric surgery vs medical obesity treatment with long-term medical complications and obesity-related comorbidities. JAMA. 2018;319:291–301.
3. Schlottmann F, Herbella FAM, Patti MG. Bariatric surgery and gastroesophageal reflux. J Laparoendosc Adv Surg Tech A. 2018;28(8):953–5.
4. Madalosso CA, Gurski RR, Callegari-Jacquess SM, Navarini D, Mazzini G, Pereira MS. The impact of gastric bypass on gastroesophageal reflux disease in morbidly obese patients. Ann Surg. 2016;263:110–6.

Robotic McKeown Esophagectomy

Lorna A. Evans and Enrique Fernando Elli

Abstract McKeown esophagectomy is a key surgical approach for the treatment of esophageal cancer, involving a three-field dissection with cervical, thoracic, and abdominal phases. This procedure allows for complete tumor resection and is widely applicable for cancers located throughout the esophagus. This chapter explores the technical aspects, indications, and detailed operative procedure for the robotic-assisted McKeown esophagectomy.

Keywords McKeown esophagectomy · Esophageal cancer · Robotic surgery · Surgical oncology

Introduction

Esophageal cancer is a malignant disease that originates in the esophagus, often diagnosed at an advanced stage due to the insidious nature of its early symptoms [1]. This contributes to the disease's high mortality rate. In 2020, esophageal cancer accounted for over 544,000 deaths globally, making it the sixth leading cause of cancer-related mortality and the seventh most prevalent cancer worldwide [2]. The 5-year survival rate for patients with esophageal cancer, regardless of stage, remains approximately 20%, highlighting the aggressive nature of the disease and the challenges associated with its treatment [2].

The McKeown esophagectomy is a critical surgical approach in the treatment of esophageal malignancies, particularly for cancers located in the upper, middle, and lower regions of the esophagus at or above the carina [3]. First introduced in 1976 by Dr. McKeown in Darlington, UK, this procedure involves a three-incision

L. A. Evans · E. F. Elli (✉)
Department of Surgery, Division of Advanced Gastrointestinal and Bariatric Surgery, Mayo Clinic Florida, Jacksonville, FL, USA
e-mail: Elli.enrique@mayo.edu

F. Schlottmann, M. A. Masrur (eds.), *Endoscopic, Laparoscopic and Robotic Techniques for Foregut Disorders*, https://doi.org/10.1007/978-3-032-00811-4_32

technique with an anastomosis performed in the cervical region [4]. It combines thoracic and abdominal dissections with cervical neck anastomosis (three-field), allowing for complete tumor resection while preserving key anatomical structures.

In recent years, there has been a notable shift toward minimally invasive techniques for the surgical management of esophageal cancer [5]. Compared to the traditional open approach, minimally invasive techniques are designed to reduce the complications and risks commonly associated with more invasive surgeries, ultimately enhancing patient outcomes [6]. Robotic-assisted McKeown esophagectomy has emerged as a significant advancement, integrating the enhanced visualization, precision, and control provided by robotic technology with the traditional three-incision technique [7].

Despite its established efficacy, the McKeown esophagectomy, including its robotic-assisted version, remains a high-risk procedure with potential complications [8]. The success of the operation depends not only on the surgeon's technical skill but also on the collaboration of a multidisciplinary team, including oncologists, nutritionists, and respiratory therapists, to ensure optimal perioperative management and smooth postoperative recovery.

Indications

The McKeown esophagectomy is indicated for patients who have malignant tumors at or above the carina, and are located in the upper, middle, or lower sections of the esophagus. This procedure is particularly helpful for early-stage T1a tumors in the mid-esophagus that cannot be treated endoscopically. It is also suitable for T1b to T2 tumors without lymph node involvement.

The main contraindication to perform this procedure is distant metastasis.

Procedure Description

Thoracic Phase

Following the induction of general endotracheal anesthesia and placement of a double-lumen endotracheal tube, the patient is positioned in the left lateral decubitus position with the right side of the chest raised. The entire right chest is prepped and draped in a sterile fashion. Four 8-mm robotic thoracoscopic ports are placed in the 7th intercostal space, with an additional 12-mm assistant port placed more inferiorly. The chest is then visualized using a thoracoscope, and the robotic platform is docked.

The operation begins with division of the inferior pulmonary ligament, followed by anterior retraction of the lung to expose the operative field. The pleura is carefully opened and the esophagus, along with the surrounding periesophageal fat, is meticulously dissected from the aorta. This dissection continues toward the azygos vein using a bipolar vessel-sealer. The esophagus and its associated tissues are then carefully separated from both the right and left mainstem bronchi, with great attention paid to preserving the airway. To aid in the dissection, a gauze sling is placed around the esophagus, providing traction to facilitate circumferential dissection, which helps free both the esophagus and the paraesophageal tissues.

Next, the paraesophageal tissues are delicately separated from the pericardium and aorta. The left pleura is opened, allowing the esophagus to be fully separated from the left lung. At this stage, lymphadenectomy is performed, and the excised tissue is sent for histopathological analysis.

The azygos vein is divided using the vessel sealer, and the esophagus is further dissected toward the thoracic inlet. After ensuring hemostasis, a Penrose drain is placed around the esophagus and positioned into the thoracic inlet. Another drain is placed distally, around the esophagus at the level of the hiatus, to facilitate retrieval from the abdominal cavity later.

A 20 French chest tube is then introduced through a separate stab incision anteriorly, directed into the posterior mediastinum. The chest tube is secured in place, and the lung is reinflated under thoracoscopic guidance. Once all ports are withdrawn, the incisions are closed with absorbable sutures.

Then the abdominal phase of the operation can proceed.

Abdominal Phase

Patient Positioning and Trocar Placement

The patient is positioned supine, an intraoperative upper GI endoscopy is performed, during which pyloric dilation is carried out using an achalasia balloon for 5 min. The patient is then prepped and draped in a sterile manner. Trocar placement begins with the insertion of an 8 mm trocar at the umbilicus using the OptiView technique. After establishing a pneumoperitoneum at 15 mmHg, initial exploration of the abdominal cavity is performed, and the remaining ports are placed under direct visualization to ensure proper alignment and placement.

An additional 8 mm trocar is positioned just above the umbilicus on the left side, followed by another 8 mm trocar placed in the left upper quadrant. A 12 mm trocar is then inserted in the right lower quadrant, and a Nathanson liver retractor is carefully positioned at the epigastrium to lift and retract the left lobe of the liver. Once these steps are completed, the robotic platform is docked, preparing for the next phase of the procedure.

The dissection begins with both blunt and sharp techniques to mobilize the duodenum, including the second and third portions, ensuring that a complete Kocher maneuver is carried out for optimal exposure. Next, the gastrocolic ligament is divided with the vessel sealer to facilitate access to the lesser sac. The greater curvature is mobilized while preserving the gastroepiploic artery at its origin (Fig. 1). The integrity of the artery is confirmed using indocyanine green (ICG) angiography. The dissection continues with the division of the short gastric vessels, extending up to the gastroesophageal junction.

The posterior attachments are carefully divided, allowing the left crus to be identified and fully dissected, which exposes the left side of the esophagus. The gastrohepatic ligament is then dissected (Fig. 2). The pars flaccida is then opened, and the fat pad between the liver and the right crus is removed. The dissection continues, with both the pars flaccida and pars condensa being excised up to the hepatic artery.

The right crus is identified and dissected away from the esophagus. As the dissection progresses a retroesophageal window is created (Fig. 3). A Penrose drain is passed around the distal esophagus to maintain traction (Fig. 4). The distal esophagus is dissected circumferentially and then mobilized (Fig. 5).

Fig. 1 Dissection of the greater curvature of the stomach preserving the gastroepiploic artery

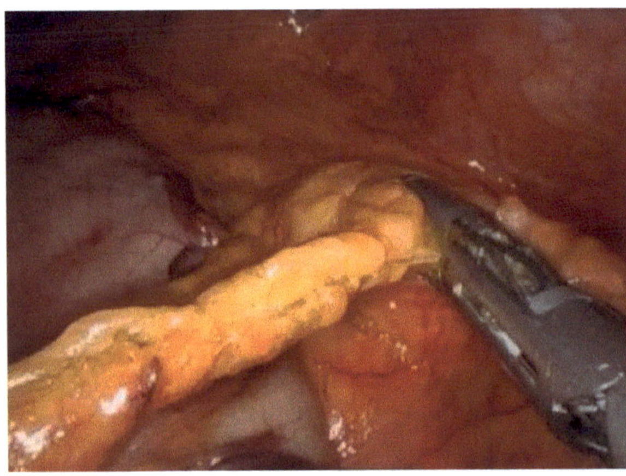

Fig. 2 Gastrohepatic ligament dissection

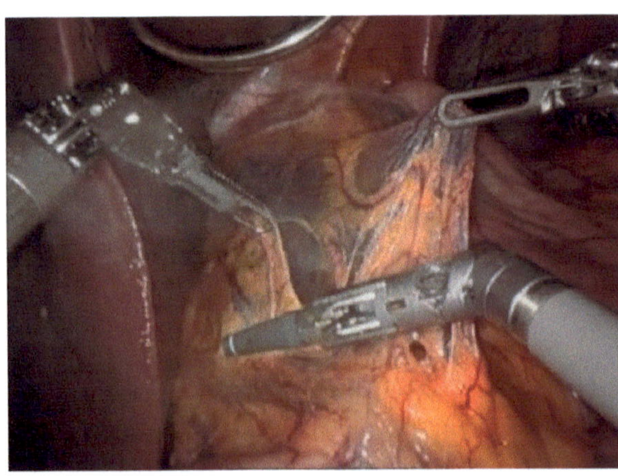

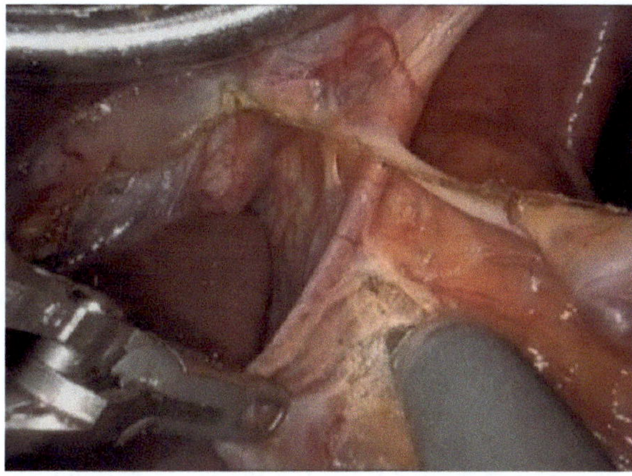

Fig. 3 Right crus dissection off the esophagus

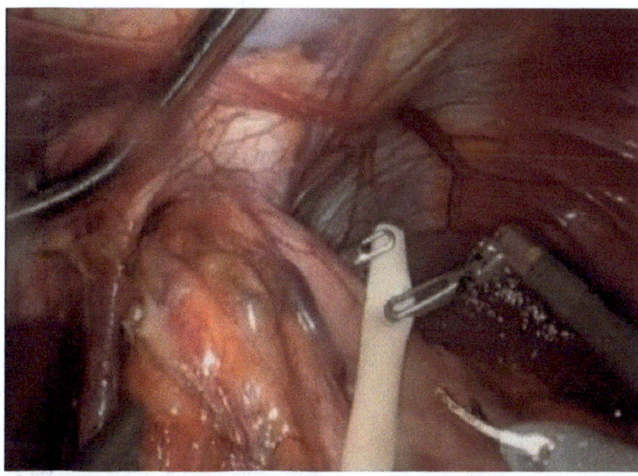

Fig. 4 Penrose drain around the distal esophagus

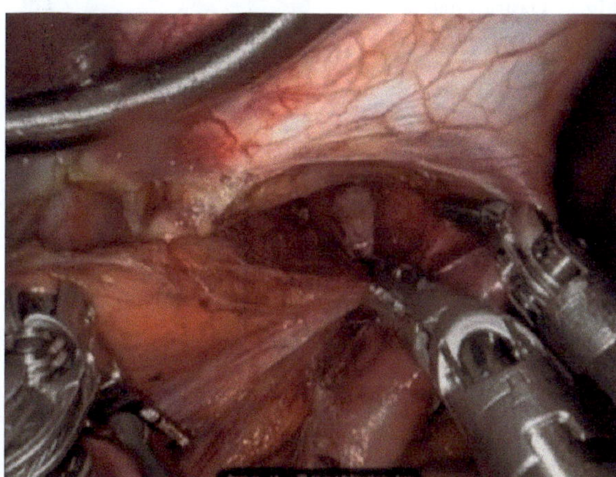

Fig. 5 Circumferential dissection of the esophagus

The left gastric artery is skeletonized and divided using a robotic stapler white load (Fig. 6).

At the incisura, the junction between the right and left gastric arteries is identified. Approximately 5 cm from the pylorus, the gastric conduit is constructed using robotic staplers. The process begins with the firing of a green staple load, followed by four blue robotic staplers to complete the construction of the conduit. To facilitate the mobilization of the specimen into the chest, the final 4 cm of the stomach are left attached (Figs. 7 and 8). The gastric conduit is carefully assessed to ensure it measures approximately 5 cm in width. This measurement is crucial for ensuring the conduit will be of adequate size to allow for proper anastomosis and function (Fig. 9). The stapler line of the conduit is oversewn with 3-0 silk sutures placed every 2 cm along the suture line (Fig. 10).

A laparoscopic jejunostomy is performed 40 cm from the angle of Treitz. Three silk sutures are used to anchor the jejunum to the abdominal wall, and using the

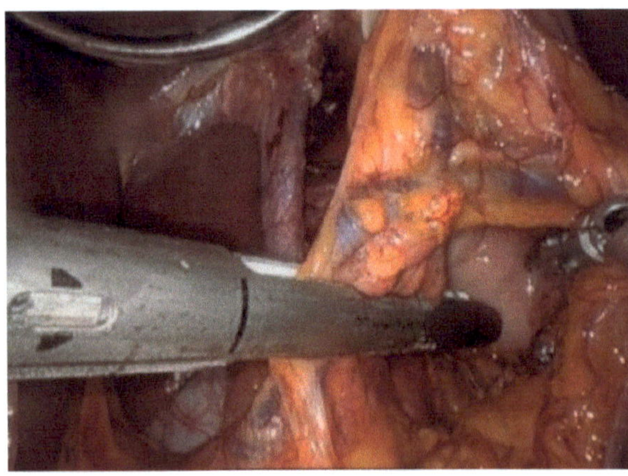

Fig. 6 Division of left gastric artery with stapler

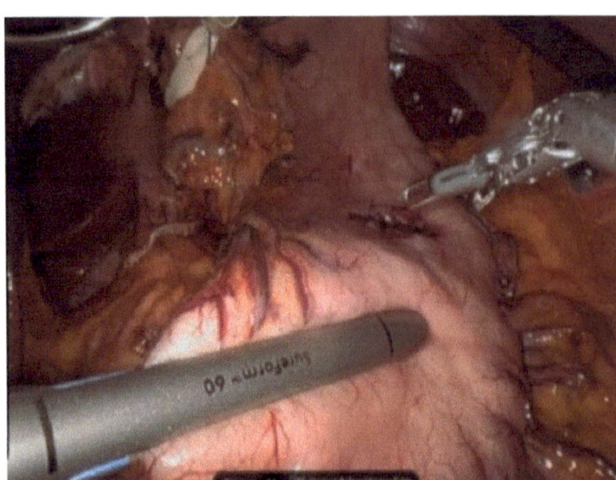

Fig. 7 Gastric conduit construction

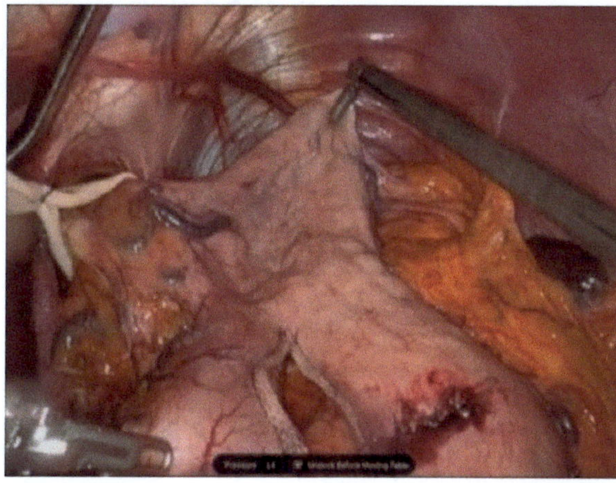

Fig. 8 Gastric conduit construction

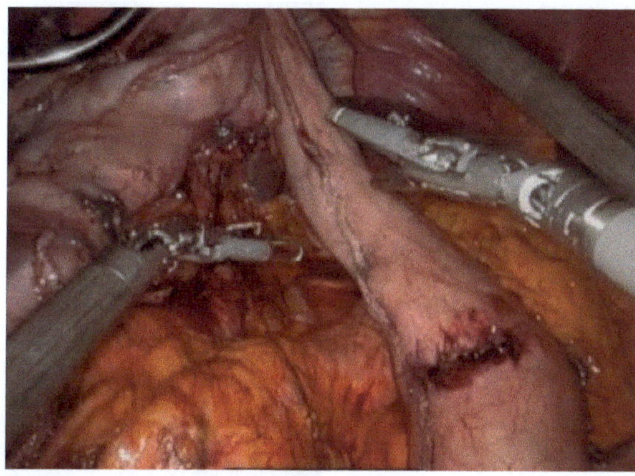

Fig. 9 Gastric conduit

Seldinger technique, a 16-French jejunostomy tube is placed. The silk sutures are tied to securely anchor the jejunostomy site, and the tube is then fixed to the skin with nylon sutures to ensure stability. To confirm that the tube is patent and functioning properly, it is flushed with saline, ensuring there are no obstructions (Fig. 11).

Hemostasis should be carefully confirmed, and the gastric conduit should be tested by advancing it toward the hiatus to ensure it passes smoothly without any resistance or complications. This step helps confirm the conduit's proper positioning and readiness for the next phase of the procedure. Prolene 3-0 sutures are placed at the midpoint of the conduit to mark the extent to which it can be safely advanced into the chest.

In order to prevent gastric outlet obstruction, 10 mL of botulinum toxin is injected into the pylorus (Fig. 12).

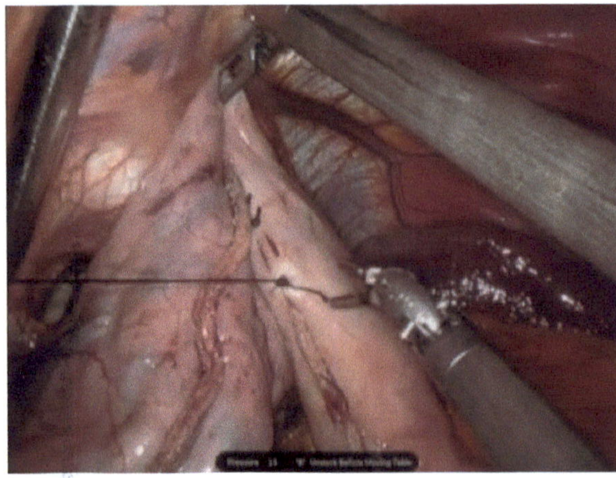

Fig. 10 Reinforcement of mechanical suture line

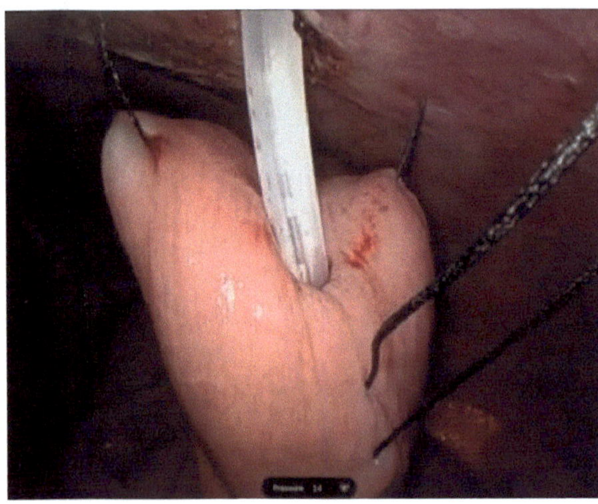

Fig. 11 Feeding jejunostomy tube

The pneumoperitoneum is evacuated, and the trocars are removed under direct visualization. The trocar sites are then closed using figure-of-eight 0 monofilament absorbable sutures.

Cervical Phase

After the gastric conduit has been created, the cervical portion of the procedure begins. The patient's neck and chest are prepped and draped in a sterile fashion.

An incision is made anterior to the left sternocleidomastoid muscle and carried through the platysma using cautery. The omohyoid muscle is divided with cautery,

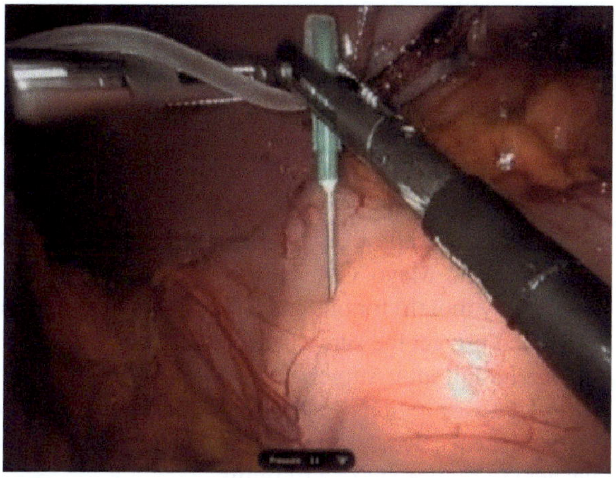

Fig. 12 Botulinum toxin injection

and the left sternocleidomastoid muscle is retracted laterally. Dissection is then extended into the tracheoesophageal groove, retracting the carotid sheath and its contents laterally. Blunt dissection is performed along the prevertebral fascia to mobilize the cervical esophagus.

The Penrose drain, placed around the esophagus at the thoracic inlet, is retrieved and used to maintain traction as dissection continues. A nasogastric tube is advanced into the esophagus by the anesthesia assistant. The thoracic esophagus and gastric conduit are then brought up to the neck incision. The sutures holding the proximal fundus to the conduit are divided, separating the two structures. The esophagus is transected approximately 2 cm below the cricoid cartilage using sharp scissors, ensuring a clean division of the tissue. Prior to this step, the nasogastric tube is pulled proximally to facilitate a clear and precise cut. Once the transection is complete, the resected specimen is sent to pathology for evaluation and to assess tumor margins.

The esophagus and conduit are then aligned, and stay sutures are placed. A transverse gastrotomy is performed along the posterior wall of the conduit. To create a posterior anastomosis between the esophagus and the stomach a medium-thickness stapler is used. The anterior wall is then aligned, and a medium-thickness 60 mm stapler is used to staple it closed. This stapling also resects the gastric tip simultaneously. Interrupted 2-0 silk sutures are placed in a Lembert fashion to imbricate the anterior staple line. Stay sutures are placed on either side of the anastomosis to secure the esophagus and conduit together.

The anastomosis is then gently reduced into the posterior mediastinum, and traction is applied to the conduit from the abdominal side to eliminate any redundancy. A 15-French round Jackson-Pratt drain is placed in the mediastinum and brought out through a separate stab incision in the left neck. The neck is then closed in layers, with absorbable interrupted sutures used for the muscle layer and skin closure achieved with staplers.

Post-operative Care

The patient is closely monitored in the Intensive Care Unit for 24–48 h. A nasogastric tube is placed for decompression and kept on suction until an upper gastrointestinal swallow study is performed. Feeding through a jejunostomy tube begins on postoperative day 1.

A contrast swallow study is typically performed on day 5 to assess for leaks. Following the Mayo Clinic esophagectomy protocol, the patient remains NPO (nothing by mouth) for one month. Proton pump inhibitors are prescribed to manage reflux and protect the surgical anastomosis.

One month after surgery, a follow-up swallow study is performed, and diet is started if no aspiration is detected. At this stage, the patient is instructed to eat small, frequent meals, avoid eating immediately before bedtime, and sleep with the head elevated to reduce the risk of reflux.

The patient is discharged once they are tolerating enteral feeds, and their pain is well-controlled. Ongoing follow-up appointments for wound care, nutritional support, and oncologic monitoring are critical to ensuring a smooth recovery and long-term success.

Conclusions

Robotic-assisted McKeown esophagectomy offers a minimally invasive approach to managing esophageal cancer, combining thoracic, abdominal, and cervical phases to achieve complete tumor resection while preserving vital structures. This complex procedure requires meticulous planning, surgical expertise, and a multidisciplinary team for optimal patient outcomes. Postoperative care plays a critical role in recovery, with early mobilization, nutrition support, and monitoring for potential complications. When performed with precision and followed by careful postoperative management, the McKeown esophagectomy can significantly improve survival rates and quality of life for patients with esophageal cancer.

Conflict of Interest Lorna A. Evans and E. Fernando Elli declare that they have no conflicts of interest.

References

1. Wang Y, Mukkamalla SKR, Singh R, Babiker HM, Lyons S. Esophageal cancer. In: StatPearls. StatPearls Publishing; 2024. http://www.ncbi.nlm.nih.gov/books/NBK459267/. Accessed 5 Nov 2024.
2. Rodriguez GM, DePuy D, Aljehani M, et al. Trends in epidemiology of esophageal cancer in the US, 1975–2018. JAMA Netw Open. 2023;6(8):e2329497. https://doi.org/10.1001/jamanetworkopen.2023.29497.

3. McKeown KK. Esophagectomy. In: Lomanto D, WTL C, Fuentes MB, editors. Mastering endo-laparoscopic and thoracoscopic surgery. Springer Nature Singapore; 2023. p. 243–50. https://doi.org/10.1007/978-981-19-3755-2_37.
4. McKeown KC. Total three-stage oesophagectomy for cancer of the oesophagus. J Br Surg. 1976;63(4):259–62. https://doi.org/10.1002/bjs.1800630403.
5. Patel S, Petrov R, Abbas A, Bakhos C. Robotic-assisted McKeown esophagectomy. J Vis Surg. 2019;5:43. https://doi.org/10.21037/jovs.2019.03.14.
6. Bencini L, Moraldi L, Bartolini I, Coratti A. Esophageal surgery in minimally invasive era. World J Gastrointest Surg. 2016;8(1):52–64. https://doi.org/10.4240/wjgs.v8.i1.52.
7. Scheese D, Ramamoorthy BU, Bane B, Puig CA, Julliard WA, Shah RD. Robotic-assisted minimally invasive esophagectomy—technical considerations and outcomes. Ann Esophagus. 2024;7:20. https://doi.org/10.21037/aoe-24-18.
8. Zheng XD, Li SC, Lu C, et al. Safety and efficacy of minimally invasive McKeown esophagectomy in 1023 consecutive esophageal cancer patients: a single-center experience. J Cardiothorac Surg. 2022;17(1):36. https://doi.org/10.1186/s13019-022-01781-2.

Gastric Cancer

Endoscopic Mucosal Resection in Early Gastroesophageal Cancer

Ashley A. Vareedayah

Abstract Endoscopic resection is a safe and effective treatment approach, and an excellent alternative to surgical resection, in the treatment of early (T1N0M0) esophageal and gastric cancer. In this chapter, we provide a brief introduction to the basic principles of endoscopic resection of upper gastrointestinal cancers.

Keywords Endoscopic resection · Esophageal cancer · Gastric cancer · Endoscopic mucosal resection · Endoscopic submucosal dissection

Introduction

The greatest and most obvious advantages of endoscopic management in early gastrointestinal (GI) cancer involve organ preservation, as well as its minimally invasive nature. Advanced techniques for endoscopic resection of GI lesions generally fall into two categories, endoscopic mucosal resection (EMR) and endoscopic submucosal dissection (ESD). Endoscopic ablative therapies (radiofrequency ablation, argon plasma coagulation, photodynamic therapy, etc) are not discussed in this chapter.

To adequately understand the nuances of the different approaches of endoscopic resection, it is important to have a grasp of the wall layers in the esophagus and stomach. When viewed with an echoendoscope, as in for a staging endoscopic ultrasound, these layers (from superficial to deep) are:

1. superficial mucosa
2. muscularis mucosa
3. submucosa

A. A. Vareedayah (✉)
Department of Medicine, Division of Gastroenterology & Hepatology, University of Illinois Hospital and Health Sciences, Chicago, IL, USA
e-mail: vareedaa@uic.edu

F. Schlottmann, M. A. Masrur (eds.), *Endoscopic, Laparoscopic and Robotic Techniques for Foregut Disorders*, https://doi.org/10.1007/978-3-032-00811-4_33

4. muscularis propria
5. adventitia or serosa

Generally accepted indications for endoscopic resection include lesions that are limited to the superficial mucosa, since these lesions are associated with extremely rare risk of lymph node metastasis. Lesions extending to muscularis mucosa and superficial submucosa (<200 μm) are also suitable for endoscopic resection, with the understanding that the risk of lymph node metastasis is slightly higher in this circumstance.

Prior to resection, careful endoscopic, and sometimes endosonographic, evaluation is essential. Endosonographic evaluation provides valuable information with respect to lesion depth, and aids in appropriate patient selection for successful R0 resection. This meticulous endoscopic evaluation includes using both high-definition white light as well as narrow-band imaging, as well as examination of the morphology, surface, and the overlying vascular pattern of the lesion for features that may suggest deeper submucosal invasion. Features suggestive of submucosal invasion, such as decrease/loss of vascular pattern, ulceration, and central depression signify poor candidacy for endoscopic resection. Another feature of deep submucosal invasion is non-lifting sign—when fluid is injected into the submucosa (technique described further below) with failure of adequate lift. A thoughtful approach in any of these above scenarios with the best interests of the patient in mind should prompt multidisciplinary discussion and referral for surgical evaluation.

In patients that are candidates for endoscopic resection, in some cases, the choice between EMR and ESD for resection is dependent on availability of endoscopic expertise. It is advisable to always employ ESD if lesion size is >20 mm, or if histology or endoscopic appearance of the lesion is suggestive of malignancy or submucosal invasion, to maximize the chance of negative horizontal and vertical margins, and R0 resection. When opting for endoscopic resection of gastrointestinal cancers, the importance of *en bloc* resection cannot be understated. En bloc resection is vital for accurate histologic assessment of resection margins.

Piecemeal EMR, a common practice in the resection of premalignant lesions, in which large, laterally spreading polyps are resected piece by piece, is not appropriate in the endoscopic management of cancer. This is due to high rate of recurrence and inability for accurate histologic evaluation.

It is important to note that despite the obvious advantage of ESD in en bloc, R0, and curative endoscopic resection of neoplastic lesions, it has not been conclusively shown that ESD is superior to EMR in avoiding additional surgery or all-cause mortality. This highlights the need for additional randomized comparative studies between the two techniques. Our general practice is to attempt en bloc resection using EMR only for lesions <20 mm in size, and to choose ESD over EMR if there is suspicion for, or biopsy-proven, cancer. There should be a low threshold for referral of these patients to high volume tertiary centers. And resection should be performed by experts with dedicated training and expertise in advanced endoscopic resection.

Procedure Description

EMR is a safe, effective, and minimally invasive technique for the resection of superficial lesions in the GI tract. EMR can be performed using one of multiple different techniques, including injection lift, suction cap, and band ligation.

The technique used most commonly involves injection of fluid, such as normal saline, into the submucosal space, to lift the lesion away from underlying muscularis propria. This helps reduce the risk of mechanical and thermal injury to the deeper layers of the GI tract. A variety of different solutions can be used, including saline, hydroxyethyl starch, dextrose, and other pre-made commercially available, precolored, submucosal injection solutions. It must be noted that the injectate is usually stained with a blue dye; in the United States, methylene blue is most commonly used. Indigo carmine is another commonly used dye. Though not absolutely necessary, this staining helps with differentiation of the submucosa (light blue after injection) from underlying muscularis propria (which appears white), and promotes easier recognition of muscular injury and perforation. Optionally, dilute epinephrine (1:10,000) may be added, to aid in local vasoconstriction and reduce the risk of intraprocedural bleeding—this is usually based on endoscopist preference. Once a fluid "cushion" is established, snare excision is performed, with or without electrocautery, referred to as hot snare or cold snare, respectively. See Fig. 1.

Cap-assisted EMR is performed after a specially designed transparent cap attachment is affixed to the tip of the endoscope. An open snare is carefully positioned circumferentially at the distal edge, within the cap. The endoscope is positioned over the target lesion, and suction is used to draw the lesion within the cap, after which electrocautery-enhanced snare resection is performed. This method can be performed with or without submucosal fluid injection. See Fig. 2.

Finally, band-ligation EMR is performed using a band-ligation device, which is attached to the distal tip of the endoscope. This technique is similar, in principle, to band ligation, a common therapy for esophageal varices. Suction is used to draw the target lesion into the cap, after which a band is deployed at the base of the newly created pseudopolyp. This tissue is then resected using a snare. See Fig. 3.

One of the advantages of EMR is ease of use and wide availability. EMR is associated with a much shorter learning curve, and compared to ESD, the procedure duration is significantly lower.

Additionally, rates of adverse events, namely bleeding and perforation, are low. Bleeding is the most common adverse event associated with EMR. Rates of

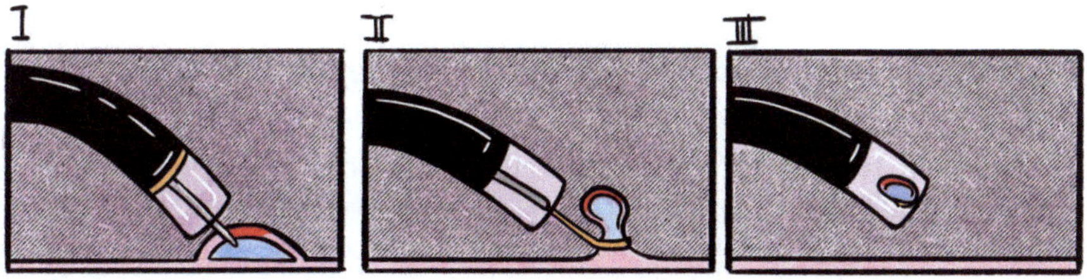

Fig. 1 Injection-lift Endoscopic Mucosal Resection. (Illustration by Bruno Cantú)

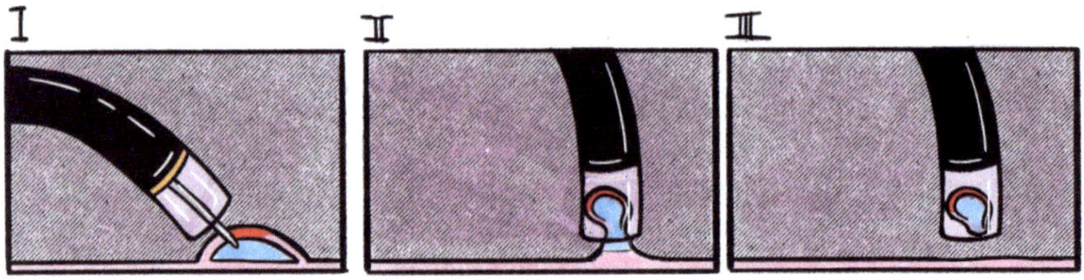

Fig. 2 Cap-assisted EMR. (Illustration by Bruno Cantú)

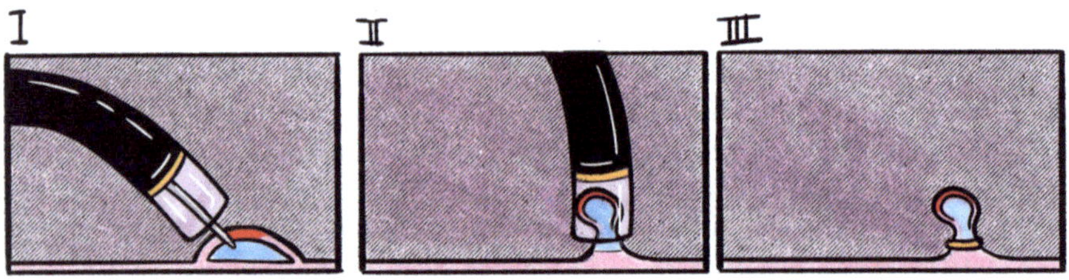

Fig. 3 Band EMR. (Illustration by Bruno Cantú)

significant bleeding after EMR in the esophagus and stomach are approximately 1% and 5%, respectively. Bleeding is generally easily managed with standard endoscopic hemostasis techniques (hemostatic clips, monopolar coagulation grasping forceps, bipolar probes, etc.). In expert hands, rates of perforation with EMR are quite low, less than 1%, in the esophagus and stomach. Immediate perforation occurs at the time of procedure, while delayed perforation is diagnosed when clinical signs / symptoms are suggestive of the diagnosis (fever, abdominal pain, and imaging findings) after completion of the procedure. Whenever possible, perforation is managed with endoscopic therapy, including clip placement and endoscopic suturing. In some cases, surgical repair is the only option.

However, the limitations to EMR are significant, with respect to management of GI cancer. EMR is associated with suboptimal histologic assessment of the specimen, due to its relatively superficial submucosal plane of transection, potential for cautery artifact at the resection margins, and higher recurrence rate, likely due to microscopic residual disease left behind after resection. Therefore, ESD is strongly recommended for resection of early cancers in the esophagus and stomach.

Endoscopic Submucosal Dissection Technique

ESD is a more specialized technique that allows for en bloc resection of superficial gastrointestinal lesions. It involves a steep learning curve associated with a specialized skill set that is not yet widely available in Western countries. ESD also involves longer procedure duration and a higher rate of adverse events, compared to EMR. In the United States, ESD is primary performed in select centers by specialized endoscopists experienced in this technique. The goal with ESD is en bloc resection, with curative intent. ESD is also preferred because noncurative resection can be easily recognized on histology, and patients can be appropriately referred for surgery.

ESD is quite distinct from EMR. First, a circumferential border around the target lesion is demarcated with thermal marking. Then, fluid is injected into the submucosal space around the lesion, as in EMR. With a special electrosurgical cutting knife, a circumferential mucosal incision is made around the lesion. Multiple different types of knives are now commercially available, each with nuanced advantages. Finally, the submucosa is carefully dissected, sometimes millimeter by millimeter, until the entire lesion is excised (Fig. 4). It is important to note that small submucosal blood vessels are inevitably encountered during dissection. These are usually prophylactically cauterized using the electrosurgical knife or endoscopic coagulation forceps, as intraprocedural bleeding can interfere with visualization of the submucosal plane and increase procedural duration and the risk of adverse events. CO_2 insufflation is recommended for all ESD procedures.

ESD is associated with numerous advantages, compared to EMR. With en bloc resection, ESD is potentially curative in early cancer. Compared to EMR, it allows for dissection deeper into the submucosal layer closer to muscularis propria, which

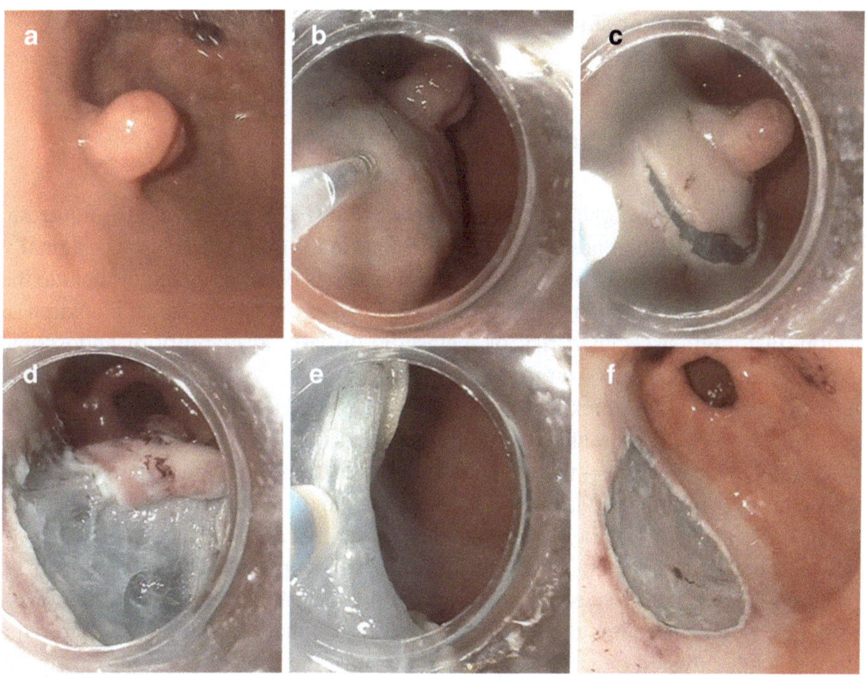

Fig. 4 Endoscopic submucosal dissection (ESD). (**a**) Gastric antrum lesion; (**b**) submucosal injection with normal saline, methylene blue, and dilute epinephrine; (**c**) circumferential mucosal incision; (**d, e**) submucosal dissection; (**f**) after successful resection

increases the likelihood of R0 resection. An important hallmark of ESD is that size is not a limiting factor. Very large lesions can be safely resected using ESD, in en bloc fashion. ESD is also associated with a significantly lower rate of recurrence. Therefore, ESD is indicated and an excellent option for the treatment of nodular Barrett's esophagus and associated high-grade dysplasia/intramucosal carcinoma, esophageal adenocarcinoma, esophageal squamous cell carcinoma, and gastric cancer.

We must note a few disadvantages to ESD. First, the risk of adverse events, such as bleeding, perforation, and stricture formation, are significantly higher, than in EMR. Bleeding rates range from 2% to 10% in esophagus and stomach. Perforation rates range from 3% to 5% in the esophagus and stomach, and these rates can be higher with ESD in the duodenum and colon.

When obtaining informed consent for esophageal ESD, it is important to explain the potential risks of stricture formation as well. Risk of stricture after esophageal ESD is more likely if the resection defect involves >50% of the circumference of the esophagus. These strictures are generally managed with endoscopic methods, including endoscopic balloon dilation, and in some cases, injection of steroid therapy. This can often require multiple endoscopic treatment sessions.

Another disadvantage is that, as of now, there is no standardized curriculum in North America for training in ESD. The learning curve is steep and generally requires dedicated training in addition to that provided during a General Gastroenterology fellowship.

Full Thickness Resection

Device-assisted endoscopic full thickness resection (FTR) is a novel technique that allows for focal full thickness resection of lesions in the GI tract. This was originally designed for resection of colon lesions, but its use has been expanded to include the stomach and duodenum. Considerations include layer of origin, size and location of lesion, histology, associated risk of metastatic disease, availability of endoscopic expertise, and the patient's surgical risk.

Device-assisted full thickness resection is performed as follows: first, the periphery of the lesion is demarcated, using thermal marking. An integrated full-thickness resection device (FTRD)—which includes a large, transparent plastic cap, an over-the-scope clip, and snare—is affixed to the distal end of an endoscope, and advanced to the lesion. Given the bulky size of the device, it can be difficult, at times, to advance the endoscope to the target lesion. Endoscopic balloon dilation can be required to facilitate successful advancement of the endoscope and full-thickness resection device through the upper and lower esophageal sphincters. After the device is maneuvered over the target lesion, a grasping forceps is used to grasp the tissue and gently pull it within the cap. Adjuvant use of suction may be helpful to coax target tissue within the device. The FTRD clip is then deployed, and the

Fig. 5 Endoscopic device assisted FTR

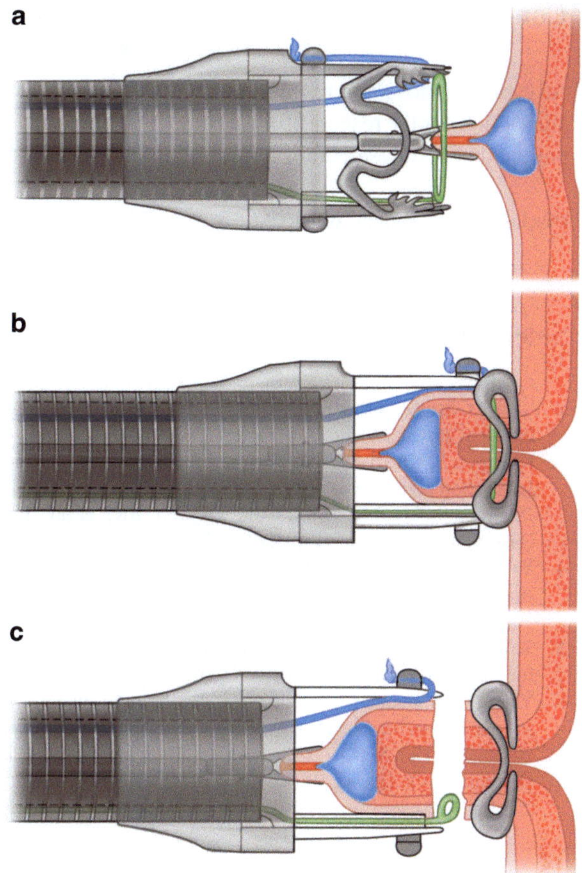

integrated snare is used to resect the invaginated tissue, with the aid of electrocautery (Fig. 5).

This approach has been shown to be safe and effective but a major limitation of endoscopic device-assisted FTR is lesion size. Since successful R0 resection is entirely dependent on the volume of tissue that can be drawn into the device cap, it is recommended that use of the FTRD be limited to lesions ≤2 cm in diameter. Device-assisted full thickness resection is performed only in the stomach, duodenum, and colorectum.

Conclusion

Advanced endoscopic resection techniques are a safe and effective minimally invasive option for the resection of early (T1N0M0) gastrointestinal cancers. Appropriate patient and lesion selection is paramount, as is endoscopic expertise.

Disclosure No conflicts of interest

Selected Readings

1. Lian J, Chen S, Zhang Y, et al. A meta-analysis of endoscopic submucosal dissection and EMR for early gastric cancer. Gastrointest Endosc. 2012;76:763–70.
2. Kitagawa Y, Uno T, Oyama T, et al. Esophageal cancer practice guidelines 2017 edited by the Japan esophageal society: part 2. Esophagus. 2019;16:25–43.
3. Committee AT, Maple JT, Abu Dayyeh BK, et al. Endoscopic submucosal dissection. Gastrointest Endosc. 2015;81:1311–25.
4. Yanai Y, Yokoi C, Watanabe K, et al. Endoscopic resection for gastrointestinal tumors (esophageal, gastric, colorectal tumors): Japanese standard and future prospects. Glob Health Med. 2021;3:365–70.
5. Thiruvengadam SS, Fung BM, Barakat MT, et al. Endoscopic mucosal resection: best practices for gastrointestinal endoscopists. Gastroenterol Hepatol (N Y). 2022;18:133–44.
6. Yang D, Othman M, Draganov PV. Endoscopic mucosal resection vs endoscopic submucosal dissection for Barrett's esophagus and colorectal neoplasia. Clin Gastroenterol Hepatol. 2019;17:1019–28.
7. Committee AT, Hwang JH, Konda V, et al. Endoscopic mucosal resection. Gastrointest Endosc. 2015;82:215–26.

Endoscopic Submucosal Dissection (ESD) in Gastric Cancer

Mark A. Solinski, Anthony J. Kang, Kevin P. Shah, and Abdul A. Aadam

Abstract Gastric Cancer is the fifth most common cancer and third leading cause of cancer death worldwide. Endoscopic submucosal dissection is an effective, non-invasive option for removal of early gastric neoplasms. In this chapter, each step of endoscopic submucosal dissection with intraprocedural images is described.

Keywords Endoscopic submucosal dissection · Gastric neoplasia · Early gastric cancer · Node negative tumor

Introduction

Gastric Cancer is the fifth most common cancer and third leading cause of cancer death worldwide. Endoscopic submucosal dissection (ESD) is an effective, non-invasive option for removal of early gastric neoplasms. In this chapter, we describe each step of endoscopic submucosal dissection with intraprocedural images. Indications for ESD are found in Table 1 [1–6].

M. A. Solinski · A. J. Kang · K. P. Shah · A. A. Aadam (✉)
Division of Gastroenterology & Hepatology, Northwestern Feinberg School of Medicine, Chicago, IL, USA
e-mail: abdul.aadam@northwestern.edu

F. Schlottmann, M. A. Masrur (eds.), *Endoscopic, Laparoscopic and Robotic Techniques for Foregut Disorders*, https://doi.org/10.1007/978-3-032-00811-4_34

Table 1 Absolute and expanded indications for ESD based on Japanese guidelines

Absolute indication for ESD	A differentiated-type adenocarcinoma without ulcerative findings [UL(−)], of which the depth of invasion is clinically diagnosed as T1a and the diameter is ≤2 cm.
Expanded indication for ESD	Tumors clinically diagnosed as T1a and: (a) Of differentiated-type, UL(−),but >2 cm in diameter. (b) Of differentiated-type, UL(+), and ≤3 cm in diameter. (c) Of undifferentiated-type, UL(−),and ≤2 cm in diameter.

UL Ulcerative findings

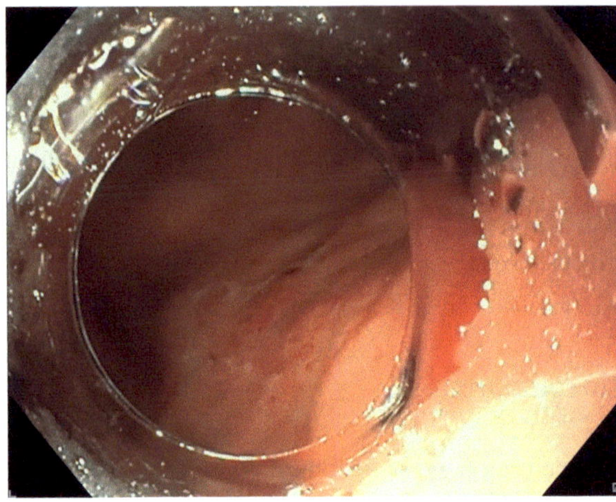

Fig. 1 Gastric tumor visualized under white light

Procedure Description

Patient Positioning and preparation

The patient is placed in left lateral position for this procedure. The patient should be placed under monitored anesthesia care or general anesthesia with endotracheal intubation and mechanical ventilation.

Procedural Technique

Identification of and Marking Around the Lesion

The endoscope is inserted through the patient's mouth, passed through the esophagus, and into the stomach. The stomach is then insufflated using carbon dioxide. The lesion is identified using high-definition white light, near focus, and digital or dye-based chromoendoscopy (Fig. 1). Chromoendoscopy with a contrast dye such

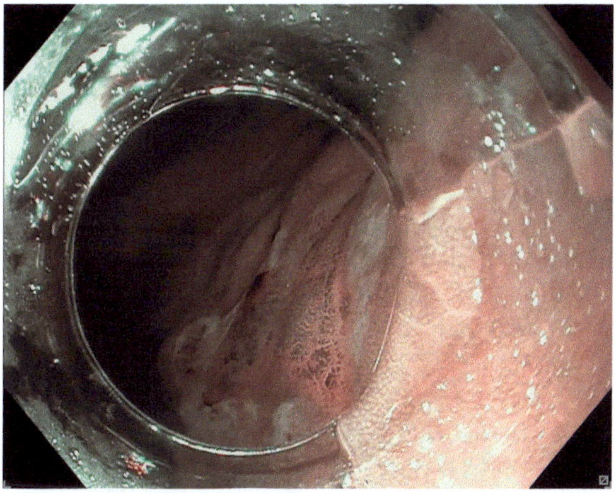

Fig. 2 Gastric tumor visualized under chromoendoscopy

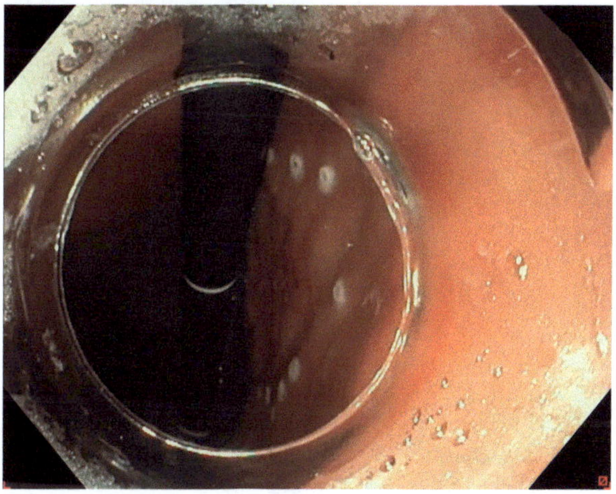

Fig. 3 Marking perimeter of the lesion using an ESD knife

as 0.25% indigo carmine or methylene blue is used to aid in determining the borders of the lesion (Fig. 2). The perimeter of the lesion plus a 5–10 mm margin of normal mucosa is then marked using an ESD knife with soft coagulation current at an interval of 2 mm per marking (Fig. 3). The margin of normal mucosa helps ensure negative margins when the lesion is removed.

Submucosal Injection

Submucosal injection is used to create a submucosal fluid buffer that lifts the lesion away from the muscularis propria to reduce the risk of perforation. A retractable injection needle or waterjet enabled knife is placed outside of the circumferential markings made in step one at the location where the first mucosal incision intends to be made (Fig. 4). The submucosal injection is directed to allow appropriate submucosal lift in a symmetric fashion around the borders of the lesion. Subsequent injections are performed throughout the duration of the procedure to ensure overall safety (Fig. 5).

Inability to lift the submucosa via this technique can be suggestive of submucosal fibrosis or invasion of the lesion into the muscularis propria. The solution used for submucosal injection varies by operator, with several proprietary solutions commercially available. Methylene blue can be added to delineate the submucosa and highlight the lesion's margins. Diluted epinephrine may lower the risk of immediate post resection bleeding.

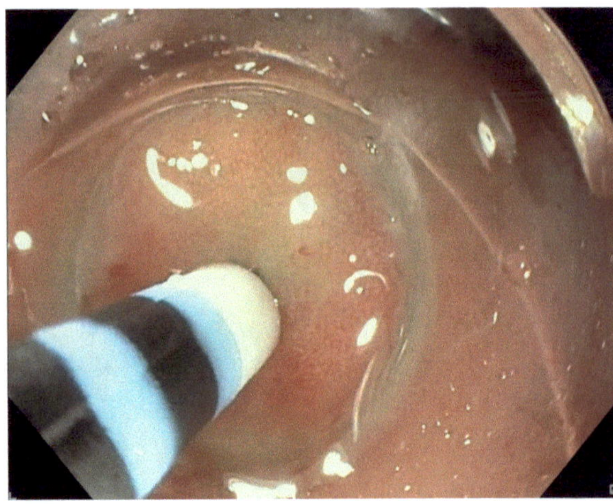

Fig. 4 Submucosal injection where the first mucosal incision intends to be made

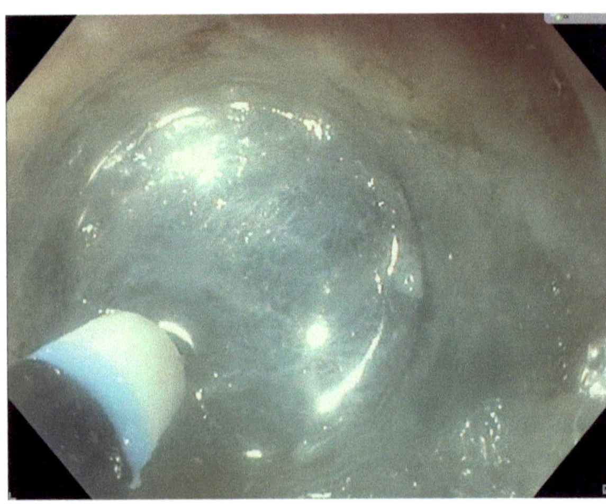

Fig. 5 Subsequent submucosal injection completed during dissection

Mucosal Incision

After the lesion is lifted with submucosal injection, the mucosa outside of the markings is circumferentially incised using an ESD knife. There are two common methods for mucosal incision: the conventional method and the pocket creation method. For the conventional method, an initial incision is made on the side that is most proximal to the mouth, or on the far side of the field in a retroflex view. A circumferential incision is then made from the far side (cranial) to the near side (caudal) (Fig. 6). For the pocket creation method, two initial incisions are made on the lateral sides of the lesion. Mucosal incision is then completed along one-third to one-half of the circumference of the lesion on the near side of the field of view. Submucosal dissection is then preformed on the near side followed by completion of the circumferential mucosal incision along the far side of the field of view (Fig. 7). A variation

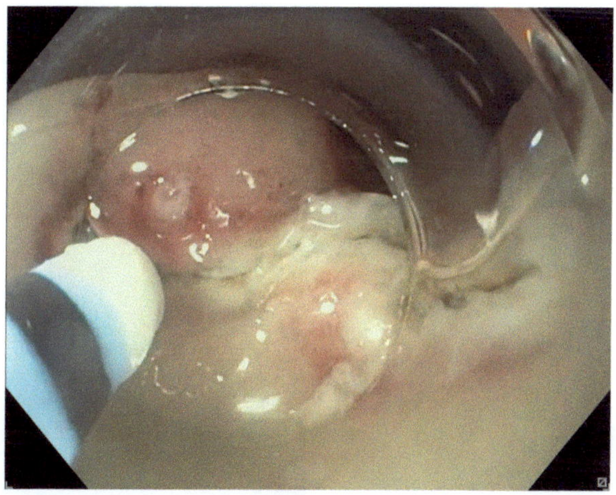

Fig. 6 Creation of circumferential incision from the far side (cranial) to the near side (caudal)

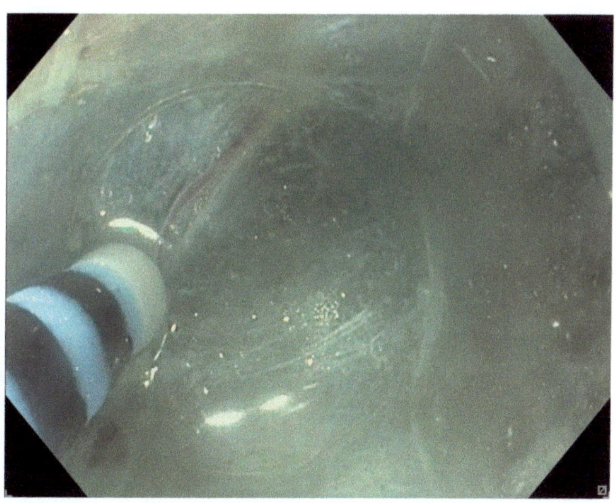

Fig. 7 Initial submucosal dissection on the near side of the lesion

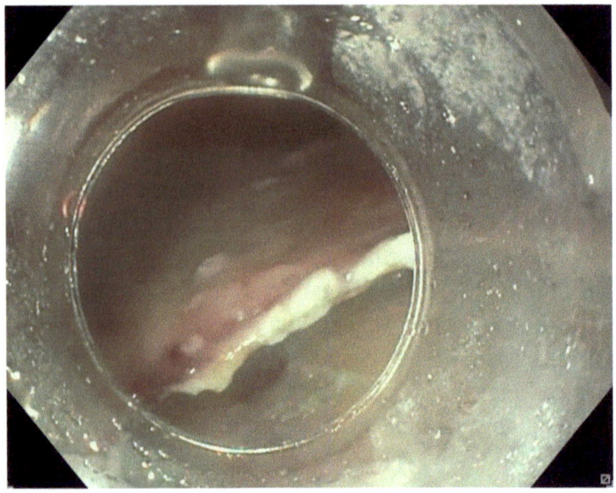

Fig. 8 Circumferential mucosal incision starting at the near side of the lesion

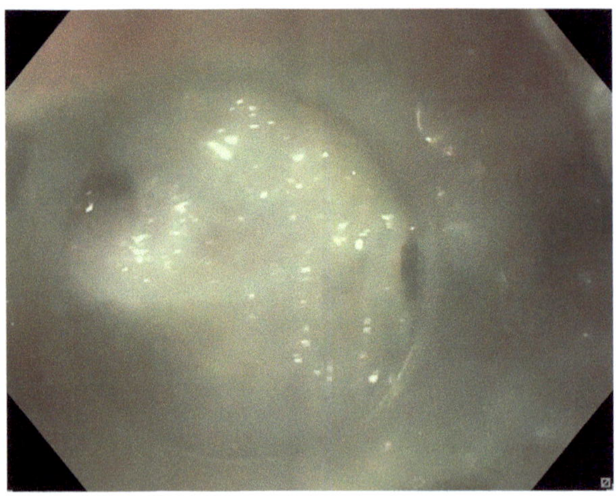

Fig. 9 Small portion of mucosa left intact to provide traction during submucosal dissection

of the near-side approach method is to initiate mucosal incision at the near side and incise the entire circumference of the lesion (Fig. 8). Some operators will leave a small amount of mucosa intact to provide traction while they perform the submucosal dissection (Fig. 9). The incision should be deep enough to get through the entirety of the mucosa and visualize the submucosa.

Submucosal Dissection

The stomach has large vessels that vertically penetrate the muscle layer and flow through the submucosa horizontally. Caution must be used to minimize intraoperative bleeding during submucosal dissection. This can be achieved using

Fig. 10 Final completion of resection

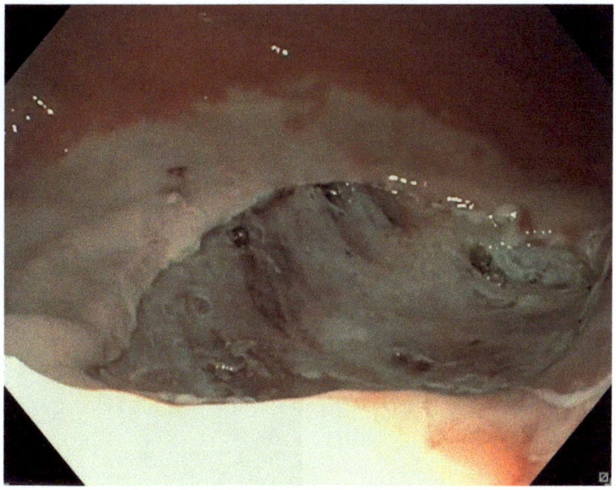

coagulation modalities such as precise sect or forced coagulation when blood vessels are visualized.

During dissection, the knife is kept parallel to the gastric wall to reduce the risk of perforation. Using the ESD knife, the submucosa is dissected fiber by fiber typically at the level of the lower 1/3 of the submucosal space to allow for negative deep margins on final histopathology. The IT knife in particular has an insulated cap that aids in minimizing risk of perforation. Use of a clear cap on the endoscope can help provide traction and improve the viewing field. Repeat submucosal injections may be necessary to allow for clear delineation of the submucosa. Treating visible vessels in advance is beneficial as bleeding will obscure the endoscopic view. Large vessels may require the use of hemostatic forceps. After the lesion is completely dissected, the lesion is removed using either suctioning the lesion into the distal attachment cap or using a retrieval net (Fig. 10).

Management of Post Resection Defect

After the specimen is removed, carefully evaluate the post-dissection wound for any defects in the muscularis propria. The resection defect can be closed using clips or endoscopic suture (Figs. 11 and 12).

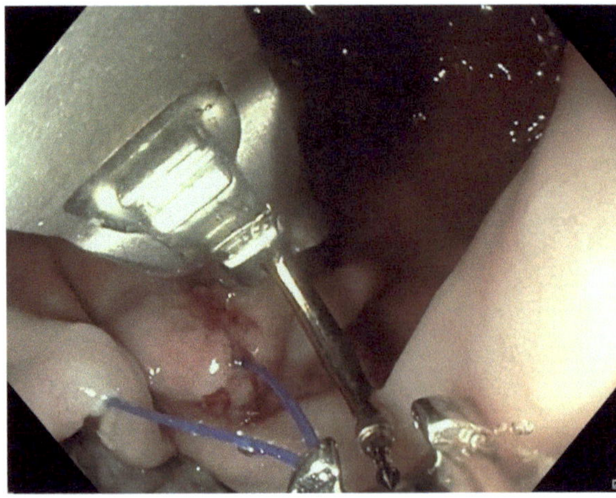

Fig. 11 Initial suture of resection defect

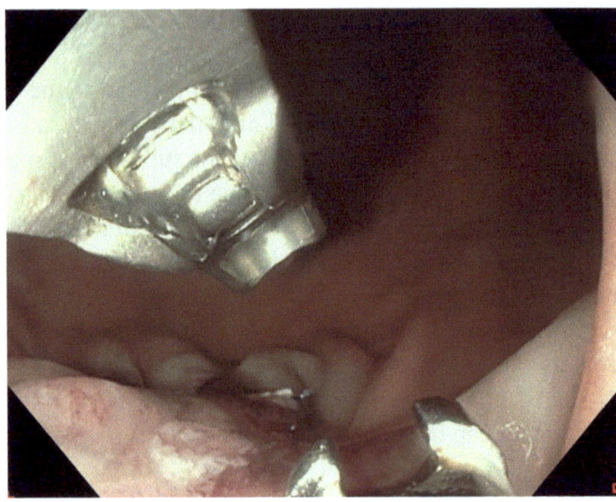

Fig. 12 Closure of resection defect with endoscopic sutures

Conclusions

Endoscopic submucosal dissection allows for en bloc resection of early gastric cancer and is a safe and effective alternative to surgical gastrectomy and piecemeal endoscopic mucosal resection. En bloc resection allows for full histopathologic analysis of the lesion as well as vertical and horizontal margins. Utilization of ESD for early gastric cancer provides potential for curative treatment while preserving their whole stomach, allowing for a higher quality of life compared to surgical gastrectomy.

Conflict of Interest Mark A. Solinski, Anthony J. Kang, Kevin P. Shah and Abdul A. Aadam declare they have no conflicts of interest.

References

1. Draganov PV, Aihara H, Karasik MS, et al. Endoscopic submucosal dissection in North America: a large prospective multicenter study. Gastroenterology. 2021;160(7):2317–27.
2. Draganov PV, Wang AY, Othman MO, Fukami N. AGA Institute clinical practice update: endoscopic submucosal dissection in the United States. Clin Gastroenterol Hepatol. 2019;17(1):16–25.
3. Hu J, Zhao Y, Ren M, et al. The comparison between endoscopic submucosal dissection and surgery in gastric cancer: a systematic review and meta-analysis. Gastroenterol Res Pract. 2018;2018:4378945.
4. Japanese Gastric Cancer Association. Japanese gastric cancer treatment guidelines 2014 (ver.4). Gastric Cancer. 2017 Jan;20(1):1–19.
5. Mori G, Nonaka S, Oda I, Abe S, Suzuki H, Yoshinaga S, Nakajima T, Saito Y. Novel strategy of endoscopic submucosal dissection using an insulation-tipped knife for early gastric cancer: near-side approach method. Endosc Int Open. 2015 Oct;3(5):E425–31.
6. Ngamruengphong S, Ferri L, Aihara H, et al. Efficacy of endoscopic submucosal dissection for superficial gastric neoplasia in a large cohort in North America. Clin Gastroenterol Hepato. 2021;19(8):1611–9.

Laparoscopic Distal Gastrectomy

Gabriel Carrizo and Pablo Omelanczuk

Abstract Subtotal gastrectomy remains the gold standard surgical treatment for various gastric pathologies, including distal gastric cancer, benign ulcers, and gastrointestinal stromal tumors of the distal stomach. The laparoscopic approach offers several advantages over traditional open surgery, including reduced postoperative pain, shorter hospital stay, and improved cosmetic outcomes. This chapter provides a detailed step-by-step description of the laparoscopic subtotal gastrectomy with Omega limb reconstruction.

Keywords Distal gastrectomy · Laparoscopic Distal gastrectomy · Gastric Cancer · Peptic ulcer disease

Introduction

Subtotal gastrectomy is a safe and effective procedure for a variety of pathologies involving the distal portion of the stomach, including neoplasia, refractory peptic ulcer disease and gastric outlet obstruction, among others [1]. Reconstruction of the gastrointestinal tract is performed simultaneously, and different techniques have been described, such as Roux-en-Y termino-lateral gastrojejunostomy or Billroth II [2].

Proper diagnostic preoperative evaluation will determine the extension of the resection, mainly dependent on oncological margins in cancer patients, as well as the concurrent lymphadenectomy. In this chapter, the technique for a laparoscopic Subtotal gastrectomy with an Omega gastrojejunostomy (Billroth II) reconstruction will be described.

G. Carrizo · P. Omelanczuk (✉)
Department of Surgery, Hospital Italiano de Mendoza, Mendoza, Argentina

F. Schlottmann, M. A. Masrur (eds.), *Endoscopic, Laparoscopic and Robotic Techniques for Foregut Disorders*, https://doi.org/10.1007/978-3-032-00811-4_35

Patient Positioning and Preparation

The patient is positioned supine in Reverse Trendelenburg position, parted legs (Lithotomy position), with both arms abducted sustained by cushioned pads. Prophylactic antibiotics and anticoagulation are administered intravenously and subcutaneously, respectively. General anesthesia is achieved, and pneumatic compression devices are placed in both lower extremities for additional thrombosis prophylaxis. Lastly, the abdomen is draped and prepped under antiseptic and aseptic conditions, from xiphoid to pubis symphysis.

Pneumoperitoneum and Port Placement

A Veress needle is placed in Palmer's point. After confirmation of correct positioning of the Veress by irrigation of sterile saline in the abdomen, insufflation starts until reaching 14–15 mmHg of intraabdominal pressure. A 5 mm trocar is placed in the left upper quadrant using Optiview. A diagnostic laparoscopy is then performed through this port, with the goal of identifying anatomic variations, distal metastases or any other condition that may alter the course of the surgery. Afterwards, the rest of the trocars are placed under direct view in the following order: a 12 mm trocar is placed in the right upper quadrant where the stapler will be introduced; the scope will be positioned left to the umbilicus trough a 10 mm trocar; lastly two 5 mm working ports will be placed in the right and left mid-abdomen. A Nathanson liver retractor is then placed subxiphoid. Once the ports are correctly placed, the instruments are introduced in the abdominal cavity under direct view (Fig. 1).

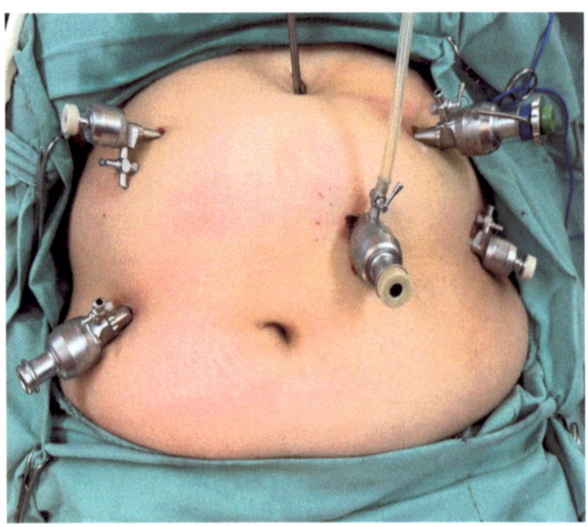

Fig. 1 Trocar placement

Procedure Description

Although pre-operative imaging evaluation is crucial beforehand, an intraoperative endoscopic evaluation is recommended for an accurate lesion location (Fig. 2). In this case, a lesion located in the body of the stomach was encountered and a subtotal gastrectomy was planned.

Dissection and Mobilization of the Proximal Stomach

The procedure begins with ultrasonic energy dissection at the level of the Angle of His and mobilization of the esophagogastric ligament (Fig. 3). Next, the lesser curve is dissected about 4–5 cm below the esophago-gastric junction and a window is achieved to access the lesser sac (Fig. 4). At this point a horizontal stapler is fired to divide the stomach (Fig. 5).

A tunnel under the fundus of the stomach is created to connect posteriorly with the Angle of his dissection (Fig. 6). This will allow for a perfect placement of a vertical stapling device and the creation of a gastric pouch of about 50 cc volume (Fig. 7). Once the gastric pouch is created, reinforcement sutures are applied over the stapled line (Fig. 8).

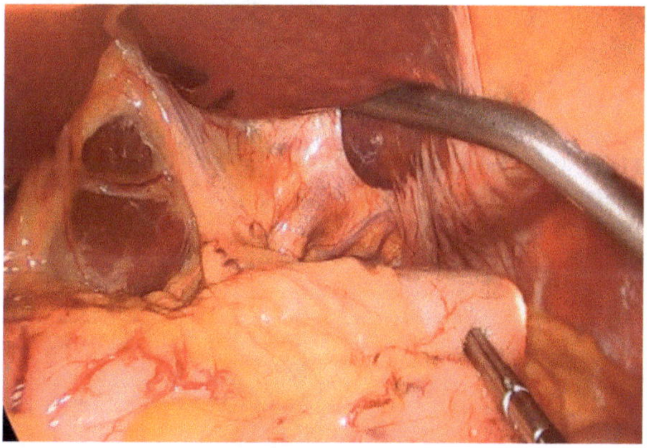

Fig. 2 Endoscopic evaluation

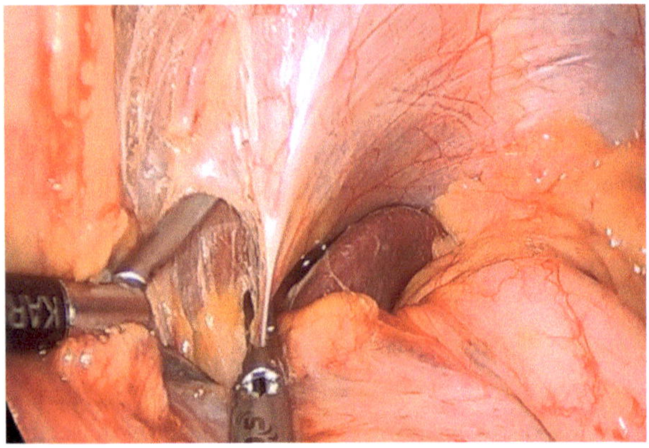

Fig. 3 Angle of His dissection

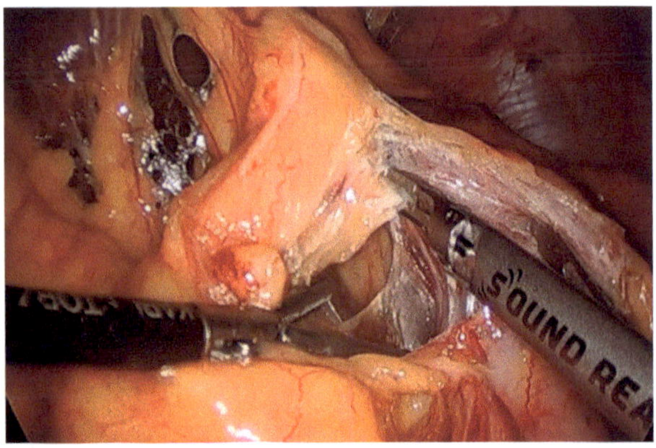

Fig. 4 Dissection of the lesser curve

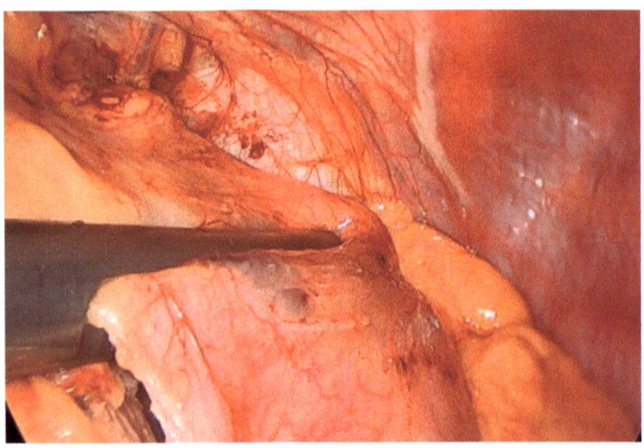

Fig. 5 Proximal gastric transection (horizontal stapling)

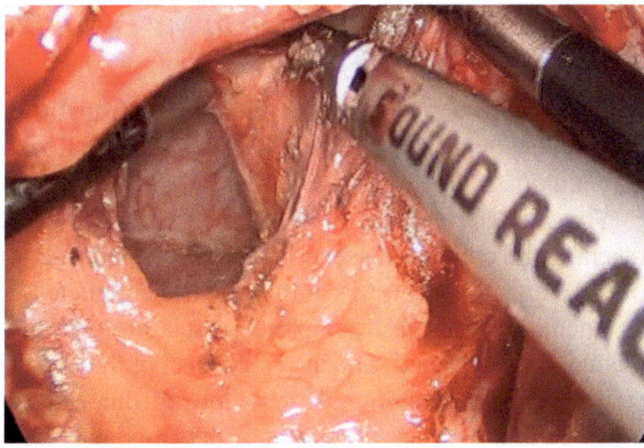

Fig. 6 Posterior gastric fundus dissection

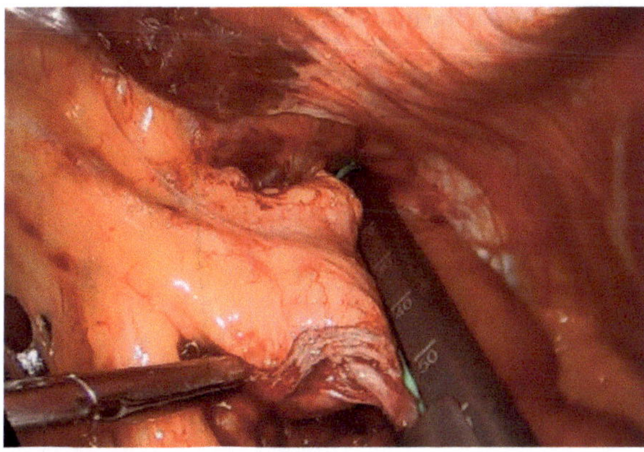

Fig. 7 Proximal gastric transection (vertical stapling)

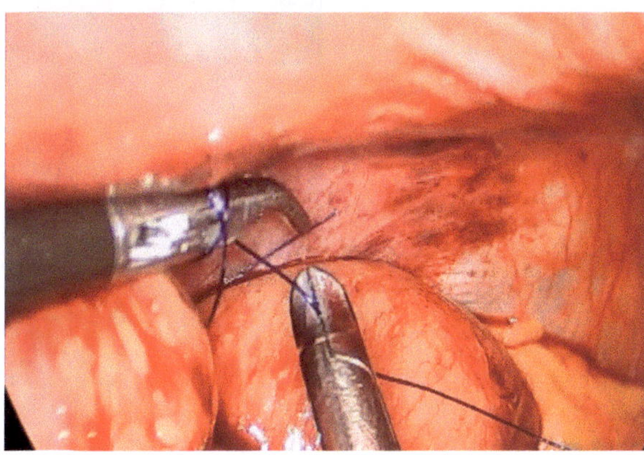

Fig. 8 Reinforcement of staple line

Dissection and Mobilization of the Distal Stomach

In this step, the greater omentum is detached from the transverse mesocolon (Fig. 9). A complete omentum resection is performed to allow for better oncological margin and outcomes.

The greater curvature of the stomach is mobilized with the omentum (Fig. 10), reaching the previous dissection at the level of the Angle of His (Fig. 11). Dissection of the lymph nodes groups at this stage is completed.

Then, the right gastroepiploic vessels are divided, and the first portion of the Duodenum is reached. The inferior aspect of the Duodenum is dissected using ultrasonic energy device (Fig. 12). Following this step, the gastrohepatic ligament is accessed and the superior aspect of the Duodenum is dissected (Fig. 13). The right gastric vessels are identified and transected. Hemostasis is confirmed. Complete mobilization of the distal stomach and proximal duodenum is achieved at this point.

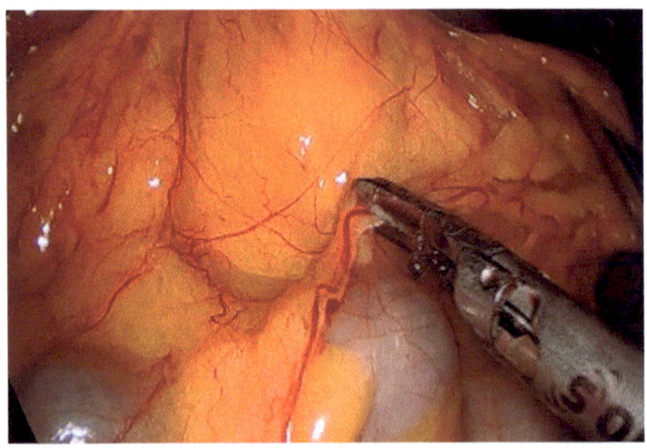

Fig. 9 Mobilization of omentum

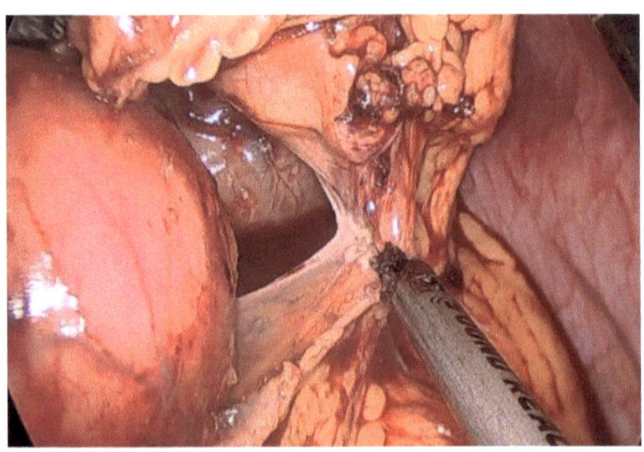

Fig. 10 Greater curve dissection

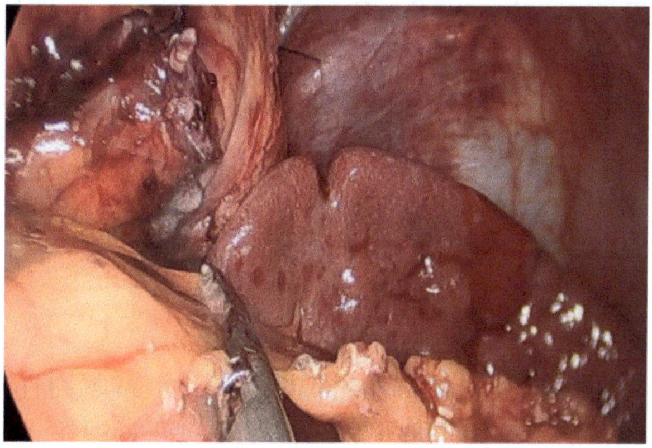

Fig. 11 Mobilization of gastric fundus

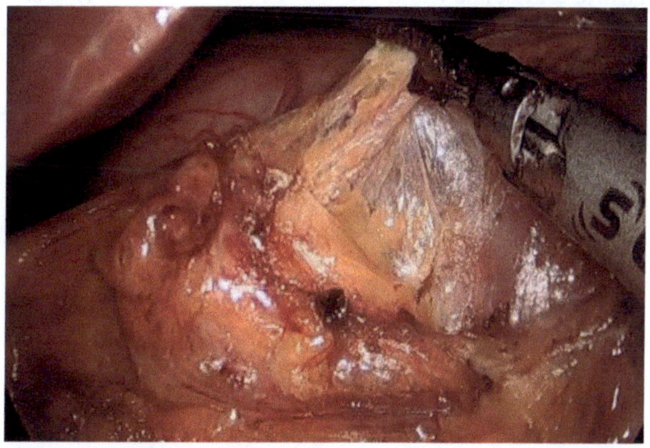

Fig. 12 Dissection of inferior aspect of the first portion of the duodenum

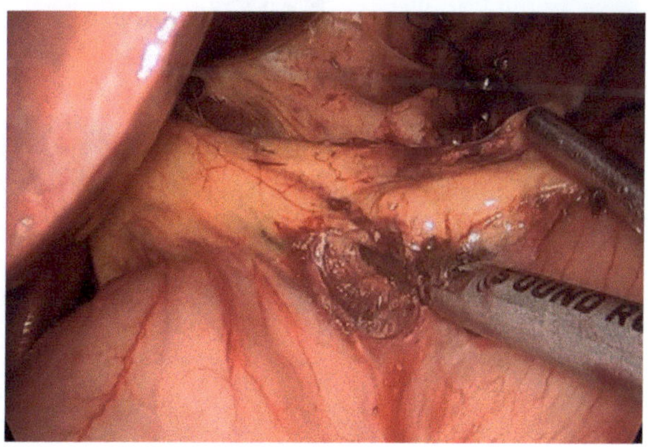

Fig. 13 Mobilization of the superior aspect of the first portion of the duodenum

Transection of the Duodenum

The next step is to transect the duodenum (Fig. 14). This is achieved using a laparoscopic green load stapler (Fig. 15). Reinforcement of the Duodenal stump stapler line is performed using absorbable stitches of 3/0 PDS (Fig. 16). Hemostasis of the stump is confirmed.

Lymphadenectomy

In oncological cases, a proximal margin of 5 cm should be maintained and a D2 lymphadenectomy with excision of at least 15 lymph nodes should be attempted for oncological safety and histopathological evaluation. Completion of Lymphadenectomy of Left gastric and celiac trunk groups (Group VII and IX) is shown in Fig. 17. The specimen should then be placed in an Endobag for posterior extraction.

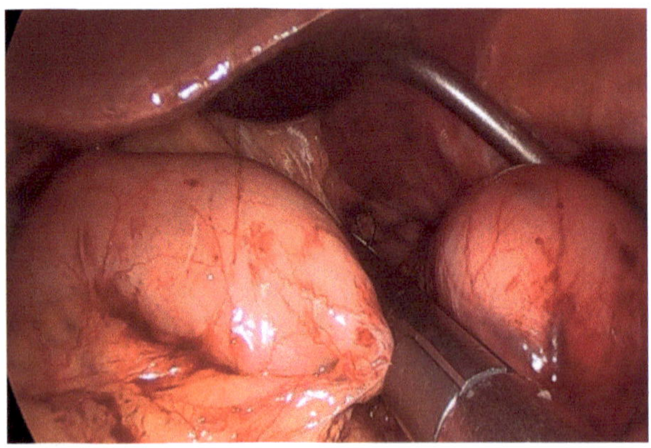

Fig. 14 Duodenal transection

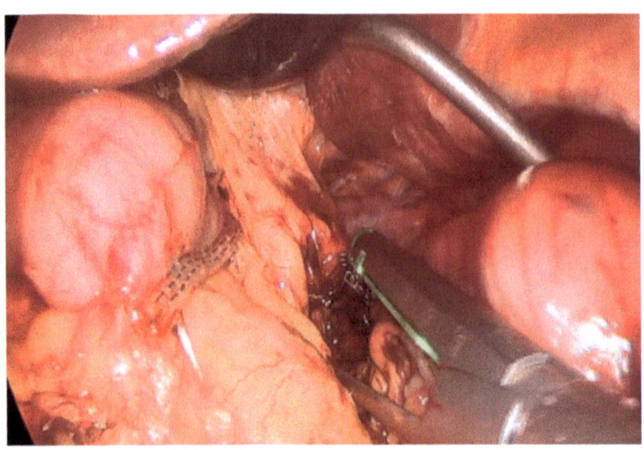

Fig. 15 Laparoscopic staple duodenal transection

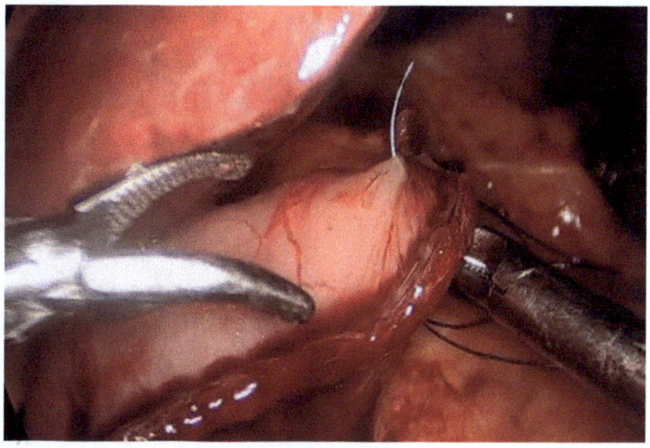

Fig. 16 Duodenal staple line reinforcement

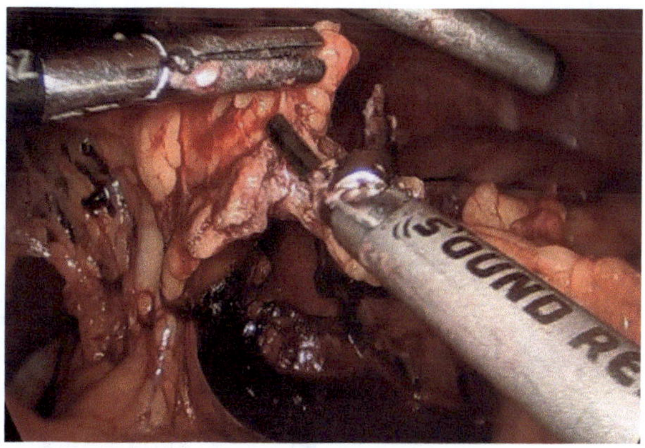

Fig. 17 Lymphadenectomy group VII and IX

Gastrojejunostomy Reconstruction

The transverse colon is retracted cephalad and the ligament of Treitz is visualized (Fig. 18). Once identified, about 60–80 cm of jejunum is run distally. This portion of the small bowel is brought up antecolic next to the gastric pouch. In this case, a gastrojejunostomy is performed in an Omega fashion (Billroth II) after an enterotomy is done (Fig. 19).

While the assistant holds the bowel in position, a gastrotomy is created using ultrasonic energy device in the posterolateral aspect of the gastric pouch. Using a blue laparoscopic linear stapler, a termino-lateral gastrojejunal anastomosis of about 3 cm is created (Fig. 20). The gastrojejunostomy opening is then closed in a double layer fashion, using 3-0 PDS (Fig. 21).

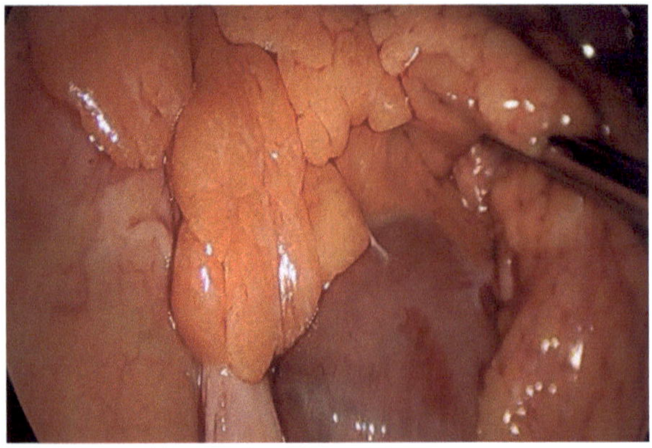

Fig. 18 Identification of Ligament of Treitz

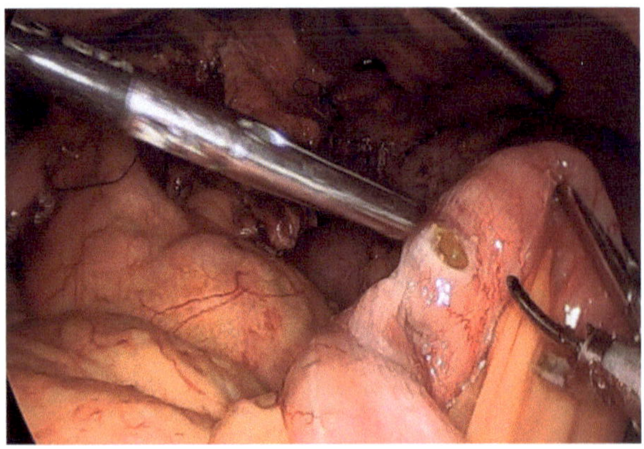

Fig. 19 Enterotomy 50 cm from Ligament of Treitz

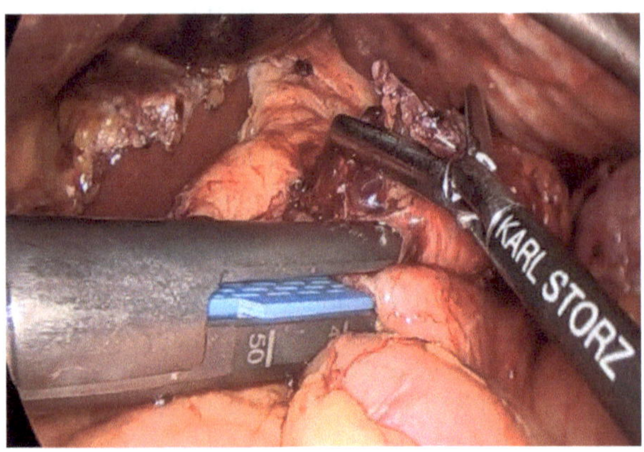

Fig. 20 Termino-lateral stapled gastro-jejunostomy

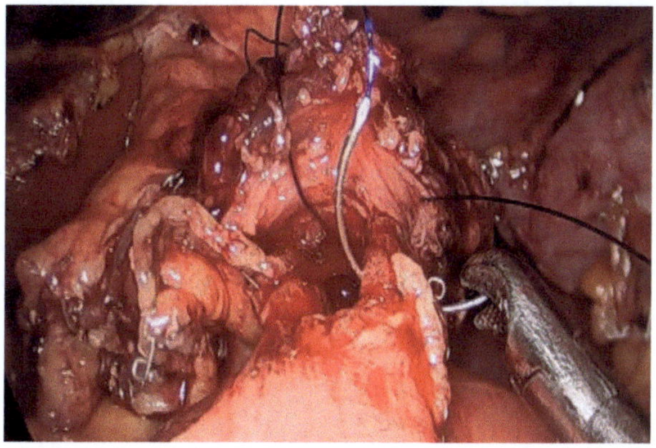

Fig. 21 Gastro-enterotomy closure

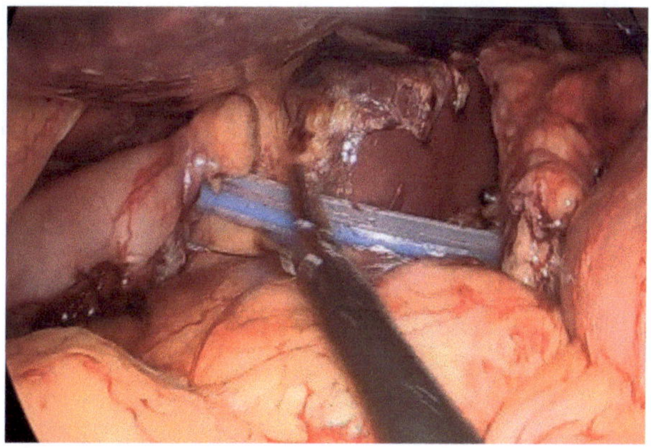

Fig. 22 Placement of drain

Leak Test

The small bowel loops are clamped, and a methylene blue test is performed through a nasogastric tube. The goal of this test is to check the integrity of the anastomosis and assess the presence of leaks.

The specimen can be removed through a 5 cm Pfannenstiel incision or a port site incision. The specimen previously placed in the Endobag, should be extracted as a single piece and the abdominal wall is closed in layers.

Final Inspection and Removal of Trocars

The peritoneal cavity is inspected one last time, hemostasis achieved, and a drain is placed posterior to the gastrojejunostomy next to the Duodenal stump (Fig. 22). All trocars are removed under direct visualization. The Nathanson liver retractor is removed. The 12 mm trocar fascia is closed using Vicryl 0 suture, and the rest of the port sites are closed with subcutaneous sutures.

Conclusions

Laparoscopic Distal/Subtotal gastrectomy represents a technically demanding yet rewarding surgical procedure. The minimally invasive approach offers numerous advantages over traditional open surgery, including reduced postoperative pain, shorter hospital stays, and improved cosmetic outcomes. By meticulously dissecting the gastric and duodenal tissues, carefully ligating vessels, and creating tension-free anastomoses, surgeons can achieve optimal functional and oncological results.

References

1. Motamiez A, Maximous D, Salem AAS, et al. surgical outcomes of laparoscopic-assisted distal gastrectomy versus totally laparoscopic distal gastrectomy Billroth I for gastric cancer. Surg Laparosc Endosc Percutan Tech. 2024;34(1):80–6. https://doi.org/10.1097/SLE.0000000000001255.
2. Lombardo F, Aiolfi A, Cavalli M, et al. Techniques for reconstruction after distal gastrectomy for cancer: updated network meta-analysis of randomized controlled trials. Langenbecks Arch Surg. 2022;407(1):75–86. https://doi.org/10.1007/s00423-021-02411-6.

Robotic Distal Gastrectomy

Beatriz Figueroa, Emiliano G. Manuelli Laos, and Mario A. Masrur

Abstract Gastric resections serve as a treatment for both benign and malignant pathologies. The extent of gastric resection and reconstruction techniques are affected by the nature of the pathology and the location or extent of the disease. Reconstruction techniques are based on the complications that may arise due to each new anatomic configuration. For pathologies involving the distal two-thirds of the stomach, distal gastrectomy with Roux-en-Y reconstruction has proven to have better overall outcomes and provide a better quality of life to patients. In this chapter we describe a robotic approach to distal gastrectomy with Roux-en-Y reconstruction.

Keywords Distal gastrectomy · Robotic surgery Roux-en-Y reconstruction · Gastric Cancer · Peptic ulcers disease

Introduction

Distal gastrectomy is the surgical intervention of choice for both early and advanced malignancies of the distal stomach, as well as for other benign pathologies particularly peptic ulcers resulting in gastric outlet obstruction or pyloric stenosis [1]. A good pre-operative evaluation including EGD and biopsies are essential to differentiate benign from malignant gastric outlet obstuctions. This will also aid determining the extend of the gastric resection (oncological margins) and associated lymphadenectomy.

B. Figueroa · E. G. Manuelli Laos · M. A. Masrur (✉)
Department of Surgery, University of Illinois at Chicago, Chicago, IL, USA
e-mail: mmasrur@uic.edu

F. Schlottmann, M. A. Masrur (eds.), *Endoscopic, Laparoscopic and Robotic Techniques for Foregut Disorders*, https://doi.org/10.1007/978-3-032-00811-4_36

Although other types of reconstructions have been described, the Roux-en-Y gastrojejunostomy offers excellent outcomes and provides better quality of life to patients [2]. This technique had become the gold standard and involves the creation of an end-to-side anastomosis between the alimentary limb of the jejunum and the gastric remnant as well as a more distal anastomosis between the alimentary limb and the biliopancreatic limb [3–5].

This chapter will provide a detailed, step-by-step approach to performing a distal gastrectomy and subsequent Roux-en-Y gastrojejunostomy utilizing a robotic surgical platform.

Procedure Description

Patient Positioning

The patient is placed supine on the operating room table with sequential compression devices in place at the bilateral lower extremities. Intravenous prophylactic antibiotics is administered prior to the induction of general anesthesia. Both arms are left abducted to 90° taking care not to overextend upper extremities and to pad all pressure points. As the patient will be placed in a steep reverse Trendelenburg position, the use a footboard at the lower end of the operating room table is recommended. After this setup is complete, the abdomen is prepped and draped in the usual sterile fashion, exposing from xiphoid to pubic symphysis.

Pneumoperitoneum and Port Placement

Pneumoperitoneum is achieved by placing a Veress needle at Palmer's point. Adequate peritoneal entry is confirmed by easy irrigation of sterile saline into abdominal cavity. After this, pneumoperitoneum of 15 mmHg is induced and a 5 mm Optiview trocar is introduced at the left upper quadrant. A diagnostic laparoscopy is performed to confirm any anatomical variations or rule out distant metastatic disease, if surgery is being performed for oncological purposes. Given no contraindications to proceed, additional trocars are placed as shown in Fig. 1, under direct visualization. The scope is placed at the umbilical level, just to the left of the midline. A 12 mm robotic trocar is placed at the right upper quadrant for robotic stapling, and an additional 8 mm robotic trocar at the left, upper flank. The assistant trocar, also an 8 mm trocar, is placed between the scope and the stapling trocar at the right lower quadrant. The Nathanson Liver Retractor is preferred and typically placed at the epigastric level. Once trocars are in place, the surgical Robot is docked laterally, and instruments are introduced under direct visualization.

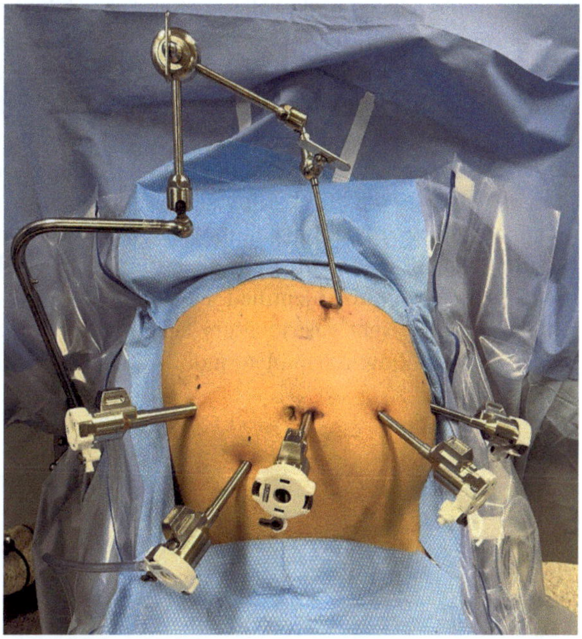

Fig. 1 Trocar placement

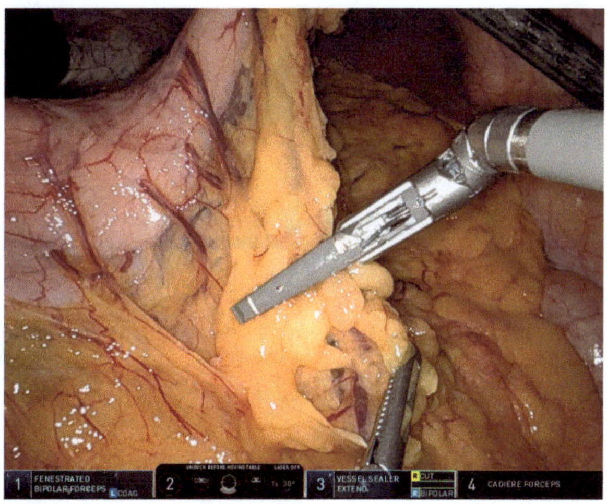

Fig. 2 Mobilization of greater curvature

Operative Technique

Mobilization of Distal Stomach and Ligation of Vessels

Dissection starts along the greater curvature of the stomach using a robotic Vessel sealer. After identifying our gastric transection line, dissection will follow the gastroepiploic arcade in a caudal fashion, up to the level of the pylorus (Fig. 2). Once this is completed, a complete dissection of the right gastroepiploic artery and vein is performed, and transection carried out at its origin. Transection of these vessels is done with Robotic Sureform™ Stapler with a white load, taking care to secure hemostasis once division is complete (Fig. 3). Using the vessels sealer device the first portion of the duodenum is mobilized at its inferior edge allowing a good exposure of this area for ulterior stapling (Fig. 4). At this point, any posterior attachments of the stomach to the retroperitoneum are taken down with vessel sealer device or monopolar hook and mobilization of the lesser curvature is continued. The gastrohepatic ligament is identified and entered in its avascular plane. The left and right gastric arteries are fully identified. Dissection continues distally using vessel sealer taking down the right gastric artery and superior Duodenal arteries (Fig. 5). This maneuver will allow a complete mobilization of the distal stomach and proximal duodenum.

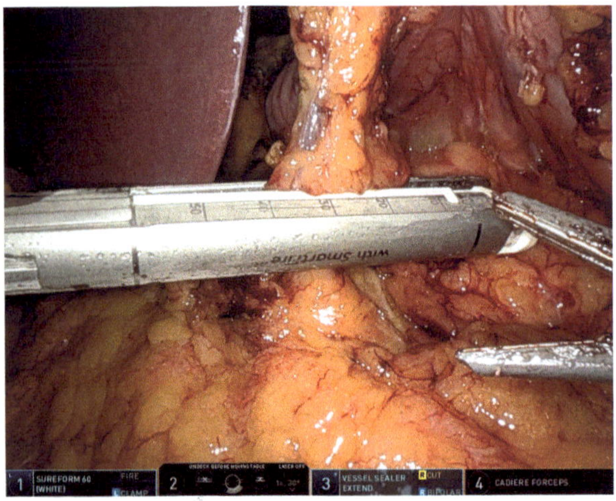

Fig. 3 Transection of right gastroepiploic artery

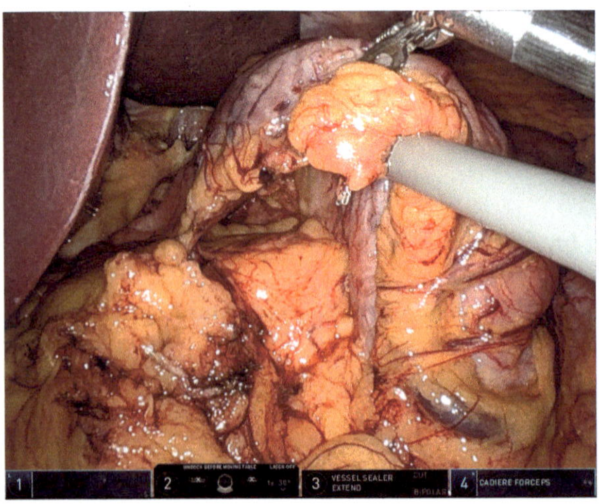

Fig. 4 Dissection of inferior aspect of the first portion of the duodenum

Duodenal Transection

After complete mobilization and vascular control of the distal stomach and duodenum, duodenal transection is performed using robotic stapler. A blue load Robotic Sureform™ Stapler with reinforcement is preferred for this step (Fig. 6). The duodenal staple line can be oversewn, as per surgeon preference. Adequate hemostasis is ensured along both staple lines. It is preferred to transect the duodenum first, as this maneuver will allow a better mobilization and stapling at the proximal margin in the stomach.

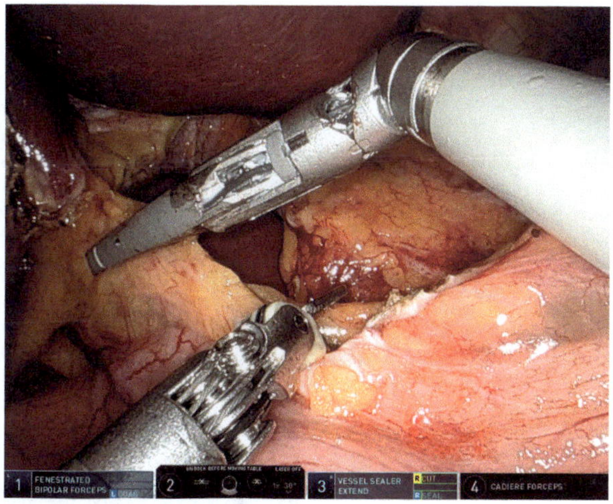

Fig. 5 Mobilization of the superior aspect of the first portion of the duodenum

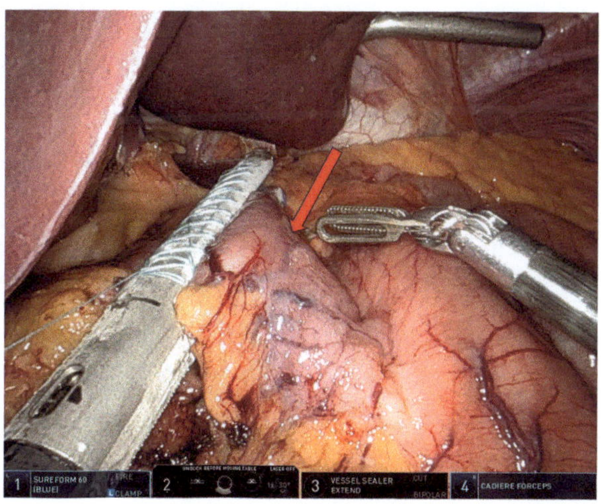

Fig. 6 Duodenal transection (*Red arrow marking Gastric Pylorus)

Proximal Gastric Transection

Using the Vessel sealer device dissection continues at the proximal edge of the lesser curve allowing a precise isolation of the vessels at this level of transection (Fig. 7).

Next, using a white robotic stapler load, the gastric arcade vessels at the transection line are taken down ensuring an adequate blood supply for the remaining proximal stomach (Fig. 8). Once this is done, a complete proximal mobilization of the proximal stomach is achieved (Fig. 9).

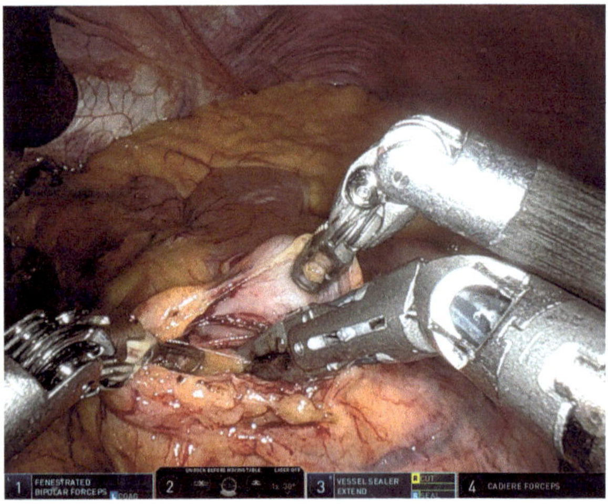

Fig. 7 Proximal dissection at the lesser curve

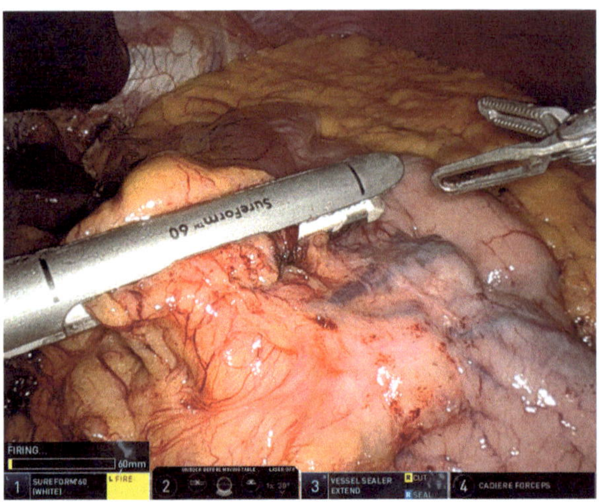

Fig. 8 Transection of gastric vessels arcade in the lesser curve

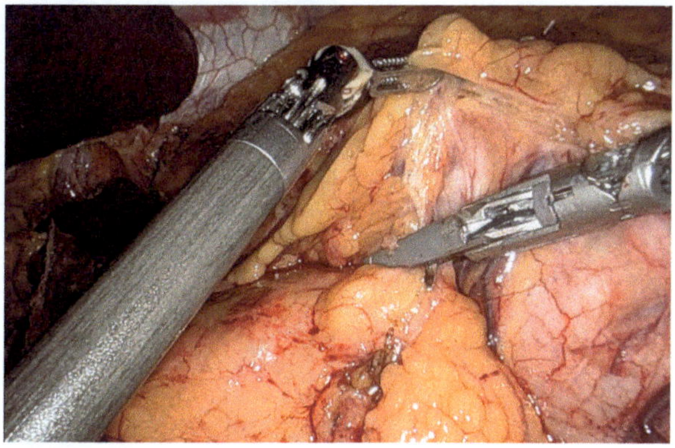

Fig. 9 Complete proximal mobilization

Proximal Gastric Transection

The line of transection at the proximal margin had been well identified at this point. Using the Robotic Sureform™ Green loads Stapler with reinforcement, the stomach is transected horizontally from medial to the lateral (Fig. 10). Once this is completed, the specimen is fully separated and placed in Endobag for subsequent extraction at completion of the procedure. Indocyanine green (ICG) is injected intra-vascularly to confirm adequate perfusion of both, remnant stomach and duodenal stump (Fig. 11).

It is important for oncological resections that surgeons ensure a margin of at least 5 cm proximal to the tumor. In addition, in oncological surgery for gastric adenocarcinoma, adequate D2 lymphadenectomy should be completed with excision of at least fifteen lymph nodes for a precise anatomo-pathology evaluation.

Roux-en-Y Reconstruction

The Roux-en-Y reconstruction is the gold standard after these operations. Other options include Billroth I and II reconstructions. Despite being more technically complex, Roux-en-Y reconstruction has persistently demonstrated a lower incidence of reflux gastritis and esophagitis, leading to better, long-term quality of life [1, 2].

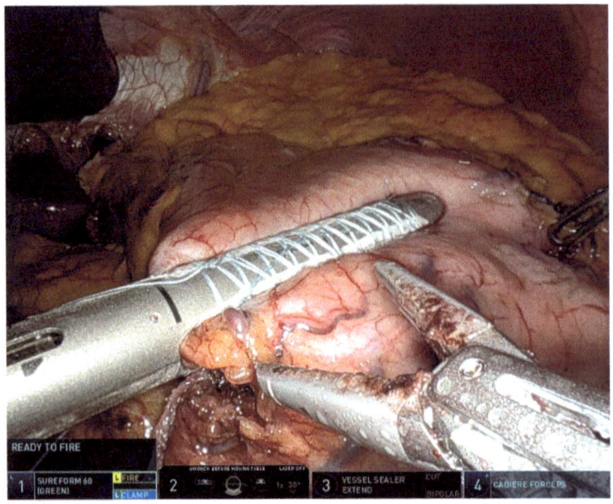

Fig. 10 Proximal Gastric transection

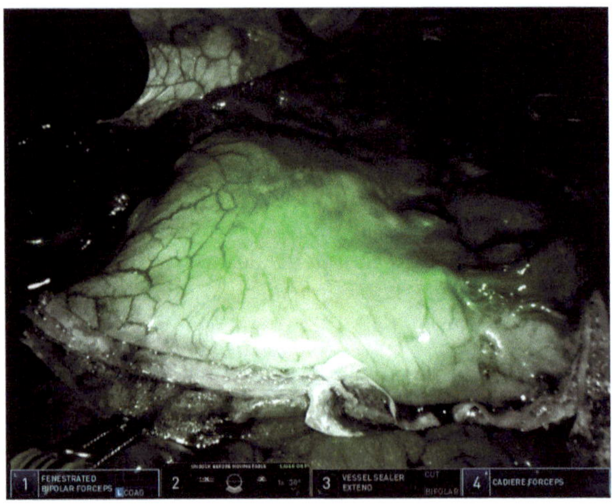

Fig. 11 ICG perfusion evaluation of Proximal Stomach margins

Division of Small Bowel and Creation of Jejuno-Jejunostomy

The first step is to identify the ligament of Treitz (LOT). The omentum is divided using vessel sealer device, this maneuver will allow better visualization and decrease tension at the gastr-jejunostomy anastomosis. To identify LOT, the transverse colon is retracted cephalad and the jejunum is run proximally until identifying the LOT, confirmed by visualizing the inferior mesenteric vein to the left of the ligament. The jejunum is then run distally between 35 and 50 cm to create our biliopancreatic (BP) limb and transection is carried at this point using a Blue load Robotic Sureform™ stapler with reinforcement (Fig. 12). The mesentery is divided further to allow a good mobilization of both stumps and ICG perfusion evaluation of the bowel stumps is performed at this time (Fig. 13).

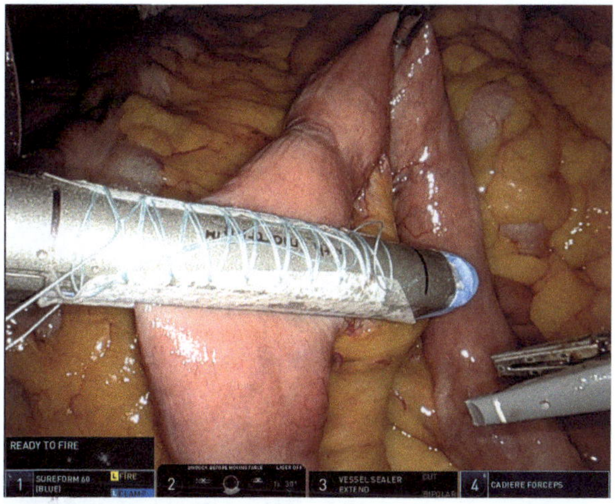

Fig. 12 Transection of jejunum 35–50 cm from Ligament of Treitz

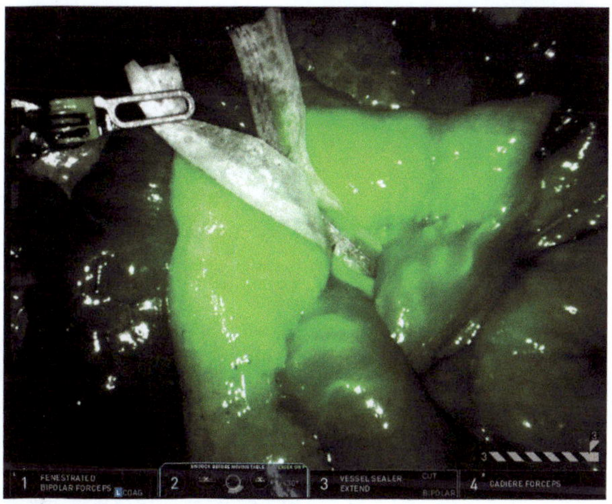

Fig. 13 ICG perfusion evaluation of the bowel stumps

Once this is completed, the BP limb is fixed into position using the fourth robotic arm (Arm 3). The distal bowel stump, which represents the Roux- or Alimentary Limb (AL), is then run distally for about 40–50 cm. At this point the AL and BP limb are jointed together using the 3th arm for the subsequent creation of the jejuno-jejunostomy (Fig. 14). Enterotomies are created with hook monopolar electrocautery in the antimesenteric border of both bowel loops, and a side-to-side anastomosis is created using a White Robotic Sureform™ Stapler load (Fig. 15). Adequate hemostasis of the staple line is confirmed and the common enterotomy is then closed in two layers using running PDS 3-0 sutures for the inner layer and interrupted PDS 3-0 sutures for our outer layer (Fig. 16).

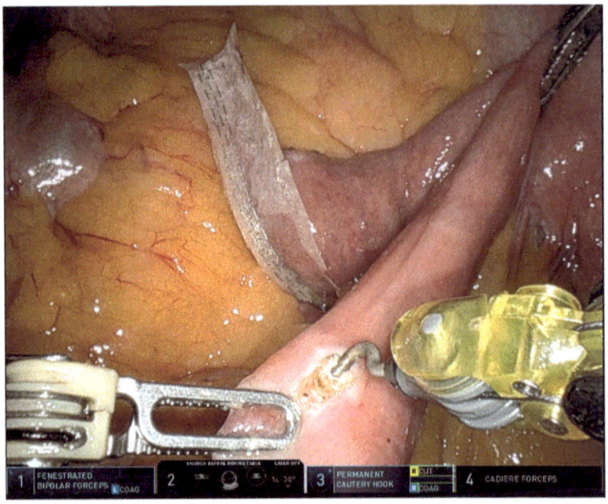

Fig. 14 Alimentary Limb and Bilio-pancreatic limb positioned for anastomosis

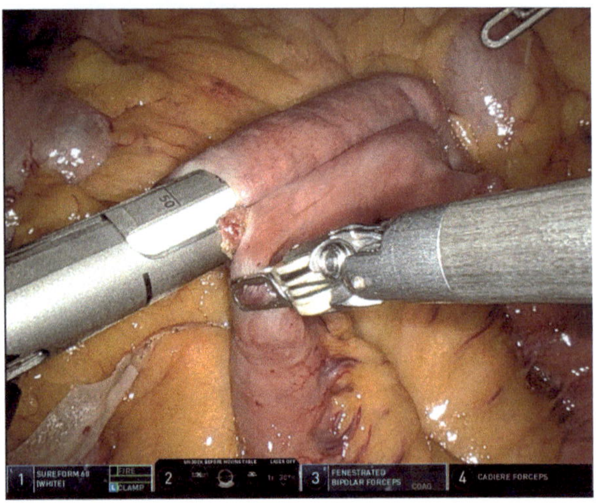

Fig. 15 Side-to-side jejuno-jejunostomy anastomosis using Robotic Stapler

Creation of Gastrojejunostomy and Closure of Mesenteric Defects

After completion of bowel anastomosis, the roux limb is brought up to the remnant stomach, assuring a tension-free anastomosis (Fig. 17). If some tension is noted, a few maneuvers can be implemented to decrease this tension. The first, the mesentery can be further divided taking care not to compromise the blood supply small bowel, alternatively the AL can be brought up retro-colic through the transverse mesocolon. The roux limb is held in position with the assisting robotic arm (arm 3). A termino-lateral stapled anastomosis for distal gastrectomy is the preferred technique, as it creates a widened anastomosis. At this point, a gastrotomy and an

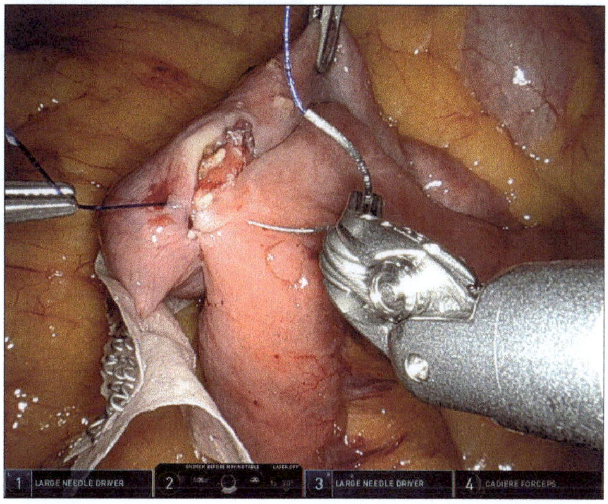

Fig. 16 Closure of enterotomies using running stitches

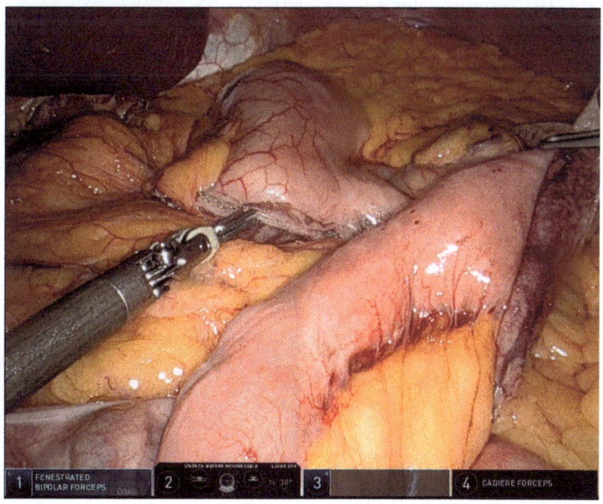

Fig. 17 Roux limb next to the remnant stomach

enterotomy is created using hook monopolar electrocautery (Fig. 18). The gastrotomy is performed in the anterior and most medial aspect of the gastric remnant and the enterotomy is created in the antimesenteric border of the bowel loop. Then, a termino-lateral stapled gastro-jejunostomy is constructed with a White Robotic Sureform™ Stapler (Fig. 19). After hemostasis is secured along the staple line, the common gastro-enterotomy is closed with a running PDS 3-0 suture and reinforced with an outer layer with interrupted 3-0 PDS sutures (Fig. 20). After this, Petersen space and mesenteric defect at jejuno-jejunostomy are both closed with unabsorbable 2-0 Polyester sutures.

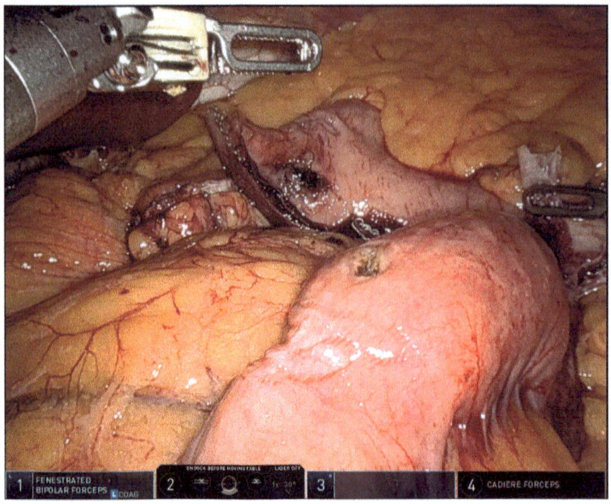

Fig. 18 Gastro-enterotomy creation

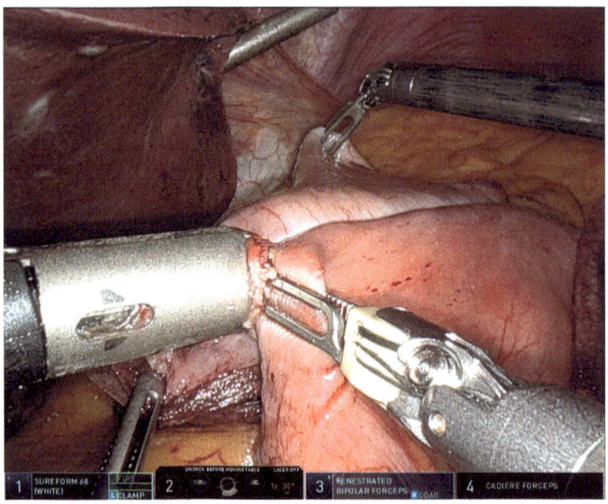

Fig. 19 Termino-lateral stapled gastro-jejunostomy using Robotic stapler

Intraoperative Endoscopy

After completion of our final anastomosis, an intraoperative endoscopy is routinely performed. The alimentary limb is clamped, and the assistant performs the upper endoscopy to confirm the patency of anastomosis as well as to identify any source of intraluminal bleeding or potential leak from anastomosis (Fig. 21). Once this is complete, we remove the liver retractor and proceed with the extraction of the specimen using a large endobag.

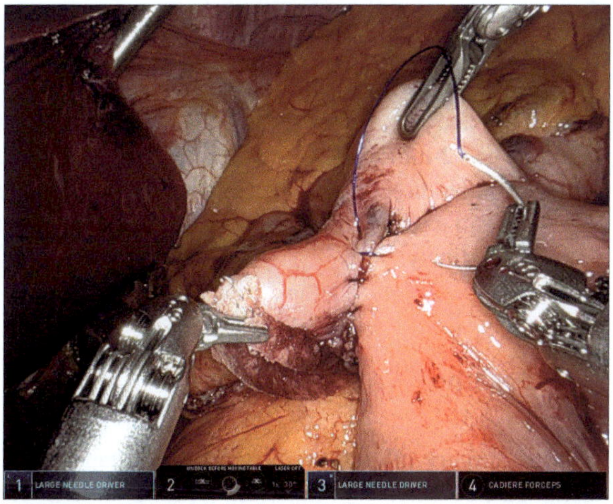

Fig. 20 Gastro-enterotomy closure

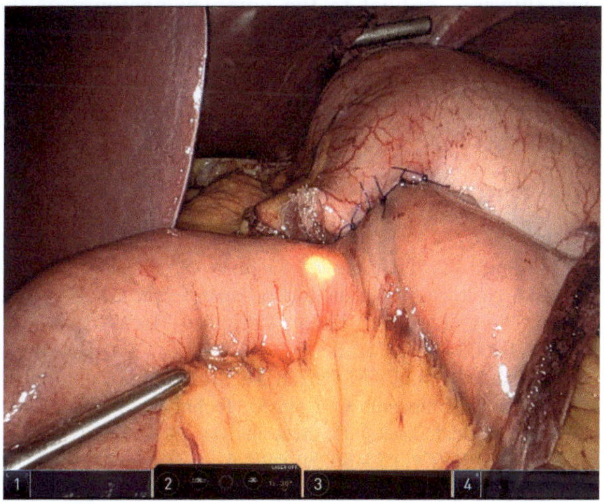

Fig. 21 Upper endoscopy showing widely patent anastomosis

Extraction of Specimen

Due to the size of the specimen, a Pfannenstiel incision is performed for its extraction. Keeping the abdomen insufflated a five-centimeter skin incision is performed two fingerbreadths above the pubic symphysis. Dissection is carried down to the fascia and this is opened using electrocautery, sparing underlying rectus muscles. Fascia is then separated from the rectus muscles superiorly and inferiorly. Midline identified rectus muscles retracted laterally, and the peritoneum entered. Once in the peritoneal cavity, the endobag is identified and the specimen is extracted intact. The closure is performed in layers and hemostasis is secured at this point.

Final Inspection and Removal of Trocars

A final inspection of the peritoneal cavity is performed. Pneumoperitoneum is again established and hemostasis along both anastomosis as well as all trocar sites is confirmed. The 12 mm trocar site fascia is closed with Vicryl 0 suture. All trocars are removed under direct visualization, the pneumoperitoneum is completely evacuated and skin at all trocar sites is closed with subcutaneous sutures. Abdominal drains are not used routinely.

Conclusions

Robotic surgery offers key technical advantages over traditional laparoscopy for distal gastrectomy, especially in treating gastric cancer. The robotic system's enhanced dexterity and 3D high-definition visualization enable precise dissection and suturing, critical in the complex anatomy of the upper abdomen. Overall, robotic instruments provide greater freedom of movement, allowing more refined maneuvers than laparoscopy.

References

1. Motamiez A, Maximous D, Salem AAS, et al. Surgical outcomes of laparoscopic-assisted distal gastrectomy versus totally laparoscopic distal gastrectomy Billroth I for gastric cancer. Surg Laparosc Endosc Percutan Tech. 2024;34(1):80–6. https://doi.org/10.1097/SLE.0000000000001255.
2. Lombardo F, Aiolfi A, Cavalli M, Mini E, Lastraioli C, Panizzo V, Lanzaro A, Bonitta G, Danelli P, Campanelli G, Bona D. Techniques for reconstruction after distal gastrectomy for cancer: updated network meta-analysis of randomized controlled trials. Langenbecks Arch Surg. 2022;407(1):75–86. https://doi.org/10.1007/s00423-021-02411-6. Epub 2022 Jan 30.
3. Dreifuss N, Bustos R, Masrur M. Roux-en-y gastric bypass. The foundation and art of robotic surgery. McGraw-Hill 2023.
4. Yang K, Zhang W, Chen Z, Chen X, Liu K, Zhao L, Hu J. Comparison of long-term quality of life between Billroth-I and Roux-en-Y anastomosis after distal gastrectomy for gastric cancer: a randomized controlled trial. Chin Med J (Engl). 2023;136(9):1074–81. https://doi.org/10.1097/CM9.0000000000002602. PMID: 37014767; PMCID: PMC10228481.
5. Zong L, Chen P. Billroth I vs. Billroth II vs. roux-en-y following distal gastrectomy: A meta-analysis based on 15 studies. Hepatogastroenterology. 2011;58(109):1413–24. https://doi.org/10.5754/hge10567.

Laparoscopic Total Gastrectomy

Camilo Boza, Ricardo Funke, and Martín Andrada

Abstract Gastric cancer is one of the malignant pathologies with the highest mortality rates worldwide. Resection surgery, combined with adequate lymphadenectomy, is one of the fundamental pillars for the treatment of the disease. In this chapter, we will describe the steps of laparoscopic total gastrectomy.

Keywords Gastric cancer · Laparoscopy · Laparoscopic total gastrectomy · Lymphadenectomy

Introduction

Gastric cancer remains one of the most lethal malignant pathologies of the digestive tract worldwide. Gastrectomy combined with an adequate lymphadenectomy, specifically D2 for advanced gastric cancer, is one of the key components in the treatment of this disease. The laparoscopic approach has proven to reduce postoperative complications and enhance recovery in high-volume centers [1, 2].

In this chapter, a description of the steps of laparoscopic total gastrectomy with representative images of the surgical technique is presented.

Procedure Description

Pacient Positioning

The patient is placed supine on the operative table with legs apart. Once general endotracheal anesthesia is achieved, sequential compression devices are placed in both legs. An orogastric tube is also inserted to decompress the stomach. A Foley

C. Boza (✉) · R. Funke · M. Andrada
Department of Surgery, Clinica MEDS, Santiago, Chile

F. Schlottmann, M. A. Masrur (eds.), *Endoscopic, Laparoscopic and Robotic Techniques for Foregut Disorders*, https://doi.org/10.1007/978-3-032-00811-4_37

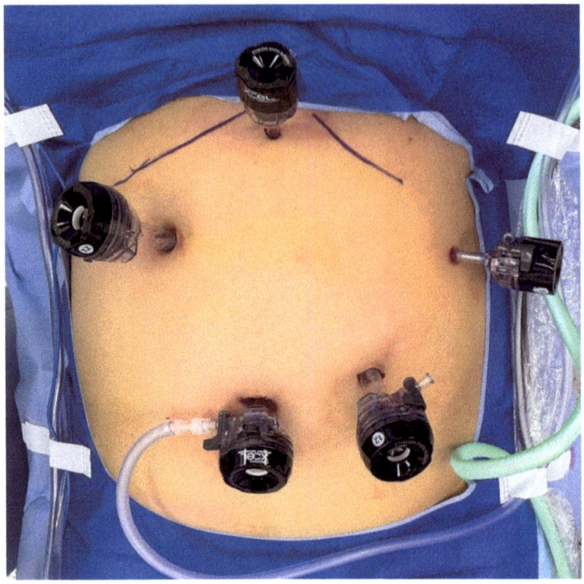

Fig. 1 Port placement

catheter is needed for the procedure. The surgeon is positioned between the legs, the first assistant to the patient's right side, and the second assistant on the left side.

Pneumoperitoneum and Port Placement

Pneumoperitoneum at 15 mmHg is created with Veress needle in the midline.

Three 12 mm trocars are used, one on the right side, one at the umbilical level and one in the left flank. One 5 mm trocars on the left side. A liver retractor is also placed through a 5-mm incision in the epigastrium (Fig. 1).

Operative Technique

Intraperitoneal Examination

During a diagnostic laparoscopy, the abdomen is explored to detect peritoneal implants or hepatic metastases. If any are found, biopsies are taken and sent for anatomopathological analysis. If the results are positive, the procedure is aborted, and the need for a palliative maneuver is determined based on the specific case (Fig. 2).

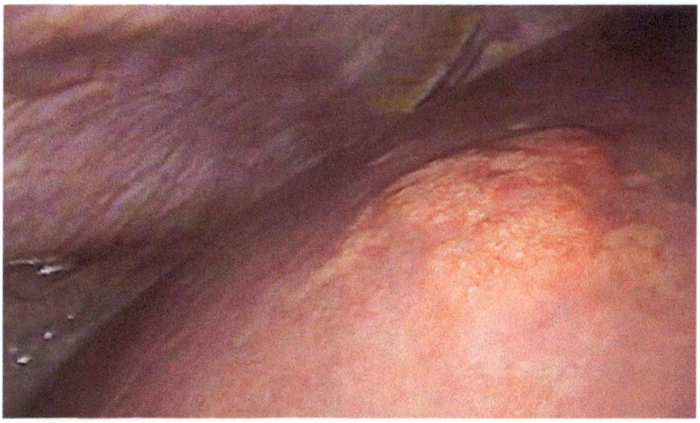

Fig. 2 Diagnostic laparoscopy and tumor identification

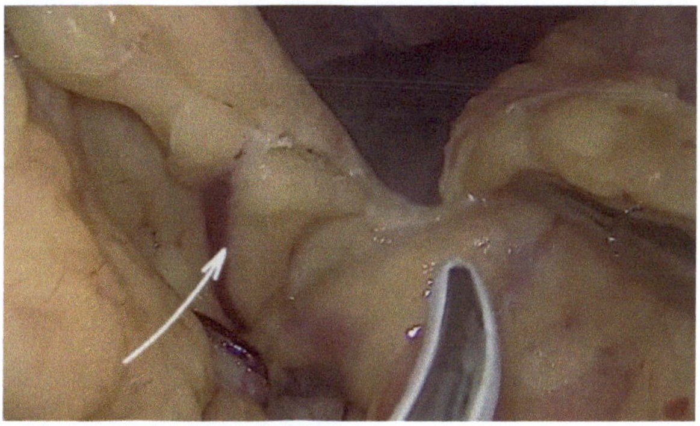

Fig. 3 Proximal dissection of gastrocolic ligament

Greater Omentum Resection and Dissection of Groups 4D and 4SB

The procedure begins with the mobilization of the greater omentum from the transverse colon. Dissection is started on the left side, reaching the left gastroepiploic vessels (Fig. 3), and then proceed in the same manner towards the right side until the duodenal arc is exposed (Fig. 4). Special caution is required in cases of previous cholecystectomy, as adhesions have to be dissected. A complete greater omentum resection is usually performed.

Dissection of Group 6 and Ligation of the Gastroepiploic Vessels

After mobilizing the omentum, the plane between the omentum and the transverse mesocolon is accessed towards the posterior surface of the stomach and continue the dissection, refining the gastroepiploic right vessel pedicle in a "V" shape. Generally, the colic and pancreatoduodenal veins can be observed over the mesocolon, heading towards Henle's trunk, where the origin of the right gastroepiploic vein is ligated (Fig. 5). After dividing this vessel, the space between the superior border of the

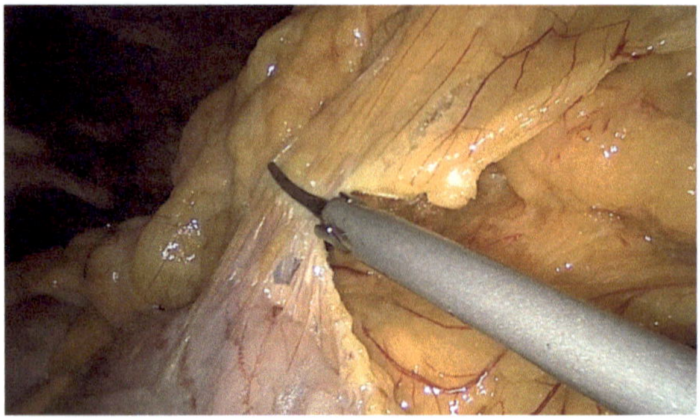

Fig. 4 Distal dissection of gastrocolic ligament

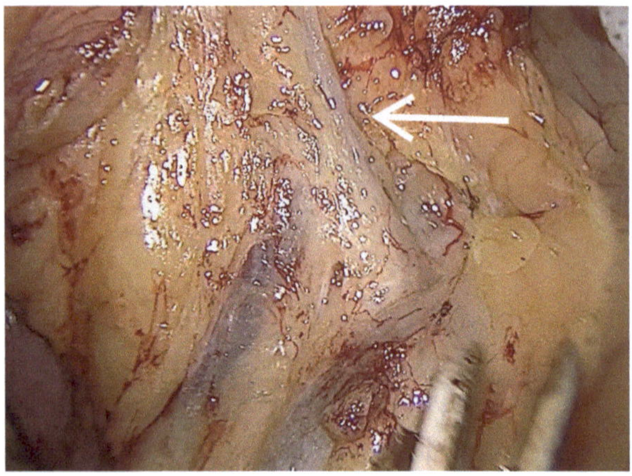

Fig. 5 Dissection of the gastroepiploic pedicle

pancreas is dissected in close relation to the duodenum, where we find the origin of the right gastroepiploic artery, that arises from the gastroduodenal artery. The artery is transected with hemolocks of stapler depending on the diameter (Fig. 6).

Dissection of Group 12, Group 5 and Duodenum Transection

The duodenum is dissected and division of the preduodenal vessels is performed by dissecting group 5 (Fig. 7). The dissection is continued on its anterior surface and follow its left branch until the hepatic pedicle dissection is completed. Typically, at this stage, the right gastric artery is ligated. Group 12 lymphadenectomy is achieved (Fig. 8). Then the duodenum is transected with a blue stapler (Fig. 9).

Dissection of Group 8 (Common Hepatic Artery) 9 and 7

Procedure continues by incising the prepancreatic peritoneum to reach the common hepatic artery, which represent a significant lymph node station (group 8) located right above it (Fig. 10). To the left of the artery, continuing the retroperitoneal

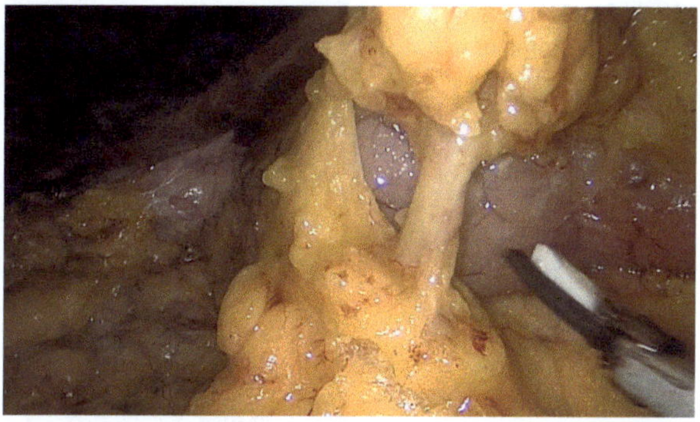

Fig. 6 Lymphadenectomy gastroepiploic artery (group 6)

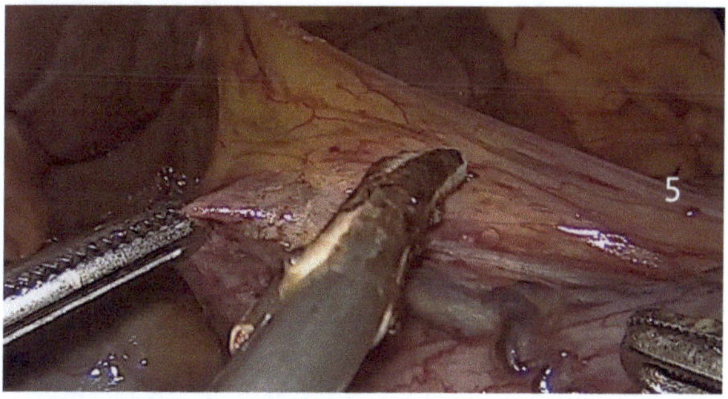

Fig. 7 Dissection of the superior aspect of the first portion of duodenum

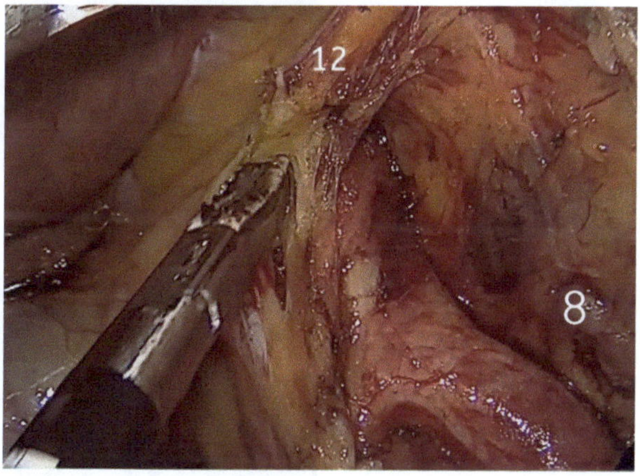

Fig. 8 Dissection of the proper hepatic artery (group 12)

dissection, we encounter the splenic artery, and between them, the left gastric vein, which leads toward the portal vein (Fig. 11). The left gastric vein is ligated as soon as it is identified to prevent bleeding. Then the left gastric artery is ligated (Fig. 12), completing the dissection of groups 9 (celiac trunk), 7 (left gastric artery), and 3 (lesser curvature).

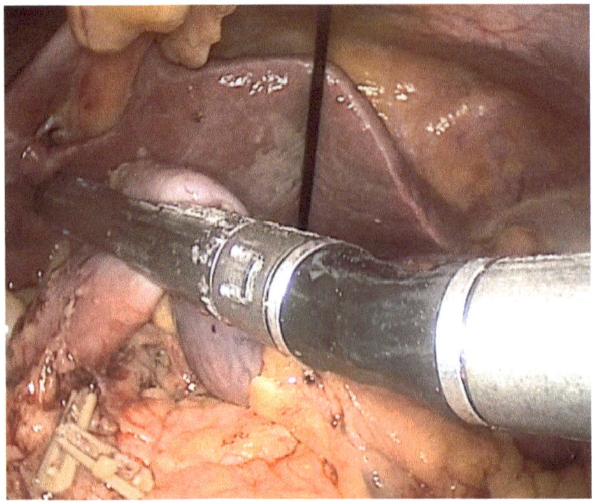

Fig. 9 Staple transection of the first portion of the duodenum

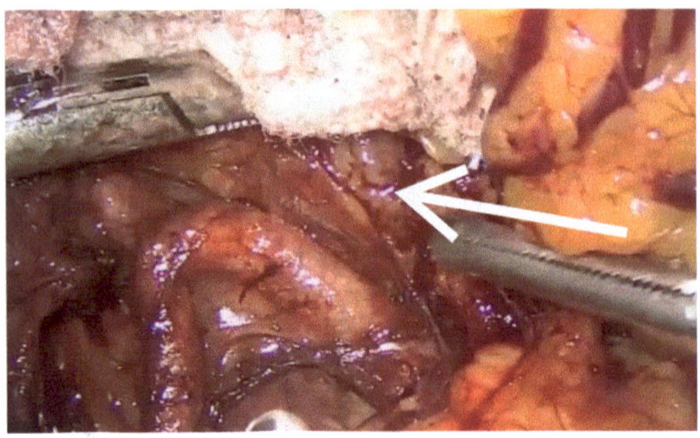

Fig. 10 Isolation of common hepatic artery (group 8)

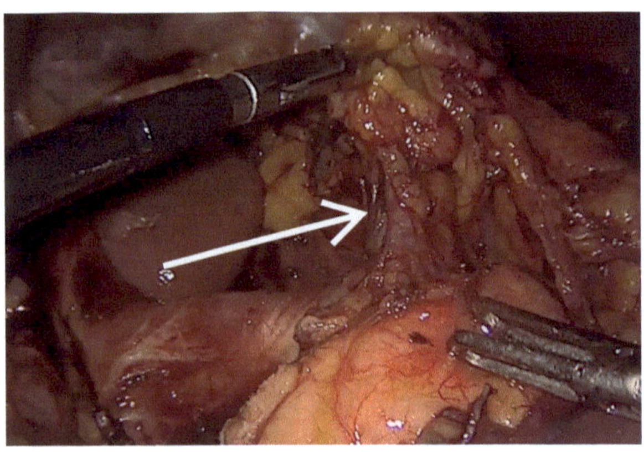

Fig. 11 Dissection of the left gastric vessels

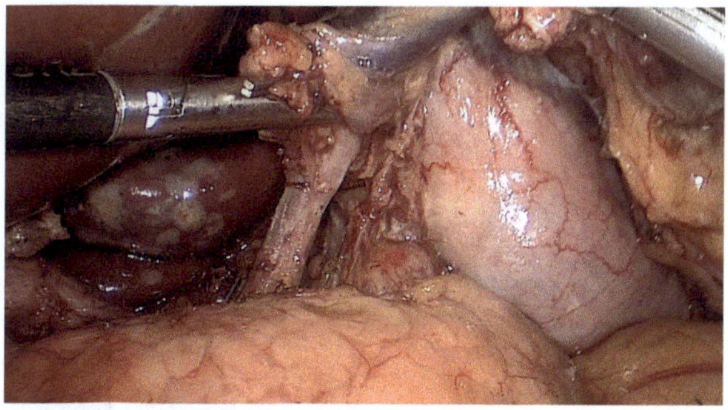

Fig. 12 Lymphadenectomy left gastric vessels

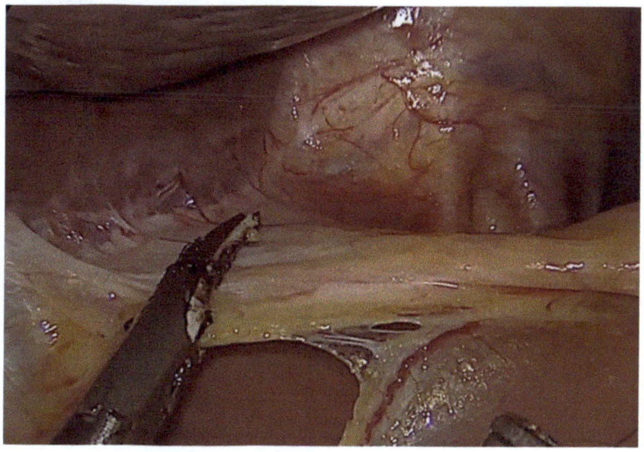

Fig. 13 Dissection of pars flaccid

Pars Flaccid and Dissection of Group 1

During this step, the opening of the lesser omentum and dissection of group 1 is performed. The right crus of the diaphragm is fully dissected (Figs. 13 and 14). In cases where the tumor is near the esophagogastric junction (Siewert II), group 20 lymphadenectomy is recommended, removing the periaortic and pericardial lymphatic tissue.

Dissection of Group 11

From this point, the splenic artery is dissected laterally until its bifurcation at the splenic hilum (Figs. 15 and 16). Dissection of the splenic hilum or group 10 is not recommended. In cases of tumors affecting the greater curvature or splenic involvement, splenectomy is recommended.

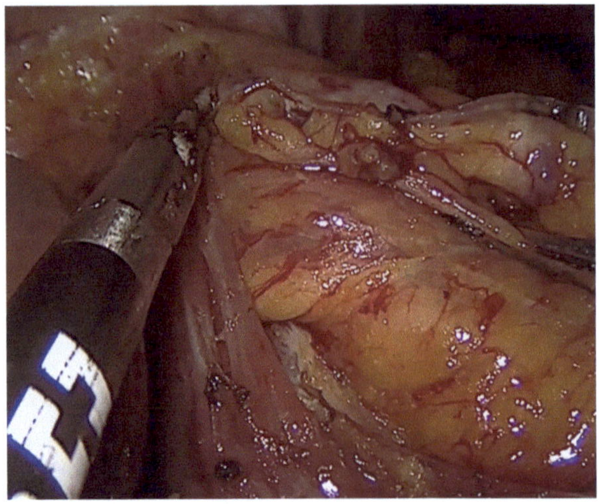

Fig. 14 Mobilization and division of the distal esophagus

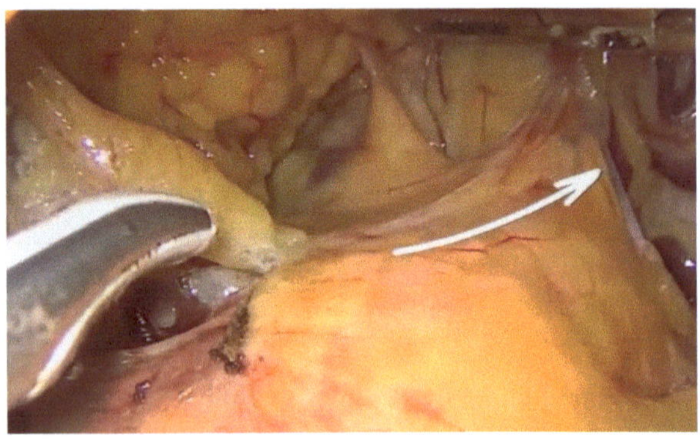

Fig. 15 Incision of pre-pancreatic peritoneum

Distal Esophageal Dissection

The left crus of the diaphragm is then dissected, leaving group 2 lymphadenectomy attached to the specimen. The distal esophagus is encircled and completely mobilized inside the mediastinum.

Esophagueal Section and Reconstruction

The esophagus is then transected with a white stapler (Fig. 17). The specimen is then removed through a small Pfannenstiel incision. Next, for the reconstruction, the jejunum is divided approximately 70 cm distal to the ligament of Treitz, using a white load stapler. Once the jejunum is divided, another 70 cm of jejunum are used to construct the Roux limb.

The alimentary limb is brought ante-colic. Routinely, the vagus nerves are sectioned (Fig. 18). The esophagojejunostomy reconstruction is done first in two

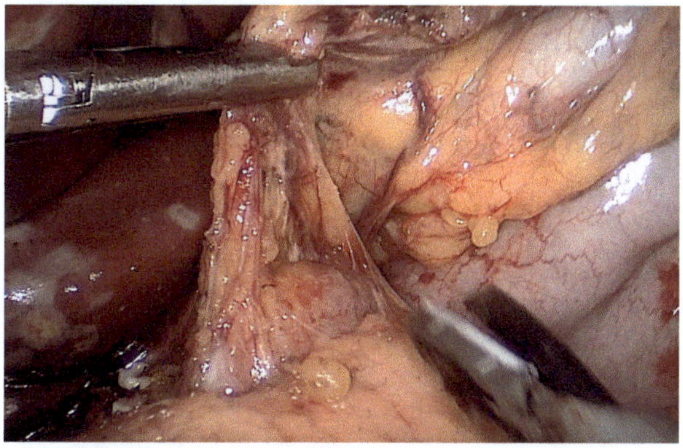

Fig. 16 Lymphadenectomy splenic artery (group 11)

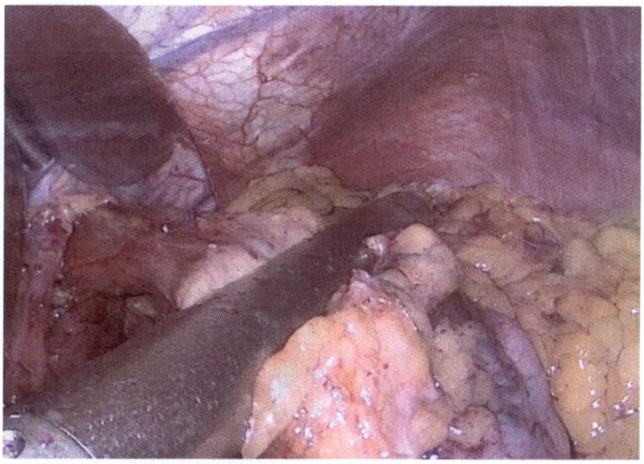

Fig. 17 Distal Esophageal transection

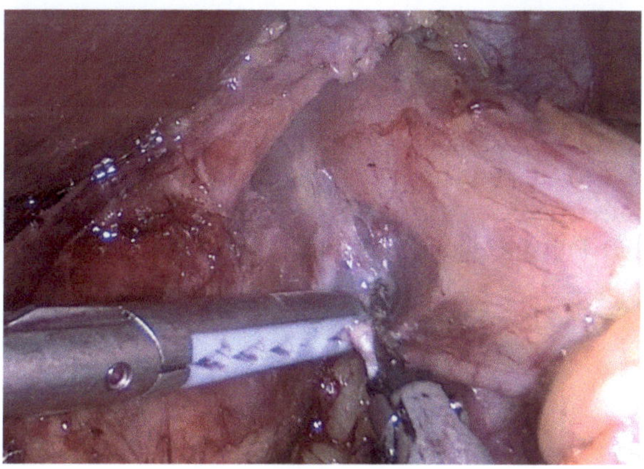

Fig. 18 Vagus nerve transection

layers. The posterior outer layer is done with 3/0 Polydioxanone suture in a running fashion (Fig. 19). Esophagostomy and enterotomy are then done with hook electrocautery, and the posterior inner layer is completed with a 3/0 Polydioxanone running suture (Figs. 20 and 21). The anterior aspect of the anastomosis is also created

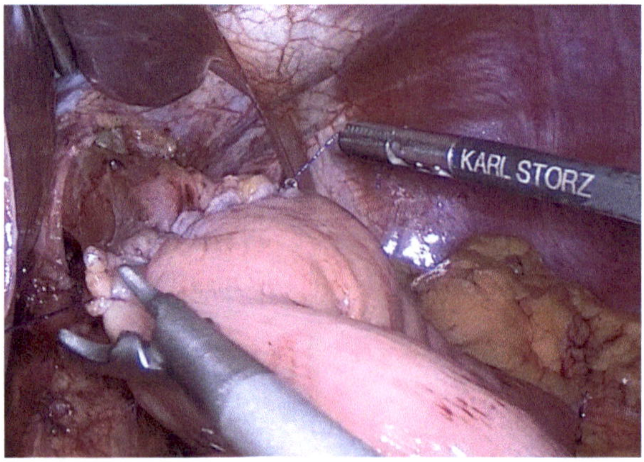

Fig. 19 Esophagojejunostomy: posterior external layer

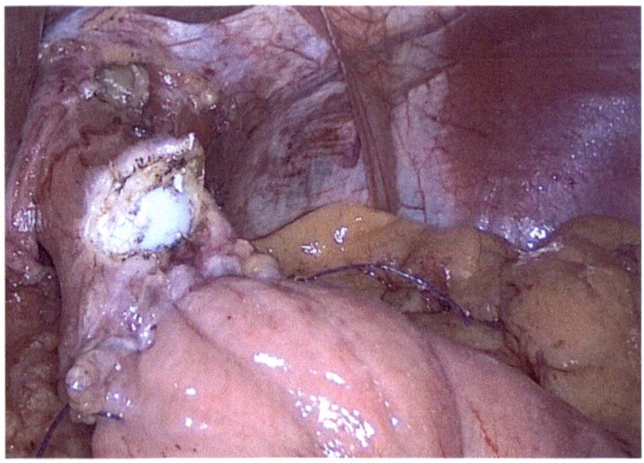

Fig. 20 Esophagostomy

with two layers of the same suture (Figs. 22 and 23). The anastomosis is then checked with methylene blue through a nasogastric tube.

Both the biliopancreatic limb and the Roux limb are approximated and two enterotomies are made with hook electrocautery. A white load stapler is then introduced into the jejunal limbs to create a side-to-side jejuno-jejunostomy (Fig. 24). A 3/0 Polydioxanone absorbable running suture is used to close the enterotomy (Fig. 25).

A drain is left in the cavity near the esophagojejunostomy.

Fig. 21 Esophagojejunostomy: posterior inner layer

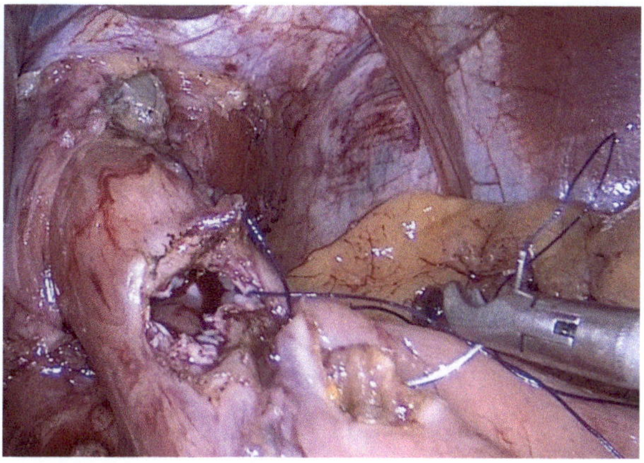

Fig. 22 Esophagojejunostomy: anterior inner layer

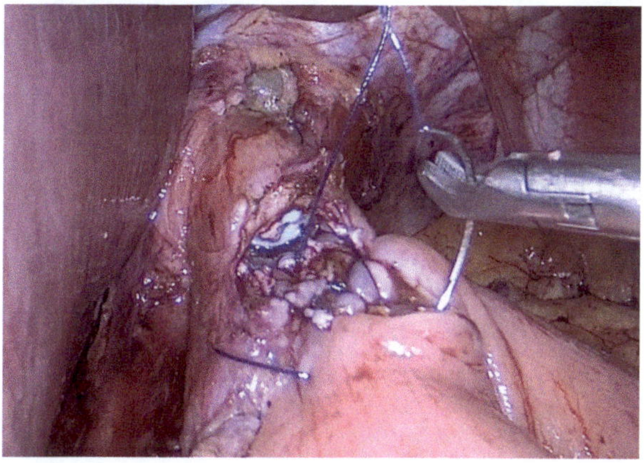

Fig. 23 Esophagojejunostomy: anterior external layer

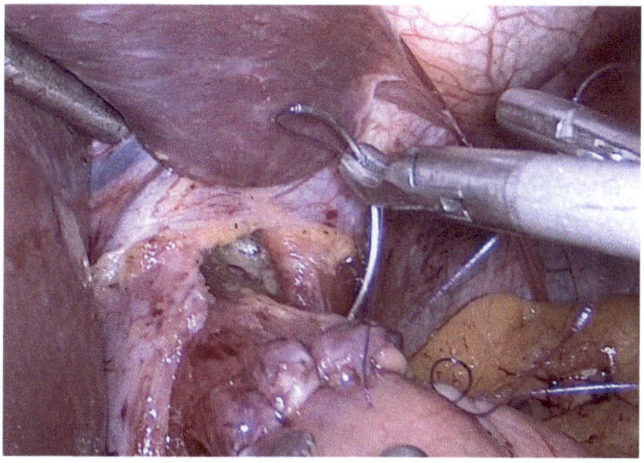

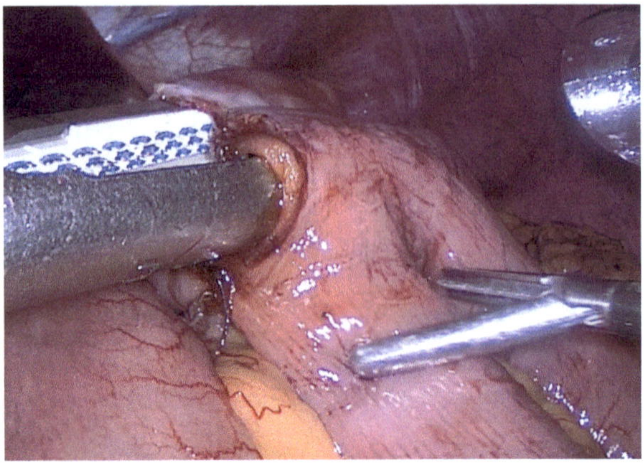

Fig. 24 Creation of the side-to-side jejuno-jejunostomy

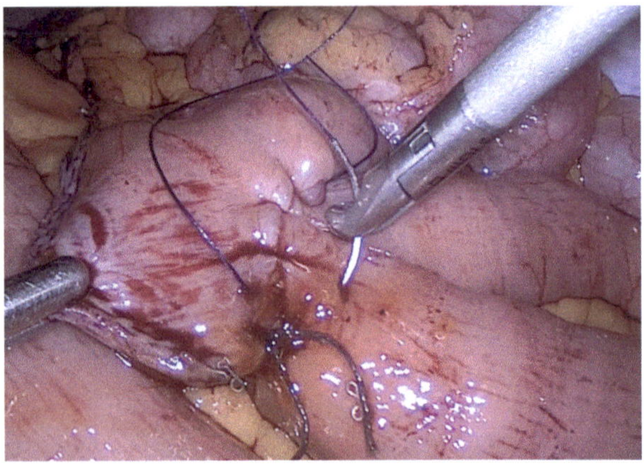

Fig. 25 Closure of jejuno-jejunostomy

Conclusions

Laparoscopic total gastrectomy with Roux-en-Y reconstruction is a feasible and effective treatment for selected patients requiring total gastric resection. Mastery of this procedure involves attention to detail, familiarity with laparoscopic techniques, and management of potential complications. Proper patient selection and perioperative care are critical for optimal outcomes.

Conflict of Interest Camilo Boza, Ricardo Funke and Martín Andrada declare that they have no conflicts of interest.

References

1. Wei Y, Yu D, Li Y, Fan C, Li G. Laparoscopic versus open gastrectomy for advanced gastric cancer: a meta-analysis based on high-quality retrospective studies and clinical randomized trials. Clin Res Hepatol Gastroenterol. 2018;42(6):577–90.
2. Liu F, Huang C, Xu Z, et al. Morbidity and mortality of laparoscopic vs open total gastrectomy for clinical stage I gastric cancer: the CLASS02 multicenter randomized clinical trial. JAMA Oncol. 2020;6(10):1590–7.

Robotic Total Gastrectomy

Patrick L. Quinn and Aslam Ejaz

Abstract Total gastrectomy is the standard of care treatment for large or proximal gastric tumors. Minimally invasive approaches offer improved recovery time without sacrificing cancer-specific outcomes compared to an open approach. In this chapter, we describe the surgical steps of a robotic total gastrectomy with accompanying intraoperative images.

Keywords Robotic surgery · Gastric cancer · Total gastrectomy · Minimally invasive

Introduction

The most common indication for total gastrectomy is gastric adenocarcinoma, which is the fifth leading cause of cancer worldwide. The worldwide incidence of gastric cancer varies greatly with more than 70% of gastric cancers occurring in the developing world and approximately 50% occurring in East Asia.

For proximal or large gastric tumors, total gastrectomy is typically utilized to achieve negative microscopic margins, offering the patient the best opportunity for long-term recurrence-free and overall survival. Additionally, total gastrectomy may be performed as a prophylactic measure for select individuals with pathogenic

P. L. Quinn
Department of Surgery, The Ohio State University, Columbus, OH, USA

A. Ejaz (✉)
Department of Surgery, Division of Surgical Oncology, University of Illinois at Chicago, Chicago, IL, USA
e-mail: aejaz@uic.edu

F. Schlottmann, M. A. Masrur (eds.), *Endoscopic, Laparoscopic and Robotic Techniques for Foregut Disorders*, https://doi.org/10.1007/978-3-032-00811-4_38

CDH1 variants who are at increased risk for developing gastric adenocarcinoma. Minimally invasive approaches have been demonstrated to be a safe and feasible option for total gastrectomy, offering improved recovery times without any difference in perioperative complications or cancer-specific outcomes compared to an open approach [1–5].

In this chapter, we describe the surgical steps involved in performing a total gastrectomy using a robotic approach.

Procedure Description

Preoperative Preparation and Patient Positioning

As part of the enhanced recovery protocol at our institution, patients are provided extensive preoperative education and counseling on exercise, nutrition, smoking and alcohol cessation, and expectations after surgery. Prior to surgery, patients receive a multi-modal pain regimen including 975 mg acetaminophen, 300 mg gabapentin, 5 mg oxycodone, and a scopolamine patch within the preoperative holding area. Patients also receive an intrathecal morphine block to assist with postoperative pain control. The patient is then brought into the operating room and placed supine on the operative table. 2 g ceftriaxone and 500 mg metronidazole are given before the incision is made as antibiotic prophylaxis. Cefazolin alone may also be used as antibiotic prophylaxis. Sequential compression devices are placed on both legs and the patient receives 5000 units of subcutaneous heparin for venous thrombosis prophylaxis. After general endotracheal anesthesia is achieved, the patient is transitioned to a split leg position, ensuring that the patient is securely strapped and pressure points are padded. A Foley catheter is then placed.

Port Placement and Docking

The abdomen is prepped and draped in the usual sterile fashion using a chlorhexidine scrub. A Veress needle is used to access the peritoneal cavity in the left upper quadrant and 15-mmHg pneumoperitoneum is established. A robotic 8-mm trocar is placed in the left abdomen using the direct Optiview technique. For cancer operations, the peritoneal cavity is then examined to rule out signs of metastases, paying close attention to tumor deposits along the falciform ligament, diaphragm, peritoneum, and liver. For patients with T2+/N+ tumors, patients would have already received a prior negative diagnostic laparoscopy prior to neoadjuvant chemotherapy administration. Two additional 8-mm ports are placed in the left lateral abdomen and right lateral abdomen in line with the initial port under direct visualization. A 12-mm robotic port is placed in the right abdomen in line with the other robotic

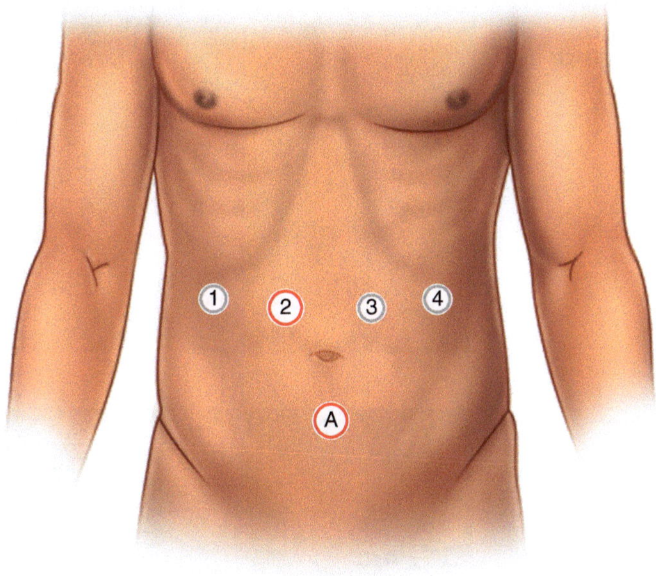

Fig. 1 Diagram of port placement. Red ports are 12 mm and black ports are 8 mm. Port A assistant port

ports. Finally, a 12-mm assistant port is placed in the lower midline below the umbilicus, a GelPOINT Mini Advanced Access Platform is placed followed by a 12-mm AirSeal port (Fig. 1).

The patient is placed in the reverse Trendelenburg position and the surgical robot is docked. The robotic camera is placed in port 3, with the following instruments placed in the other ports: tip-up fenestrated grasper (1), fenestrated bipolar forceps (2), and vessel sealer (4).

Resection and D2 Lymphadenectomy

To begin, the lesser sac is entered by opening the gastrocolic ligament (Fig. 2). Dissection is carried along the greater curvature towards the cardia to mobilize the body of the stomach. Dissection is then directed toward the origin of the gastroepiploic vein and artery (Fig. 3). Ligation at the origin ensures that all gastroepiploic lymph nodes are included within the specimen. The vessels can be ligated individually with robotic clips and vessel sealer, or the pedicle can be taken with a vascular load stapler (Fig. 4).

The distal stomach and first portion of the duodenum are mobilized off the head of the pancreas. Careful attention is paid to include station 5 and 6 nodes. The omentum and pancreatic attachments are dissected off the duodenum to visualize

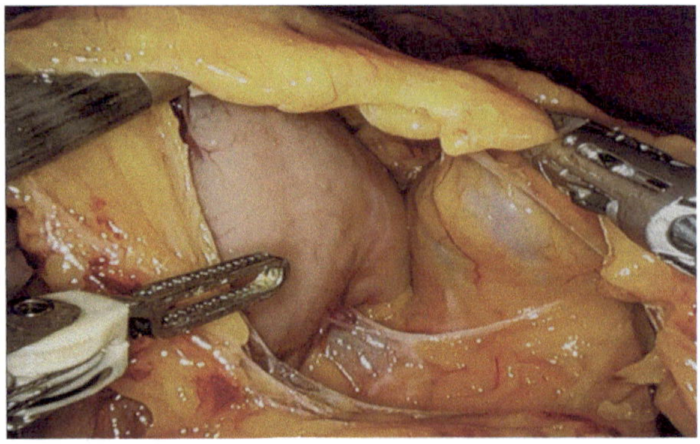

Fig. 2 Dissection of gastrocolic ligament, stomach left, colon right

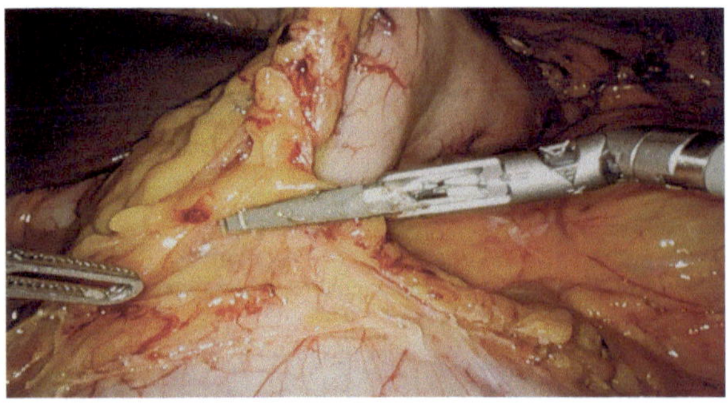

Fig. 3 Dissection of gastrocolic ligament towards gastroepiploic vein and artery

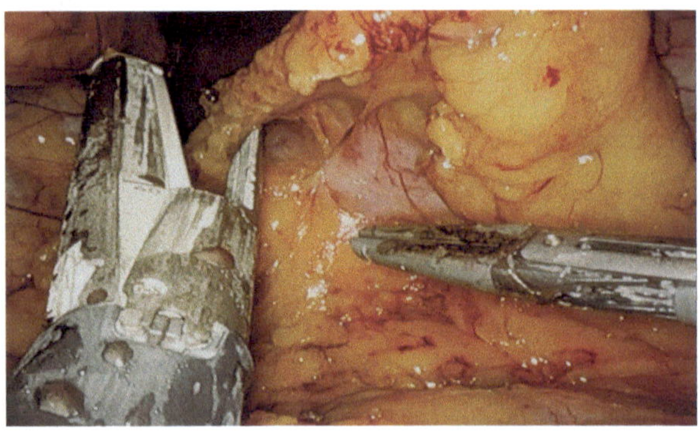

Fig. 4 Ligation of gastroepiploic pedicle

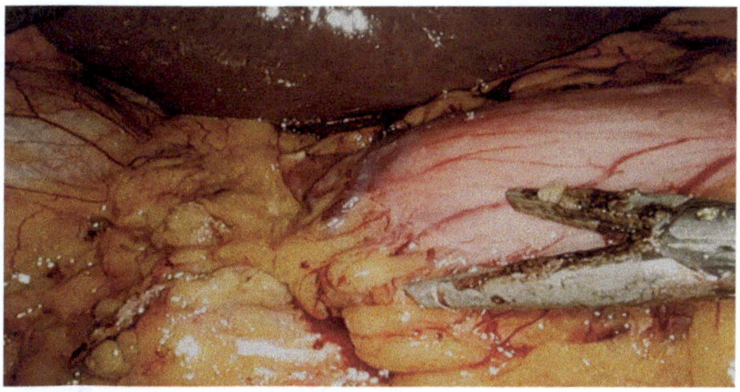

Fig. 5 Dissection of the distal stomach and proximal duodenum for ligation

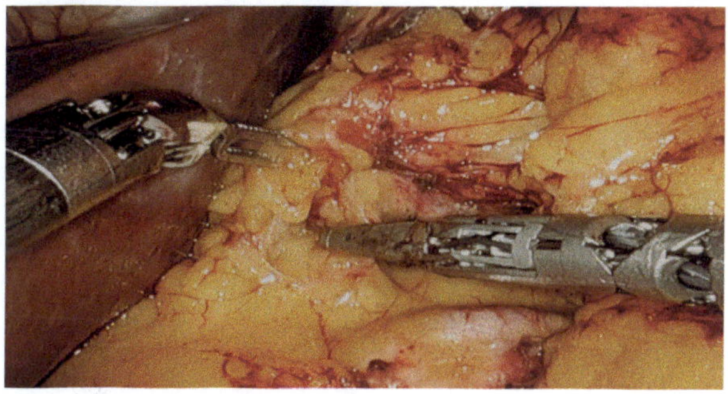

Fig. 6 Dissection of the posterior stomach. The stomach is retracted to the left upper quadrant out of the frame, splenic artery is in view

the right gastric artery and allow for a window underneath the duodenum 2 cm distal to the pylorus (Fig. 5). The right gastric artery is taken with the vessel sealer device at its origin from the common hepatic artery. The duodenum is divided using a 60-mm robotic linear stapler (2.5–3.5 mm staple height depending on tissue thickness). Bleeding at the staple line can be controlled by electrocautery or reinforcing sutures.

Dissection then continues along the gastrohepatic ligament towards the origin of the left gastric vein and artery (Fig. 6). The left gastric artery and vein are skeletonized and then divided at its origin with a vascular stapler (station 7) (Fig. 7). The common hepatic artery lymph nodes (station 8a), hepatoduoodenal ligament nodes (station 12a), and proximal splenic artery lymph nodes (station 11p) can also be harvested during this portion of the dissection. Dissection is carried towards to crus with the pars flaccida being divided widely to incorporate the lesser omental lymph nodes (station 3a and 3b) within the specimen (Fig. 8).

Attention is then turned to further mobilization of the posterior stomach off the pancreatic and retroperitoneal attachments. The short gastric vessels are carefully divided up past the cardia using the energy device, ensuring the preservation of the spleen (Fig. 9). Station 4d, 4sb, and 4sa nodes are included in this dissection. An umbilical tape (1/8 in) is used to encircle the distal esophagus to help provide tension for the dissection of the phrenoesophageal ligament and dissection of the esophagus off of the crura (Fig. 10). The esophagus is mobilized to allow for sufficient intra-abdominal length and a clear transection margin. Once adequately mobilized, the distal esophagus is divided with the robotic linear stapler with careful

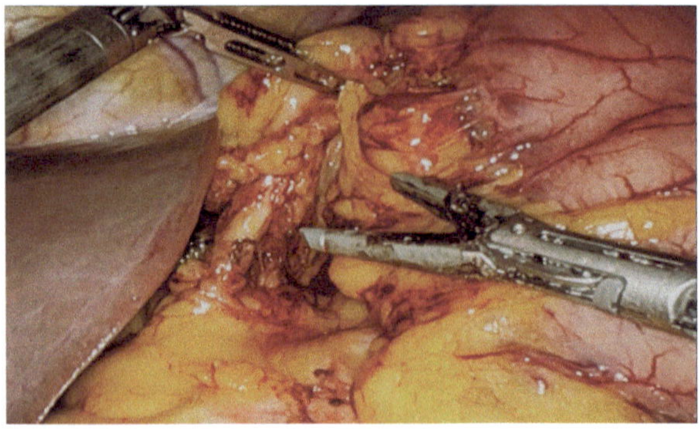

Fig. 7 Isolation of the left gastric vein and artery

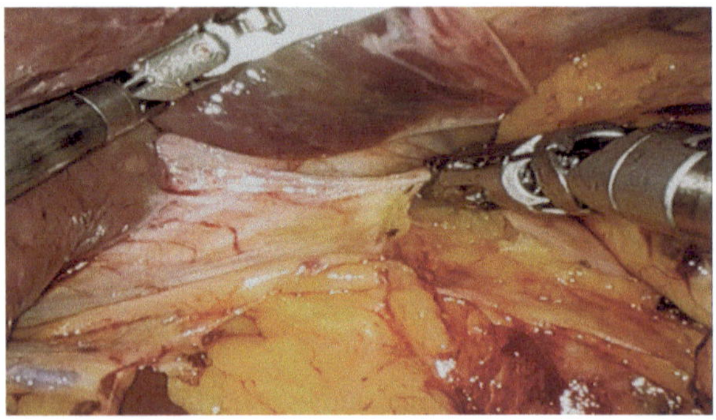

Fig. 8 Division of the pars flaccida

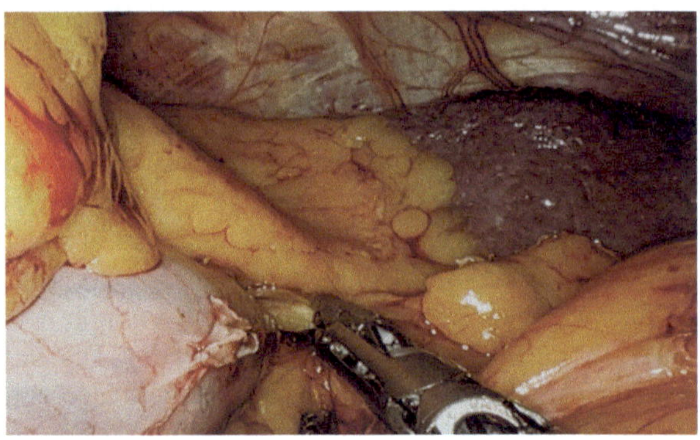

Fig. 9 Ligation of the short gastric vessels

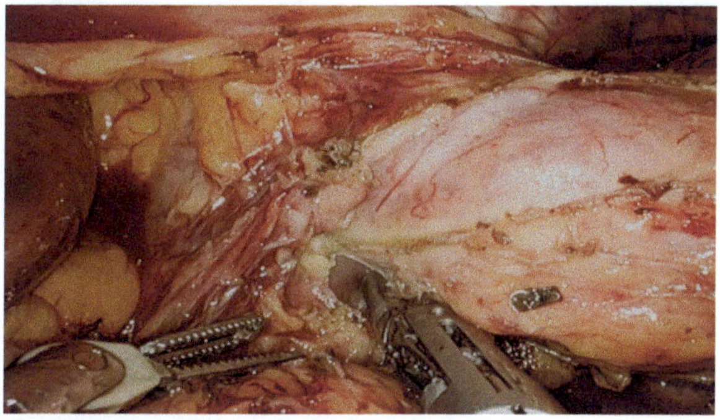

Fig. 10 Mobilization of the distal esophagus, umbilical tape (out of frame) used to provide traction of the esophagus to the right

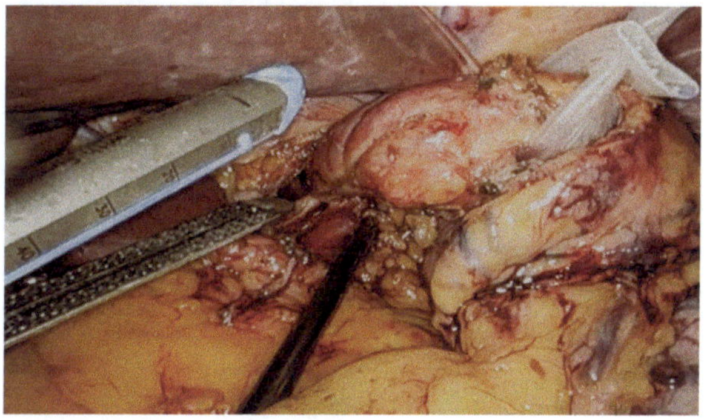

Fig. 11 Division of the distal esophagus

attention paid to avoid the spleen when positioning the stapler (Fig. 11). Stations 9–11 lymph nodes can also be harvested at this time. The specimen is then placed in an endocatch and set aside. The area is then inspected for hemostasis.

Reconstruction

The transverse colon is retracted superiorly to identify the ligament of Treitz. Approximately 25–30 cm distal to the ligament of Treitz, the jejunum is divided using the robotic linear stapler, and its mesentery is partially divided using the energy device (Fig. 12). An additional 45 cm is measured from the jejunum's division to create the jejuno-jejunostomy. A stay suture is used to approximate the bowel to be anastomosed and monopolar curved scissors are used to make two enterotomies (Fig. 13). A 60-mm linear robotic stapler is then used to create a side-to-side anastomosis. The common channel is closed using two running 3-0 v-loc sutures. Each suture is placed at a corner of the common channel, with a continuous suture using full-thickness bites as the inner layer, and continuous lembert sutures using seromuscular bites as the outer layer (Figs. 14, 15, and 16).

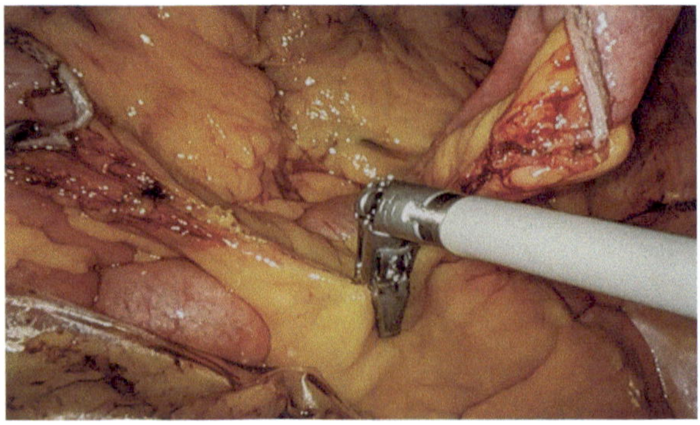

Fig. 12 Division of jejunal mesentery of roux limb

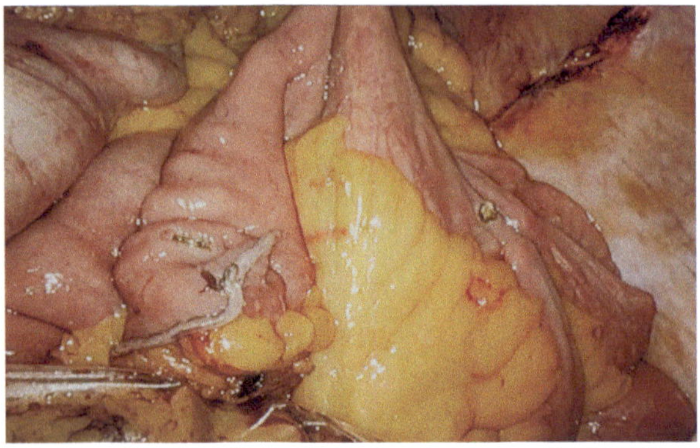

Fig. 13 Creation of jejuno-jejunostomy

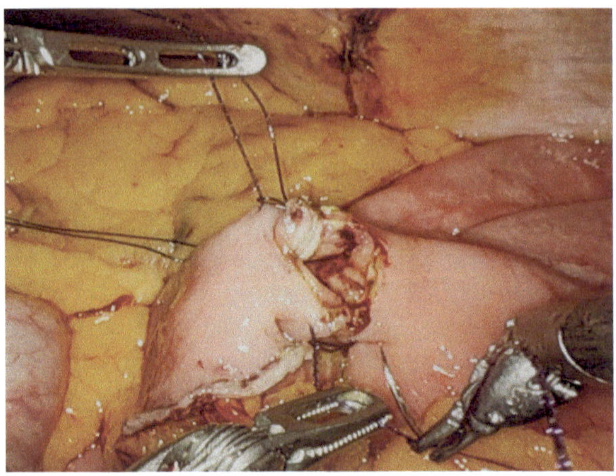

Fig. 14 Closure of jejuno-jejunostomy – first layer

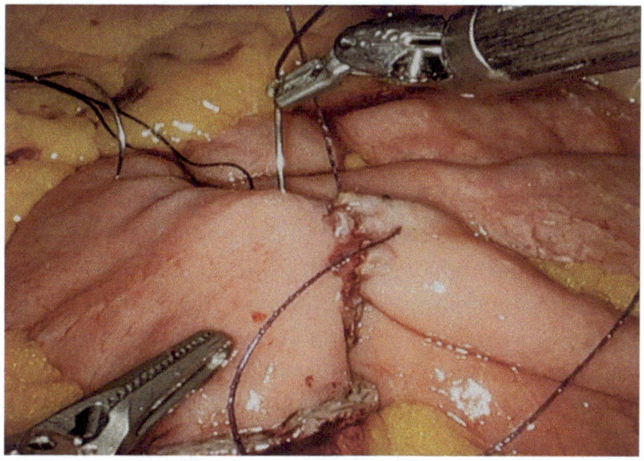

Fig. 15 Closure of jejuno-jejunostomy – second layer

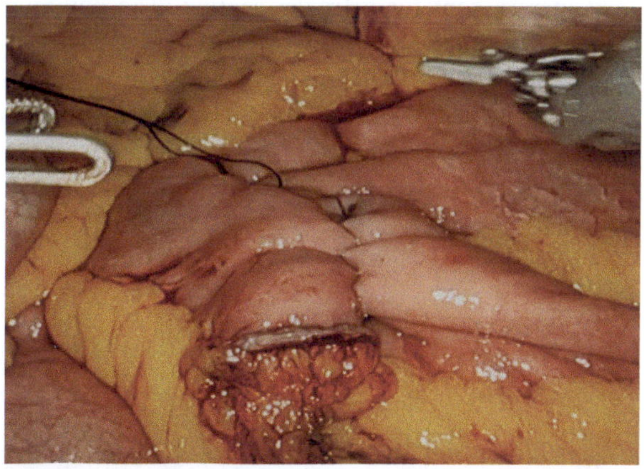

Fig. 16 Completed jejuno-jejunostomy

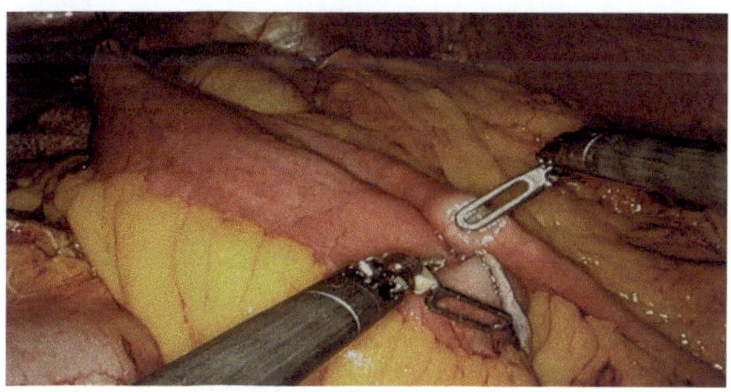

Fig. 17 Creation of the jejunal pouch

Next, a jejunal pouch is performed to aid in postoperative feeding and nutritional status, though the utility of this practice is debated. The jejunal pouch is created by measuring approximately 10 cm distal from the stapled end of the roux limb and placing a stay suture. The roux limb is then folded to create a side-to-side anastomosis (Fig. 17). Two enterotomies are made using the monopolar curved scissors and multiple loads of the robotic linear stapler are used to create the pouch.

Attention is then turned to the stapled end of the distal esophagus. The jejunal pouch is brought ante colic, although a retrocolic route may be necessary to achieve a tension-free orientation. An EEA OrVil is passed through the mouth and an esophagostomy is made superior to the staple line. The anvil is then pulled through the esophagostomy (Fig. 18). Using the assistant's gelport, an EEA stapler (25–3.5mm) is advanced through the common channel of the jejunal pouch, and an antecolic esophagojejunostomy is created (Fig. 19). The stapler is fired and checked to ensure that there are two complete tissue doughnuts, with the esophageal margin sent for a frozen section. The common enterotomy of the jejunal pouch is closed in a similar fashion as described above using two 3-0 v-loc sutures (Fig. 20). Alternative options for creating the esophago-jejunostomy include hand-sewn and linear stapler techniques. The patient is then placed in the Trendelenburg

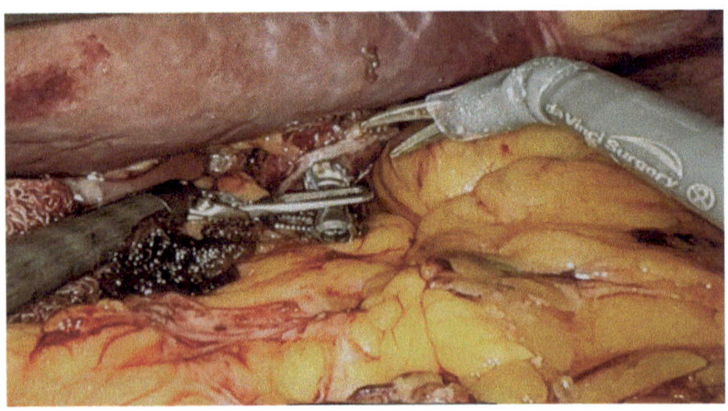

Fig. 18 Anvil pulled through the distal esophagus

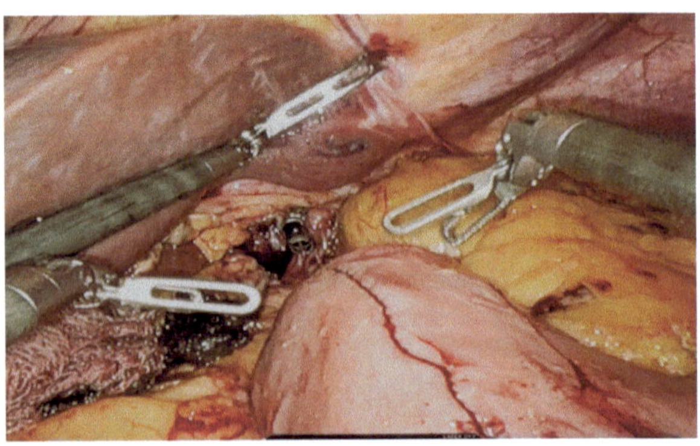

Fig. 19 Creation of esophagojejunostomy

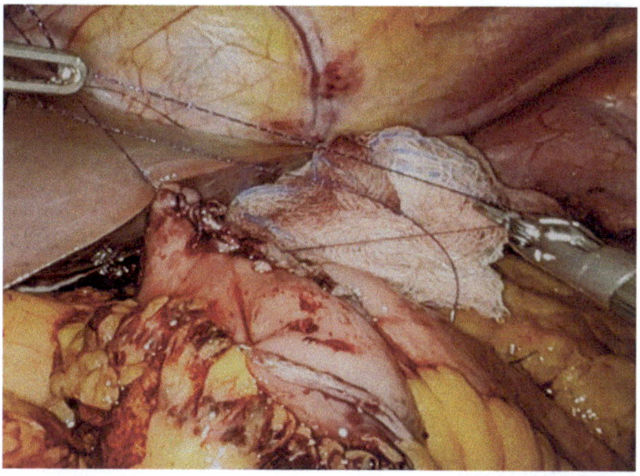

Fig. 20 Closure of common enterotomy of the jejunal pouch

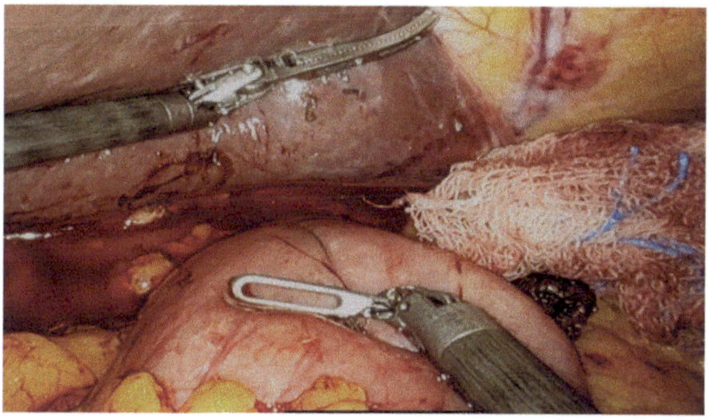

Fig. 21 Performing leak test of esophagojejunostomy anastomosis

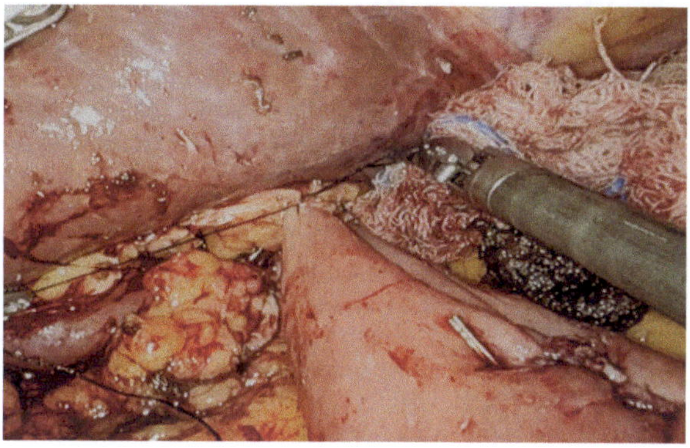

Fig. 22 Pedicled omental flap over esophagojejunostomy anastomosis

position, and an esophagogastroduodenoscopy (EGD) is performed to ensure that the esophagojejunostomy (EJ) anastomosis is widely patent and that there is no air leak from the anastomosis (Fig. 21). Reinforcement sutures are applied, if necessary (Fig. 22).

Closure

The fluid used from the leak test is suctioned out and hemostasis is confirmed. The specimen is extracted through the assistant port. Under direct visualization, a 19 Fr Blake drain is placed anterior to the duodenal stump and posterior to the EJ anastomosis. The 12-mm robotic port site and the 12-mm assistant port fascia are closed using interrupted #1 polydioxanone sutures (PDS). The other trocars are then removed under visualization and the pneumoperitoneum is evacuated. The trocar sites are closed with subcutaneous stitches using a 4-0 monofilament suture and skin adhesive.

Conclusions

In a complex operation such as the total gastrectomy, the robotic approach allows for greater maneuverability and visualization over a laparoscopic approach. While the procedure is still primarily performed at specialized centers, there is growing literature to support its safety and disseminated use when clinically appropriate.

Disclosure The authors have nothing to disclose.

References

1. Zheng-Yan L, Feng Q, Yan S, et al. Learning curve of robotic distal and total gastrectomy. Br J Surg. 2021;108(9):1126–32.
2. Chen QY, Zhong Q, Liu ZY, et al. Surgical outcomes, technical performance, and surgery burden of robotic total gastrectomy for locally advanced gastric cancer: a prospective study. Ann Surg. 2022;276(5):e434–43.
3. Wang ZK, Lin JX, Wang FH, et al. Robotic spleen-preserving total gastrectomy shows better short-term advantages: a comparative study with laparoscopic surgery. Surg Endosc. 2022;36(11):8639–50.
4. Wei Y, Yu D, Li Y, Fan C, Li G. Laparoscopic versus open gastrectomy for advanced gastric cancer: a meta-analysis based on high-quality retrospective studies and clinical randomized trials. Clin Res Hepatol Gastroenterol. 2018;42(6):577–90.
5. Liu F, Huang C, Xu Z, et al. Morbidity and mortality of laparoscopic vs open total gastrectomy for clinical stage I gastric cancer: the CLASS02 multicenter randomized clinical trial. JAMA Oncol. 2020;6(10):1590–7.

Correction to: Endoscopic, Laparoscopic and Robotic Techniques for Foregut Disorders

Francisco Schlottmann and Mario A. Masrur

Correction to:
F. Schlottmann, M. A. Masrur (eds.), *Endoscopic, Laparoscopic and Robotic Techniques for Foregut Disorders*, https://doi.org/10.1007/978-3-032-00811-4

In the original version of the book, the following corrections are to be incorporated:

In Chap. 33, Figs. 1, 2, and 3 have to be replaced with the new figures provided by the author.

In Chaps. 2 and 36, the last name of Emiliano G. Manuelli Laos was unfortunately published with an error.

The book has now been updated with these changes.

The updated version of this book can be found at
https://doi.org/10.1007/978-3-032-00811-4

F. Schlottmann, M. A. Masrur (eds.), *Endoscopic, Laparoscopic and Robotic Techniques for Foregut Disorders*, https://doi.org/10.1007/978-3-032-00811-4_39

MIX
Papier aus verantwortungsvollen Quellen
Paper from responsible sources
FSC® C105338

If you have any concerns about our products,
you can contact us on
ProductSafety@springernature.com

In case Publisher is established outside the EU,
the EU authorized representative is:
Springer Nature Customer Service Center GmbH
Europaplatz 3, 69115 Heidelberg, Germany

Printed by Libri Plureos GmbH
in Hamburg, Germany